AF661157

IATRO-CHEMISTRY
OF
ĀYURVEDA
(RASA ŚĀSTRA)

Selected Books on AYURVEDA

- Alchemy and Metallic Medicines in Ayurveda/**Vaidya Bhagwan Dash**
- Ayurvedic System of Medicine (The) or an Exposition in English of Hindu Medicine as Occurring in Charka, Sucruta, Bagbhata, and other authoritative works, ancient and modern, in Sanskrit/**Kaviraj Nagendranath Sen Gupta** (set of 2 vols)
- Complete Herbal and English Physician Enlarged/ **Nicholas Culpeper** (with a Prologue by **Vaidya Bhagwan Dash**)
- Domestic Materia Medica
- Handbook of Ayurveda(A)/**Vaidya Bhagwan Dash** and **Acharya Manfred M. Junius**
- Massage Therapy in Ayurveda (*Pancakarma Therapy of Ayurveda Series No. 1*)/**Vaidya Bhagwan Dash**
- आयुर्वेदिक निदेशिका/**वैद्य भगवान दाश**
- आयुर्वेद का सैधान्तिक अध्ययन/**वैद्य भगवान दाश एवं कु० कन्चन गुप्ता**

Todarananda-Ayurveda Saukhyam Series

- Materia Medica of Ayurveda:/**Vaidya Bhagwan Dash** and **LaliteshKashyap**
- Basic Principles of Ayurveda:/**Vaidya Bhagwan Dash** and **Lalitesh Kashyap**
- Diagnosis and Treatment of Diseases in Ayurveda Part One/**Vaidya Bhagwan Dash** and **Lalitesh Kashyap**
- Diagnosis and Treatment of Diseases in Ayurveda Part Two/**Vaidya Bhagwan Dash** and **Lalitesh Kashyap**
- Diagnosis and Treatment of Diseases in Ayurveda Part Three/ **Vaidya Bhagwan Dash** and **Lalitesh Kashyap**
- Diagnosis and Treatment of Diseases in Ayurveda Part Four/**Vaidya Bhagwan Dash** and **Lalitesh Kashyap**
- Diagnosis and Treatment of Diseases in Ayurveda Part Five/**Vaidya Bhagwan Dash** and **Lalitesh Kashyap**
- Five Specialised Therapies of Ayurveda *(Panca Karma)*/**Vaidya Bhagwan Dash** and **Lalitesh Kashyap**
- Iatro-Chemistry of Ayurveda *(Rasa Sastra)* /**Vaidya Bhagwan Dash** and **Lalitesh Kashyap**

IATRO-CHEMISTRY
OF
ĀYURVEDA
(RASA ŚĀSTRA)

BASED ON
ĀYURVEDA SAUKHYAṂ OF ṬOḌARĀNANDA

VAIDYA BHAGWAN DASH
D.A.M.S., H.P.A., M.A., Ph.D.
Former Deputy Adviser (Āyurveda)
Ministry of Health and Family Welfare
Govt. of India
and
Ex-Consultant in Traditional Medicine
World Health Organisation (1979)

VAIDYA LALITESH KASHYAP
B.I.M.S., Ph.D
Medical Superintendent
Ayurvedic Hospital
Central Govt. Health Services
New Delhi.

CONCEPT PUBLISHING COMPANY, NEW DELHI - 110059

All rights reserved. No part of this work may be reproduced, stored in a retrieval system, or transmitted in any form or by any means, electronic, mechanical, photocopying, microfilming, recording or otherwise, without the prior written permission of the copyright owner and the publisher.

ISBN 81-7022-527-2 (NO. 9)
ISBN 81-7022-024-6 (Set)

First Published 1994
Reprinted 2002

© Vaidya Bhagwan Dash (*b.*1934)
Vaidya (Miss) Lalitesh Kashyap (*b.*1939)

Published and Published by
Ashok Kumar Mittal
Concept Publishing Company
A/15-16, Commercial Block, Mohan Garden
New Delhi-110059 (India)

Phones: 5648039, 5649024
Fax: 091-(11)-5648053
E-mail: publishing@conceptpub.com

PREFACE

In Ayurvedic therapeutics, three categories of ingredients are used, viz, (1) herbal products, (2) animal products, and (3) metals including minerals, gems and costly stones. In the classical age, herbal products were extensively used in all the eight specialised branches of ayurveda including surgery. Metals and minerals were used as therapeutic agents but less frequently. During the post-classical age, practice of surgery and *pañca-karma* (five specialised therapies) was discouraged because of temporal vicissitudes. To cure these surgical ailments and to cure such obstinate diseases for which *pañca-karma* therapies were being administered earlier, intensive as well as extensive research was carried out by ayurvedic physicians as a result of which potent and safe remedies were explored from processed metals including minerals and costly stones. Apart from their therapeutic efficacy in minute doses, these remedies were found very effective for the preservation and promotion of positive health and prevention of diseases. They were found to be very effective as rejuvenating agents (*rasāyana)* and aphrodisiacs. The primary aim of ayurveda is to maintain the positive health of a person the next objective being the cure of manifested diseases. For a person to be called healthy, according to ayurveda, he should not only be free from physical ailments, but also he should be mentally happy and spiritually elevated. Metals, etc., catered to all these three requirements, viz., physical, mental and spiritual, and therefore, they became very popular among the physicians. Popularity of these metallic preparations has continued uninterrupted till the present age inasmuch, as a new specialised branch (in addition to eight specialised branches described in classics) took its birth. This is called *Rasaśāstra* or latro-chemistry.

In the forefront of these metals was mercury. Because of its miraculous rejuvenating and therapeutic effects, it was alluded to be the seed of Lord Śiva. To make this metal free from toxicity and therapeutically potent, sixteen different and consecutive steps (*saṃskāras)* were evolved. At the end of these sixteen *saṃskāras,* the processed mercury has to be tested to ensure its rejuvenating effects on human beings. This test, which is the seventeenth step, is carried out on ordinary metals to which the processed mercury is added in minute quantity and further processed. By this, the ordinary metal gets transmuted into noble metal i.e. gold or silver. Now the rejuvenating effect of mercury is ensured and it can be administered to human beings not only for rejuvenation but also for attaining salvation while still alive *(jīvan-mukta)*. Before that, the body of the individual should be purified by the administration of various types of elimination (*saṃśodhana*) therapies. This constitutes the last i.e. 18th step *(saṃskāra)*.

It will be seen from the above that the transmutation of base metals to gold and silver is only a method employed to test the efficacy of processed mercury. Thus, alchemy which is considered in the West as a myth, is a fact of reality according to ayurveda. Several saint-physicians adept in this technique have demonstrated their ability in public (for details - vide pp 7-10 of the author's *Alchemy and Metallic Medicines in Ayurveda* published by Concept, New Delhi in 1986). To prevent, unscrupulous and antisocial persons from getting this knowledge, the exact description of these are camouflaged in written texts, and the exact technique is communicated orally only to trusted disciples after examining them carefully. But it should be clearly understood that alchemy was not the primary aim of these saints; it is only a step to ascertain the ability of processed mercury to rejuvenate the body. Details of these eighteen steps are elaborated in this text, of course in a cryptic manner to prevent their misuse, and these details have given added importance to this last volume of *Ṭoḍarānanda Āyurveda-saukhyaṃ* Series.

Earlier volumes in this series have dealt with different topics like Materia Medica, Basic Principles, Diagnosis and Treatment of different categories of diseases and *Pañca karma*. The present volume deals with different types of metals, etc., used in ayurvedic therapeutics including alchemy, thus making the whole series a veritable repository and encyclopaedia of ayurveda.

The first chapter of this volume deals with the explanation of various technical terms *(paribhāṣā)* including weights and measures used in Ayurvedic pharmaceutics in general and those used in *rasaśāstra* in particular. This provides an elaborate description of various types of weights and measures prevalent in India before this work was compiled. It includes dosage of drugs, use of ripe and unripe fruits, different pharmaceutical processes involved in preparing various categories of recipes, food and drinks, various types of poison, approved substitutes and description of pestle and mortar. In ancient days, services of physician were requistioned in the houses of rich people for preparing medicines. The shares of these prepared medicines to which the physician is entitled because of his labour are also described in this chapter.

The second chapter deals with various types of physical, chemical and pharmacological impurities in mercury. Eighteen different steps (*saṃskāras*) of mercury and the instruments and equipments required for that purpose are elaborated in detail in this chapter. The method of extracting mercury from different ores like cinnabar, special recipes like *Rasa-sindūra* and *Rasa karpūra*, and the type of women (*kākinī*) who are to be engaged for assisting in the processing of mercury are described. Sulphur is required to be used in these preparations in liquid form. The process to be followed for reducing sulphur into liquid form is, therefore, described here in detail. Mica with special reference to mythological origin, to its varieties, relative merits of its different types, methods of purification and calcination is described in detail.

The third chapter deals with the metals specially used for the purpose of rejuvenation. Gold with special reference to its varieties, relative merits, adverse effect in impure form, methods of purification, different methods of preparing gold-*bhasma*, its therapeutic excellence, storage and properties, is described in detail. Similarly the varieties, mythological origin, methods of purification and calcination, and properties of other metals like silver, copper, tin, lead, bronze, iron, zinc and *maṇḍūra* (rust of iron) are described. In this connection, references from several contemporary texts (which are not available at present) are compiled.

The fourth chapter deals with subsidiary metals, gems and costly stones with reference to their physical characteristics, impurities, methods of purification and preparation of *bhasma*, and extraction of *sattva* (metallic essence). The notable items described in this chapter are copper pyrite, varieties of copper sulphate, drug used for collyrium like galena, fine oxide and stybnite, *śilājatu* (mineral pitch), calamine, orpiment, realgar, bismuth, tourmaline, diamond, borax, arsenic, iron sulphate, alum, ruby, pearl, coral, emerald, topaz, sapphire, cinnamon stone and cat's eye. This chapter also includes the description of different categories of herbs, milk, urine, water, poisons and *sattvas* extracted from plants. Methods of preparing these metals, minerals and ores in liquid form and their mixtures are elaborated in this chapter. Gems and costly stones are also described in this chapter with special refrence to their characteristics, method of examination, purification, calcination etc. In addition, methods of extracting oils from different types of seeds and plants are also mentioned in this chapter.

At the end, following indices and appendix are given to facilitate the reference of research workers :

Index I Names of Books and Authors quoted in this book.

Index II Names of Recipes described in the text.

Index III Pharmaceutical Processes described in the book.

Index IV List of processing-methods of metals, minerals, gems, etc. described in the text.

Index V Names of Plants, etc., described in the text.

Index VI Glossary of Technical terms.

Appendix Tables of Weights & Measurements according to *Kāliṅga* and *Māgadha* Schools.

For the specific features of *Rasa śāstra,* its historical background and physico-chemical as well as philosophical concepts, readers are advised to consult the following books :

1. Dash, Bhagwan : Alchemy and Metallic Medicines in Ayurveda, New Delhi : Concept Publishing Co., 1986.
2. Ray, P. : History of Chemistry in Ancient and Medieval India incorporating the History of Hindu Chemistry by Acharya Prafulla Chandra Ray, Calcutta : Indian Chemical Society, 1956.
3. Seal, Brajendra Nath : The Positive Sciences of The Ancient Hindus, Delhi : Motilal Banarasi Dass, 1958.
4. Sharma, P.V. : Āyurveda Kā Vaijñānika Itihāsa : Scientific History of Ayurveda (in Hindi), Varanasi : Chaukhambha Orientalia, 1981.
5. Dvivedi, Vasudeva Mulasbunkara : Pārada Vijñānīyam (in Hindi), : Datiya : Śarmā Āyurveda Mandira, 1969.
6. Mishra, Siddhinandan : Āyurvedīya Rasaśāstra (in Hindi), Varanasi: Chaukhambha Orientalia, 1992.

It is for the first time that this valuable work is printed after editing and English translations with indices. Several such Ayurvedic manuscripts are lying scattered in libraries and individual collections. Their publication will be of immense value to the suffering humanity.

The authors will draw immense satisfaction if these volumes will be of help to Ayurvedic physicians, physicians of modern medicine, scientists, students and indologists to further the realm of knowledge in the fields of medicine and biology.

Dt.24.3.94

BHAGWAN DASH
LALITESH KASHYAP

ACKNOWLEDGEMENTS

The first volume of this work was published in 1980 and it took us almost fifteen years to complete this series of nine volumes. During the course of our work we have received help from several quarters - Ayurvedic physicians, Sanskrit scholars and archaeologists. We are grateful to all of them. Kumari Kanchan Gupta, M.A. M. Ed., was of constant help for the preparation of these volumes. May Lord Dhanvantari bless her with good health and happiness in life. Prashant K. Dash & Ku. Pratima Dash, though studying in schools were of immense help in the preparation of these volumes. We bless them for their prosperity in the life ahead. Last but not the least, we are highly obliged to Concept Publishing Company for undertaking the publication of this work.

BHAGWAN DASH
LALITESH KASHYAP

INDO-ROMANIC EQUIVALENTS OF DEVNĀGARĪ

अ	a	क	ka	ढ	ḍha	र	ra
आ	ā	ख	kha	ण	ṇa	ल	la
इ	i	ग	ga	त	ta	व	va
ई	ī	घ	gha	थ	tha	श	śa
उ	u	ङ	ṅa	द	da	ष	ṣa
ऊ	ū	च	ca	ध	dha	स	sa
ऋ	ṛ	छ	cha	न	na	ह	ha
ए	e	ज	ja	प	pa		
ऐ	ai	झ	jha	फ	pha		
ओ	o	ञ	ña	ब	ba		
औ	au	ट	ṭa	भ	bha		
अं	ṁ/ṃ	ठ	ṭha	म	ma		
अः	ḥ	ड	ḍa	य	ya		

CONTENTS

Numbers in square brackets indicate the verse no. of the concerned chapter.

CHAPTER-I
EXPLANATION OF TECHNICAL TERMS

अथ परिमाण-परिभाषा
(WEIGHTS AND MEASUREMENTS)

विना[1] चन्द्रिकया चन्द्रः प्रतापेन विना रविः ।
विनाऽपि रोचिषा तद्वद्वैद्य स्यात्परिभाषया ॥१॥

Importance of Technical Terms

As the moon looks lustureless without the (cooling) moon-light and as the sun appears dull without its hot rays, similarly a physician becomes ineffective if he is without the knowledge of various technical terms.

"मानं च द्विविधं प्रोक्तं कलिङ्गं मागधं तथा ।
कलिङ्गान्मागधं श्रेष्ठमिति मानविदो विदुः ॥२॥

[योगरत्नाकर : मानपरिभाषा : पृष्ठ २१]

कलिङ्गं सौश्रुतं मानं मागधं चरकोदितम् ॥३॥

Weights and Measures of Different Types

Weights and measures are of two types, viz., *Kāliṅga* (which was prevalent in the ancient state of *Kaliṅga* = present Orissa in the Eastern Coast of India) and *Māgadha* (which was prevalent in the ancient state of *Magadha*=present Bihar in the North India). The latter (*māgadha*) is better than the former (*kāliṅga*). *Kālinga* type is followed or adopted by *Suśruta* (belonging to the school of surgery) and *Māgadha* type of weights and measurements are followed by *Caraka* (belonging to the school of medicine).

अथ शाङ्गर्धरात्
"न मानेन विना युक्तिर्द्रव्याणां जायते क्वचित् ।
अतः प्रयोगकार्यार्थं मानमत्रोच्यते मया ।।४।।

According to Śārṅgadhara

Without [the knowledge of] weights and measurements, appropriate combination of ingredients [in a recipe] is not possible. Therefore, for applied therapeutics the weights and measurements will be explained by me (Śārṅgadhara) [which are as follows :]

त्रसरेणुर्बुधैः[४] प्रोक्तस्त्रिंशता परमाणुभिः ।
त्रसरेणुस्तु पर्यायनाम्ना वंशी निगद्यते ।।५।।
जालान्तरगतैः सूर्यकरैर्वंशी विलोक्यते ।
षड्वंशीभिर्मरीचिः स्यात्ताभिः षड्भिस्तु राजिका ।।६।।
तिसृभि राजिकाभिश्च सर्षपः प्रोच्यते बुधैः ।
यवोऽष्टसर्षपैः प्रोक्तो गुञ्जा स्यात्तच्चतुष्टयम् ।।७।।
षड्भिश्च रक्तिकाभिः स्यान्माषको हेमधान्यकौ ।
माषैश्चतुर्भिः शाणः[५] स्याद् धरणः स निगद्यते ।।८।।
टङ्कः स एव कथितस्तद्द्वयं कोल उच्यते ।
क्षुद्रमो[६] वटकश्चैव द्रङ्क्षणः स निगद्यते ।।९।।
कोलद्वयं च कर्षः स्यात्स प्रोक्तः पाणिमानिका ।
अक्षं[७] पिचुः पाणितलं किंचित्पाणिश्च तिन्दुकम् ।।१०।।
विडालपदकं चैव तथा षोडशिका मता ।

कर्मध्य[८] हंसपदं सुवर्णं कवलग्रहः ।।११।।
उदुम्बरं च पर्यायैः कर्ष एव निगद्यते ।
स्यात्कर्षाभ्यामर्धपलं शुक्तिरष्टमिका तथा ।।१२।।
शुक्तिभ्यां च पलं ज्ञेयं मुष्टिराम्रं चतुर्थिका ।
प्रकुञ्चः[९] षोडशी बिल्वं पलमेवात्र कीर्त्यते[१०] ।।१३।।
पलाभ्यां प्रसृतिर्ज्ञेया प्रसृतश्च[११] निगद्यते ।
प्रसृतिभ्यामञ्जलिः स्यात्कुडवोऽर्धशरावकः[१२] ।।१४।।
अष्टमानं[१३] च स[१४] ज्ञेयः कुडवाभ्यां च मानिका ।
शरावोऽष्टपलं तद्वज्ज्ञेयमत्र विचक्षणैः ।।१५।।
शरावाभ्यां भवेत्प्रस्थश्चतुःप्रस्थैस्तथाढकम् ।
भाजनं कंसं पात्रं च चतुःषष्टिपलं[१५] च तत् ।।१६।।
चतुर्भिराढकैर्द्रोणः कलशो नल्वणोऽर्मणः ।
उन्मानश्च घटो राशिर्द्रोणपर्यायसंज्ञकः[१६] ।।१७।।
द्रोणाभ्यां शूर्पकुम्भौ च चतुःषष्टिशरावकः ।
शूर्पाभ्यां च भवेद् द्रोणी वाहो गोणी च सा स्मृता ।।१८।।
द्रोणीचतुष्टयं खारी कथिता सूक्ष्मबुद्धिभिः ।
चतुःसहस्रपलिका षण्णवत्यधिका च[१७] सा ।।१९।।
पलानां द्विसहस्रं च भार एकः प्रकीर्तितः ।
तुला पलशतं ज्ञेया सर्वत्रैवैष निश्चयः[१८] ।।२०।।

Elaboration of Weights & Measures

(1) According to the Wise, thirty *paramāṇu-s* (atoms) constitute one *trasareṇu* and its synonym is *vaṃśī*. When a beam of sun-rays comes to a dark room through a hole or window, the suspended particle seen in this beam of rays called *vaṃśī*.

(2) Six *vaṃśī*-s constitute one *marīci*.

(3) Six *marīci*-s constitute one *rājikā*.

(4) Three *rājikā-s* constitute one *sarṣapa*.

(5) Eight *sarṣapa-s* constitute one *yava*.

(6) Four *yava-s* constitute one *guñjā*.

(7) **Six** ***guñjā-s*** (*raktikā-s*) constitute one *māṣa* which is synonymous

with *hema* and *dhānyaka*.

(8) Four *māṣa-s* constitute one *sāṇa* which is synonymous with *dharaṇa* and *ṭaṅka*.

(9) Two *ṭaṅka-s* constitute one *kola* and it is synonymous with *kṣudra-mo(ko),vaṭaka* and *draṅkṣaṇa*.

(10) Two *kola-s* constitute one *karṣa* and its synonyms are *pāṇimānikā, akṣa, picu, pāṇitala, kiñcitpāṇi, tinduka, viḍālapadaka, ṣoḍaśikā, karamadhya, haṃsapada, suvarṇa, kavalagraha* and *udumbara*.

(11) Two *karṣa-s* constitute one *ardha pala* and its synonyms are *śukti* and *aṣṭamikā*.

(12) Two *śukti-s* constitute one *pala* and its synonyms are *muṣṭi, āmra, caturthikā, prakuñca, ṣoḍaśī* and *bilva*.

(13) Two *pala-s* constitute one *prasrti* or *prasṛta*.

(14) Two *prasṛti-s* constitute one *añjali*. Its synonyms are *kuḍava, ardha-śarāvaka* and *aṣṭamāna*.

(15) Two *kuḍava-s* constitute one *mānikā*. Its synonyms are *śarāva* and *aṣṭapala*.

(16) Two *śarāva-s* constitute one *prastha*.

(17) Four *prastha-s* constitute one *āḍhaka*. Its synonyms are *bhājana, kaṃsa, pātra* and *catuḥ-ṣaṣṭi-pala*.

(18) Four *āḍhaka-s* constitute one *droṇa*. Its synonyms are *kalaśa, nalvaṇa, armaṇa, unmāna, ghaṭa* and *rāśi*.

(19) Two *droṇa-s* constitute one *śūrpa*. Its synonyms are *kuṃbha* and *catuḥ-ṣaṣṭi-śarāvaka*.

(20) Two *śūrpa-s* constitute one *droṇī*. Its synonyms are *vāha* and *goṇī*.

(21) Four *droṇī-s* constitute one *khārī*. It is equivalent to 4096 *pala-s*.

(22) Two thousand *pala-s* constitute one *bhāra*.

(23) One hundred *pala-s* constitute one *tulā*.

These units of weights and measurements are universally accepted.

माषटङ्काक्षबिल्वानि कुडवः प्रस्थमाढकम् ।
राशिर्गोणी खारिकेति यथोत्तरचतुर्गुणाः ।।२१।।

Māṣa, ṭaṅka, akṣa, bilva, kuḍava, prastha, āḍhaka, rāśi, go(au)ṇī and *khārī* - each one of these succeeding units are four times of the preceding ones i.e. four of the preceding ones constitute one unit of succeeding ones.

[मानपरिभाषा]

गुञ्जादिमानमारभ्य यावत्स्यात्कुडवस्थितिः ।
द्रवार्द्रशुष्कद्रव्याणां तावन्मानं समं मतम् ।।२२।।

Weight of Wet and Dry Substances

From *guñjā* upto *kuḍava,* both the wet and dry substances are to be taken in similar quantities. [By implication, if a substance is described in the text to be taken in the quantity of one *guñjā* or multiple thereof, then the substance is to be taken according to the prescribed weight irrespective of the physical nature of the drug (whether it is wet or dry). This rule is to be followed upto *kuḍava* or multiple thereof.]

प्रस्थादिमानमारभ्य द्विगुणं तद्‌द्रवार्द्रयोः ।
मानं तथा तुलायास्तु द्विगुणं न क्वचित्स्मृतम् ।।२३।।

If a wet substance or a liquid is described to be taken in the quantity of *prastha* or multiple thereof, then in actual practice such substances are to be taken in double the quantity. [However, in the case of dry substances doubling of the quantity is not necessary. Doubling of the quantity of wet and liquid substances is necessary because of their moisture content. If in a recipe, such wet drugs are added in double the quantity, then therapeutically they will as effective as the dry drugs.] If a drug is mentioned in the text to be used in the quantity of *tulā,* then it should never be doubled even if it is a wet drug.

मृद्‌वृक्षवेणुलोहादेर्भाण्डं यच्चतुरङ्गुलम् ।
विस्तीर्णं च तथोच्चं च तन्मानं कुडवं वदेत् ।।२४।।

Size (Volume) of Kuḍava

The unit of *kuḍava* is used for weight and volume of measurement. For the latter, a cylindrical cup is prepared of mud, wood, bamboo, iron, etc. This cup should have internal diameter and height of four *aṅgula-s* (finger breadth = about ½ inch) each.

Note: This statement is repeated later in verse no. 68.

[योगपरिभाषा]
यदौषधं तु प्रथमं यस्य योगस्य कथ्यते ।
तन्नाम्नैव स योगो हि कथ्यतेऽत्र विनिश्चयः ।।२५।।

।। इति मागधपरिभाषा ।।

Naming a Recipe

A recipe consists of several drugs. The name of the drug appearing in the beginning of the recipe is used for naming the recipe. This rule is generally followed [notwithstanding some recipes which are named differently].

Thus, ends the description of *Māgadha* type of weights and measurements.

[मात्रापरिभाषा]
स्थितिर्नास्त्येव मात्रायाः कालमग्निं वयो[१९] बलम् ।
प्रकृतिं दोषदेशौ[२०] च दृष्ट्वा मात्रां प्रकल्पयेत् ।।२६।।

Dosage of Recipes

It is not possible to prescribe a fixed dose of medicines [uniformly for all patients]. Dosage of medicines varies depending upon the following factors :

(1) *Kāla* or time including the season when the drug is administered.
(2) *Agni* or the power of digestion of the patient.
(3) *Vayas* or the age of the patient.
(4) *Bala* or the strength of the patient.
(5) *Prakṛti* or the physical constitution of the patient.
(6) *Doṣa* or the nature of the *doṣa* involved in the causation of the disease.
(7) *Deśa* or the nature of the habitation of the patient.

A suitable dose of a medicine is to be fixed [by the physician] keeping the above points in view.

यतो मन्दाग्नयो ह्रस्वा हीनसत्त्वा नराः कलौ ।
अतस्तु मात्रा तद्योग्या प्रोच्यते सुज्ञसंमता ।।२७।।

Need for Reducing Dose

During the present *kali* age, human beings have low power of digestion, they are of short stature and they have low vitality. Therefore, the appropriate dose of medicines for the present day human beings, as suggested by the wise physicians, will be described [hereafter].

[कलिङ्गमानम्]
यवो द्वादशभिर्गौरसर्षपैः प्रोच्यते बुधैः ।
यवद्वयेन गुञ्जा स्यात्त्रिगुञ्जो बल्ल उच्यते ।।२८।।
माषो गुञ्जाभिरष्टाभिः सप्तभिर्वा भवेत्क्वचित् ।
स्याच्चतुर्माषकैः शाणः स निष्कष्टङ्क एव च ।।२९।।
गद्याणो माषकैः षड्भिः कर्षः स्याद् दशमाषकः ।
चतुःकर्षैः पलं प्रोक्तं दशशाणमितं बुधैः ।
चतुष्पलैश्च कुडवं प्रस्थाद्याः पूर्ववन्मताः ।।३०।।

Kāliṅga Type of Weights ad Measurements

Hereafter, the *kāliṅga* type of weights and measurements will be described :

(1) Twelve *gaura sarṣapa* (white mustard seed) constitute one *yava* (grain of barley).
(2) Two *yava-s* constitute one *guñjā* [seed of *Abrus precatorius*].
(3) Three *guñjā-s* constitute one *balla*.
(4) Eight or seven *guñjā-s* constitute one *māṣa*.
(5) Four *māṣa-s* constitute one *śāṇa*. Its synonyms are *niṣka* and *ṭaṅka*.
(6) Six *māṣa-s* constitute one *gadyāṇa*.
(7) Ten *māṣa-s* constitute one *karṣa*.
(8) Four *karṣa-s* constitute one *pala*. It is equivalent to ten *śāṇa-s*.
(9) Four *pala-s* constitute one *kuḍava*.

Subsequent units of weights and measurements are in accordance with the *Māgadha* school.

कलिङ्गं मागधं चेति द्विविधं मानमुच्यते ।
कलिङ्गान्मागधं श्रेष्ठं मानं मानविदो विदुः ।।३१।।

।। इति कलिङ्गपरिभाषा ।।

This verse is repetition of verse no. 2.

Thus, ends the explanation of *kāliṅga* type of weights and measures.

[औषधपरिभाषा]

नवान्येव हि योज्यानि द्रव्याण्यखिलकर्मसु ।

विना विडङ्गकृष्णाभ्यां गुडधान्याज्यमाक्षिकैः ।।३२।।

Selection of Drugs

In general, drugs which are freshly collected should be used in therapeutics (recipes). The exceptions are *viḍaṅga* (*Embelia ribes*) *kṛṣṇā* (*Piper longum*), *guḍa* (jaggery), *dhānya* (careals and pulses), *ājya* (ghee) and *mākṣika* (honey) [which are therapeutically more effective when used after preservation for sometime].

गुडूची कुटजो वासा कूष्माण्डश्च शतावरी ।

अश्वगन्धा सहचरी शतपुष्पा प्रसारिणी ।

प्रयोक्तव्या सदैवार्द्रा द्विगुणा नैव कारयेत् ।।३४।।

Drugs to be Used in Wet-Form

Guḍūcī, *kuṭaja*, *vāsā*, *kūṣmāṇḍa*, *śatāvarī*, *aśvagandhā*, *sahacarī*, *śatapuṣpā* and *prasāriṇī* should always be used in wet-form and their quantity should not be doubled [as mentioned in verse no. 23].

शुष्कं नवीनं द्रव्यं[२१] च योज्यं सकलकर्मसु ।

आर्द्रं च द्विगुणं युञ्ज्यादेष सर्वत्र निश्चयः ।।३५।।

General Rule

However, the general rule is to use a dry drug only when it is freshly collected and dried, and all wet drugs are to be used in double the prescribed quantity in all recipes barring the exceptions described before.

कालेऽनुक्ते प्रभातं स्यादङ्गेऽनुक्ते जटा भवेत् ।

भागेऽनुक्ते तु साम्यं स्यात्पात्रेऽनुक्ते[२२] च मृन्मयम् ।।३५।।

एकमप्यौषधयोगे यस्मिन्यत्पुनरुच्यते ।
मानतो द्विगुणं प्रोक्तं[23] तद्द्रव्यं तत्त्वदर्शिभिः ।।३६।।

Unspecified Time, etc.

(1) When no time is specified [in the text for taking medicine or collecting herbs], then it should be done during the morning.
(2) When the part of a plant [to be used in a recipe] is not specified [in the text] then the root [of the plant] is to be used.
(3) When the proportion [in which different ingredients of recipe are to be added] is not specified [in the text], then all the ingredients are to be taken in equal quantities.
(4) When the nature of the pot [which is to be used for cooking a medicinal potion] is not specified [in the text] then mud-pot is to be used.
(5) If in a recipe the same ingredient is mentioned twice then this ingredient is to be used in double the quantity.

चूर्णस्नेहासवालेहाः प्रायशश्चन्दनान्विताः ।
कषायलेपयोः प्रायः[24] युज्यते रक्तचन्दनम् ।।३७।।

Use of Candana

Candana is of the two types, viz., white and red. If in a recipe of powder or medicated ghee or *āsava* (alcoholic preparation) or linctus the type of *candana* is not specified then white variety of *candana* is to be used. If, however, the recipe is a decoction or *lepa* (ointment for external use), then the red variety of *candana* should be used.

गुणहीनं भवेद्वर्षादूर्ध्वं तद्रूपमौषधम् ।
मासद्वयात्तथा चूर्णं हीनवीर्यत्वमाप्नुयात्[25] ।।३८।।
हीनत्वं गुटिकालेहौ लभेते वत्सरात्परम् ।
'हीनाः[26] स्युर्घृततैलाद्याश्चतुर्मासाधिकास्तथा[27] ।।३९।।
औषधयो लघुपाकाः स्युर्निर्वीर्याः वत्सरात्परम्' ।
पुराणाः स्युर्गुणैर्युक्ता आसवा धातवो रसाः ।।४०।।

Self-life of Different Categories of Preparations

(1) Raw-drugs generally lose their potency in one year after their collection.

(2) A medicinal recipe in powder form loses its potency after two months.

(3) A medicinal recipe in the form of pills and linctus (jam or marmaled) loses its potency in four months.

(4) After one year raw-drugs become light for digestion and they lose their potency.

(5) But in the case of *āsava-s* (alcoholic preparations), *dhātu-s* (metallic and mineral preparations) and *rasa-s* (recipes containing mercury), the older the recipe the better the therapeutic effect.

व्याधेरयुक्तं यद्द्रव्यं गणोक्तमपि तत्त्यजेत् ।
अनुक्तमपि यद्युक्तं योजयेत्तत्र तद्बुधः ।।४१।।
।। इति युक्तायुक्तविचार ।।
[शार्ङ्गधर : प्रथमखण्ड : १:१४-५४]

Modification of Recipes

If in a recipe or groups of drugs, an ingredient is found to be unsuitable for a disease, then such an ingredient should be discarded [and the recipe for that disease should be prepared excluding such inappropriate ingredients]. If, however, in a recipe, a drug appropriate for a disease is not included, then the physician may add that ingredient to the recipe.

Thus, ends the description of appropriate and inappropriate ingredients in a recipe.

'वज्राभावे तु[२८] वैक्रान्तं स्वर्णाभावे तु माक्षिकम् ।
हेममाक्षिकजं सत्त्वं मृतहेमसमं गुणैः ।।४२।।
विमलमाक्षिकं ज्ञेयं ध्रुवं रजतवद्गुणैः ।
मुक्ताभावे क्षिपेन्नूनं मुक्ताशुक्ति च तद्गुणम् ।।४३।।
अभावेऽभ्रकसत्त्वस्य कान्तलोहं च योजयेत् ।
कांताभावे तीक्ष्णलोहं इत्युक्तं रसदर्प्पणे ।।४४।।
अभावे मधुनो योज्यो गुडो जीर्णश्च तद्गुणः ।

सिताभावे भवेत् खण्डं शाल्यभावे च षष्टिकः ।।४५।।
असंभवे तु द्राक्षायाः प्रदेयं काश्मरीफलम् ।
वृक्षाम्लं न भवेत्तत्र दाडिमाम्लं प्रयोजयेत् ।।४६।।
वेतसाम्लस्य चाभावे हरिमन्थाम्लमादिशेत् ।
अभावे चन्दनस्यापि मेलयेद्रक्तचन्दनम् ।।४७।।
अभावे सति पित्तानां रसाद्यैर्भावनाविधौ ।
विषमुष्टिकषायेण तद्गुणाश्चैव भावयेत् ।।४८।।

Substitutes

(1) The physician may use *vaikrānta* in the place of *vajra* (diamond) and *[svarṇa] mākṣika* in the place of *svarṇa* (gold).

(2) The *sattva* (essence) of *svarṇa mākṣika* is similar to gold-*bhasma* in properties. Similarly, the *sattva* of *vimala mākṣika* is certainly like silver in properties.

(3) If pearl is not available, then in its place *muktā-śukti* (pearl oyester), which has similar properties, may be used.

(4) If *abhraka-sattva* is not available, then in its place *kānta lauha* may be used in a recipe.

(5) According to the text '*Rasa-darpaṇa*', if *kānta-lauha* is not available, then in its place *tīkṣṇa-lauha* may be used.

(6) If honey is not available, then old jaggery having similar properties may be used in its place in a recipe.

(7) If *sitā* (crystal sugar) is not available, then in its place *khaṇḍa* (a type of brown sugar) may be used in the recipe.

(8) If *śāli* type of rice is not avialable then in its place *ṣaṣṭika* type of rice may be used.

(9) If *drākṣā* is not available, then in its place, *kāśmarī*-fruit may be used.

(10) If *vṛkṣāmla* is not available, then in its place sour variety of *dāḍima* may be used.

(11) If *vetasāmla* is not available, then in its place *harimanthāmla* may be used.

(12) If [white variety of] *candana* is not available then in its place

red variety of *candana* should be added to a recipe.

(13) If the ingredients of a recipe are described to be impregenated with juices and biles of animals, and if such biles (*pitta*) are not available, then in their places, the recipe should be impregnated with the decoction of *viṣamuṣṭi* which has similar properties.

गोरक्षमतात्

मेदा-जीवक-काकोलीद्वंद्वाभावे प्रयोजयेत् ।
यष्टीविदार्यश्वगंधाबलावरीवाराहीकान्[९] ॥४९॥

According to Gorakṣa

If *medā*, *mahā-medā*, *jīvaka*, *ṛṣabhaka*, *kākolī* and *kṣīra-kākolī* are not available, then in their places *yaṣṭī*, *vidārī*, *aśvagandhā*, *balā*, *śatāvarī* and *vārāhīkanda* should respectively be used.

वैद्यालंकारात्

फलमाममपुष्टं च त्यजेद्बिल्वादृते सदा ।
द्राक्षाबिल्वशिवादीनां फलं शुष्कं गुणोत्तरम् ॥५०॥

According to Vaidyālaṅkāra

The physician should always discard fruits which are unripe and immature excepting *bilva* [in which latter is more useful when it is unripe and immature]. Fruits of *drākṣā*, *bilva*, *śivā*, etc., are more useful when these are dry.

रसदर्पणात्

त्रुटिः स्यादणुभिः षड्भिस्तैर्लिक्षा षड्भिरीरिता ।
ताभिः षड्भिर्भवेद्यूका षड्यूकास्तु रजः स्मृतम् ॥५१॥

Weights and Measures

According to Rasa-darpaṇa

(1) Six *aṇu-s* (atoms) constitute one *truṭi*.
(2) Six *truṭi-s* constitute one *likṣā*.
(3) Six *likṣā-s* constitute one *yūkā*.
(4) Six *yūkā-s* constitute one *rajas*.

चिन्तामणिः[३०]

जालान्तरगतैः सूर्यकरैर्वंशी विलोक्यते ।
तस्य नामान्तरं ज्ञेयं त्रसरेणु रजस्तथा ॥५२॥

Weights and Measures : According to Cintāmaṇi

The suspended material visible in a beam of sun-rays coming into a dark-room through a hole or window is called *vaṃśī* (unit of weight). Its synonyms are *trasareṇu* and *rajas*.

कृष्णात्रेयात्

त्रिरजोभिश्च सिकता ताभिः षोडशभिर्बुधः[३१] ।
सर्षपश्च[३२] भवेद्गौरस्ते चाष्टौ तण्डुलं विदुः ॥५३॥
तद् द्वयं धान्यमाषः स्यात् तद् द्वयं[३३] रक्तिका मता ।
'रक्तिका[३४] त्रितयेनापि बल्लः प्रोक्तो विशारदैः' ॥५४॥
चतुर्भिरण्डिका ज्ञेया षड्भिर्बल्लः प्रकीर्तितः ।
पक्वगुञ्जाफलैस्तुल्यैरष्टाभिर्माषकः स्मृतः ॥५५॥
रक्तिकापञ्चभिर्माषः षड्भिर्वा सप्तभिस्त्रिभिः ।
दशभिर्वा भवेदत्र प्रोत्तमाधममध्यमाः ।
अण्डिका चापि निर्दिष्टा क्वचिन्माषद्वये[३५] नवे ॥५६॥
चतुर्भिर्माषकैः शाणस्त्रिभिर्वात्रियसंमतम्[३६] ।
गद्याणो[३७] माषकैः षड्भिः शाणाभ्यां द्रंक्षणो मतः ।
कोलश्च वटकश्चैव स[३८] भवेत्क्षुद्रसंज्ञकः ॥५७॥

Weights and Measures : According to Kṛṣṇātreya

(1) Three *raja-s* constitute one *sikatā*.

(2) Sixteen *sikatā-s* constitute one *gaura sarṣapa*.

(3) Eight *gaurasarṣapa-s* constitute one *taṇḍula*.

(4) Two *taṇḍula-s* constitute one *dhānya-māṣa*.

(5) Two *dhānya-māṣa-s* constitute one *raktikā*.

(6) Three *raktikā-s* constitute one *balla*.

(7) Four *raktikā-s* constitute one *aṇḍikā* and six of these constitute one *balla* (?)

(8) Eight seeds of ripe *guñjā* (*raktikā*) are equivalent to one *māṣa*.

(9) In practice, different types of *māṣa* are used inasmuch as five or six or seven or three or ten *raktikā-s* constitute one *māṣa*. Accordingly, these different units of *māṣa* are treated as superior, medium or inferior types.

(10) At times, another unit of weight called *aṇḍikā* is used and it is constituted of two *māṣa-s*.

(11) Four *māṣa-s* constitute one *śāṇa*. According to Ātreya, three *māṣa-s* constitute one *śāṇa*.

(12) Six *māṣa-s* constitute one *gadyāṇa*.

(13) Two *śāṇa-s* constitute one *draṅkṣaṇa* and its synonyms are *kola*, *vaṭaka* and *kṣudra*.

रसार्णवात्[३९]

त्रिभिः शाणैर्भवेत्तोला षड्भिर्गद्याणकं विदुः ।।५८ ।।

According to Rasārṇava

Three *sāṇa-s* constitute one *tolā* and six *sāṇa-s* constitute one *gadyāṇaka*.

कृष्णात्रेयः

शाणैश्चतुर्भिः कर्षः स्यादक्षं पाणितलं विदुः[४०] ।
पिचुः सुवर्णकं किञ्चित् विडालपदकं तथा ।।५९ ।।
उदुम्बरं हंसपादं करमध्यं च तिन्दुकम् ।
कवलग्रहः पाणिकश्च[४१] स प्रोक्तः पाणिमालिका ।।६० ।।

।। इति कर्षनाम ।।

Karṣa and Its Synonyms
According to Kṛṣṇātreya

Four *śāṇa-s* constitute one *karṣa*. Its synonyms are *akṣa*, *pāṇitala*, *picu*, *suvarṇaka*, *viḍāla-padaka*, *udumbara*, *haṃsa-pāda*, *kara-madhya*, *tinduka*, *kavalagraha*, *pāṇika* and *pāṇi-mālikā*.

वृद्धहारीतः[४२]

पाने बस्तौ तथाभ्यङ्गे शुक्तिरर्धपलेन च ।

भवेत्तैलस्य पाके[४३] च इति मे निश्चिता मतिः ॥६१॥

According to Vṛddha Hārīta

One *śukti* is equivalent to half of a *pala* and this rule is applicable to the recipes used for *pāna* (potion used for drinking), *basti* (recipe used for medicated enema), *abhyaṅga* (massage) and *taila pāka* (cooking a medicated oil).

प्रदेशिन्या निमग्ने द्वे पर्वणी गतितोऽखिलम् ।

नस्यादिषु तु[४४] विज्ञेयो भिषग्भिर्बिन्दुसंज्ञकः ॥६२॥

॥विन्दुमात्रा[४५]॥

विन्दुभिश्चाष्टभिः शाणः प्रोक्तश्चेति भिषक्तमैः ।

द्वात्रिंशद्विन्दुभिश्चात्र शुक्तिश्चैव विधीयते ।

द्वे शुक्ती पाणिशुक्तिश्च नस्यकर्मणि पूजिता ॥६३॥

॥ शुक्तिद्वयनाम[४६] ॥

Measurement of a Drop

If two proglotids of the index finger are fully immersed into oil and taken out, the oil that comes down from the finger is equivalent to one drop *(bindu.)* This unit of measurement is used for the administration of inhalation therapy, etc. Eight such drops (*bindu-s*) constitute one *śāṇa* and thirty two drops constitute one *śukti*. Two such *śukti-s* constitute one *pāṇi-śukti*. These units of measurements are useful for the administration of inhalation therapy.

कृष्णात्रेयः

शुक्तिभ्यां तु प्रकुञ्चः स्यात्पलं मुष्टिश्चतुर्थिका ।

रात्रं तदेव विज्ञेयं चरकाद्यैर्म्महर्षिभिः ॥६४॥

आम्रं बिल्वं पलाभ्यां स्यात्प्रसृतिः प्रसृतस्तथा ।

पलस्य दशमांशेन धरणं परिकीर्तितम् ॥६५॥

प्रसृतिभ्यामञ्जलिः स्यात्कुडवं तु च चतुष्पलम् ।
वेणुर्वृक्षायसादीनां भाण्डं यच्चतुरङ्गुलम् ॥६६॥
विस्तीर्णमथ वृत्तं च कुडवं तं विनिर्दिशेत् ॥६७॥
कुडवाभ्यां शरावः स्यान्माणिकाष्ट[४७]पलं तथा ।
चतुर्भिः कुडवः प्रस्थस्तथा सुप्तमितीरितः ॥६८॥
चतुःप्रस्थैर्भवेत्पात्रं[४८] स स्याद्भाजनमाढकम् ।
कंसं[४९] प्रस्थाष्टकं पात्रं पर्यायैः क्रमशो विदुः ॥६९॥
चतुराढकसंख्यातो द्रोणश्च परिकीर्तितः ।
कलशो नल्वणो राशिर्मणश्च परिकीर्तितः ॥७०॥
द्रोणाभ्यां सूर्पकुम्भो च चतुःषष्टिशरावकः ॥७१॥
शूर्पाच्च[५०] द्विगुणा द्रोणी वहो गोणी च सा स्मृता ।
तुला पलशतं तासां विंशतिर्भार उच्यते ॥७२॥
माषः शाणः पिचुर्बिल्वः कुडवः प्रस्थमाढकम्[५१] ।
राशिर्गोणी[५२] खारिकेति यथोत्तरं चतुर्गुणम् ॥७३॥

According to Kṛṣṇātreya

(1) Two *śukti-s* constitute one *prakuñca*. Its synonyms are *pala*, *muṣṭi* and *caturthikā*. According to great sages like Caraka, etc., this unit of weight is also called *pātra*. This is also called *āmra* and *bilva*.

(2) Two *pala-s* constitute one *prasṛti* or *prasṛta*. One tenth of a *pala* makes one *dharaṇa*.

(3) Two *prasṛti-s* constitute one *añjali*.

(4) Four *pala-s* constitute one *kuḍava*. A cup of bamboo or wood or iron, etc., which is four fingers in diameter and which is round is called *kuḍava*. [Ref. earlier verse no. 24]

(5) Two *kuḍava-s* constitute one *śarāva* or *māṇikā* and it is also called *aṣṭapala* or it is equivalent to eight *pala-s*.

(6) Four *kuḍava-s* constitute one *prastha* and it is called *supta*.

(7) Four *prastha-s* constitute one *pātra*. Its synonyms are *bhājana*, *āḍhaka* and *kaṃsa*. [Two other synonyms, viz., *prasthāṣṭaka* and

pātra mentioned here appear to be erroneous.]

(8) Four *āḍhaka-s* constitute one *droṇa*. Its synonyms are *kalaśa*, *nalvaṇa*, *rāśi* and *maṇa*.

(9) Two *droṇa-s* constitute *śūrpa-kumbha* and it is equivalent to 64 *śarāvaka-s*.

(10) Two *śūrpa-s* constitute one *droṇī*. Its synonyms are *vaha* and *goṇī*.

(11) One hundred *pala-s* constitute one *tulā*.

(12) Twenty *tulā-s* constitute one *bhāra*.

Māṣa, *śāṇa*, *picu*, *bilva*, *kuḍava*, *prastha*, *āḍhaka*, *rāśi*, *goṇī* and *khārī* - each one of the succeeding units is four times of the preceding ones, i.e. four of the preceding ones constitute one unit of the succeeding ones-[Ref. verse no. 21 above].

अथ रसार्णवात् रजपरिभाषा

षट्त्रुट्यश्चैकलिक्षा स्यात् षट्लिक्षा यूकमेव च ।
षट्यूकास्तु रजः[५३] सञ्ज्ञाः कथितास्तव सुव्रते ।।७४।।
[रसार्णव : दशमपटल : ३२]

Unit of Rajas : According to Rasārṇava

(1) Six *truṭi-s* constitute one *likṣā*.
(2) Six *likṣā-s* constitute one *yūkā*.
(3) Six *yūkā-s* constitute one *rajas*.

मतान्तरे

षड्रजः सर्षपः स[५४] स्याद्यवोऽष्टाभिस्तु सर्षपैः ।
यवद्वयेन[५५] गुंजा स्यात्षड्गुञ्जैश्चैकमाषकः ।
माषद्वादश तोलास्यादष्टौ तोला पलं भवेत्[५६] ।।७५।।

An Alternative Opinion

(1) Six *raja-s* constitute one *sarṣapa*.
(2) Eight *sarṣapa-s* constitute one *yava*.
(3) Two *yava-s* constitute one *guñjā*.
(4) Six *guñjā-s* constitute one *māṣa*.
(5) Twelve *māṣa-s* constitute one *tolā*.
(6) Eight *tolā-s* constitute one *pala*.

कृष्णात्रेयः
दशगुञ्जात्मकं माषं प्रवदन्ति चिकित्सकाः ।।७६ ।।
तत्र श्रेष्ठमध्या[५७]दिभेदान्माषकादिप्रतिपत्तौ समाधानमूह्यम् ।।७७ ।।

According to Kṛṣṇātreya

Some physicians hold the view that ten *guñjā-s* constitute one *māṣa*. Persons having different types of strength, viz., excellent strength, moderate strength etc., need medicines in different dosage. Therefore, there are differences in the units of *māṣa*, etc. This is how the controversy regarding the units of weight could be solved.

माषैर्द्वादशभिर्धान्यैर्माषकः परिकीर्त्तितः ।
'कषायादि[५८]निरूहेषु द्रव्यमानविधावपि ।।७८ ।।
ततोऽष्टादशभिर्माषैर्माषकः परिकीर्त्तितः' ।
वम्यादिरक्तमोक्षेषु माने मूत्रवसादिषु ।।७९ ।।
वमनादिषु योज्यश्च माषकश्चाष्टरक्तिकः ।
'लोहरत्नादि[५९]विषये दशरक्तिकमाषकः' ।।८० ।।
वमने च विरेके च तथा शोणितमोक्षणे ।
सार्द्धत्रयोदशपलं प्रस्थमाहुर्मनीषिणः ।।८१ ।।

Controversy Regarding Different Units of Weight

(1) Twelve *dhānya-māṣa-s* constitute one *māṣa*. This unit of weight is applicable to the ingredients used for the preparation of decoctions for *nirūha* type of medicated enema.

(2) Eighteen *dhānya-māṣa-s* constitute one *māṣa*. This unit of weight is applicable to the urine, fat (*vaṣā*), etc., used in the preparations for emetic and blood-letting therapies.

(3) Eight *rattī-s* constitute one *māṣa*. This unit of weight is applicable to the weight of raw-drugs used in the recipes for emetic therapy.

(4) Ten *rattī-s* constitute one *māṣa*. This unit of weight is applicable to the measurement of metals, gems and jewels.

(5) Thirteen and half *pala-s* constitute one *prastha*. This unit of measurement is applicable to recipes used for emetic, purgation and blood-letting therapies.

शुष्कद्रव्यस्य या मात्रा आर्द्रस्य द्विगुणा हि सा[१०] ।
शुष्कस्य गुरुतीक्ष्णत्वादर्धमानं तु योजयेत् ॥८२॥

Dry and Wet Drugs

The weight prescribed for dry-drugs (ingredients in a recipe) is doubled if these ingredients are to be used in wet-form. Dry-drugs are heavy and more potent (lit.-sharp); therefore, these are used in half of the prescribed quantity.

गोपुररक्षितः
रक्तिकादिषु मानेषु यावन्न कुडवो भवेत् ।
शुष्कार्द्रद्रव्ययोस्तावत्तुल्यं मानं प्रयोजयेत्[६१] ॥८३॥
शुष्कद्रव्येष्विदं मानं द्विगुणं तु द्रवार्द्रयोः ।
यद् द्रव्यं कुडवादूर्ध्वं प्रस्थादिश्रुतं मानतः[६२] ।
द्विगुणं न तुलामानमिति मानविदो विदुः ॥८४॥

According to Gopura-rakṣita

If an ingredient in a recipe is prescribed to be used in the units of weight from *ratti* upto *kuḍava* then irrespective of their nature, both the dry and wet-drugs are to be used in equal (same) quantities. If an ingredient in a recipe is prescribed to be taken in *kuḍava* or above it like *prastha*, then the dry-drugs are to be taken in the prescribed quantities and wet-drugs and liquids are to be taken in double of the prescribed quantities.

However, if the quantity is prescribed in *tulā*, then doubling the quantity in respect of wet drugs and liquids is not necessary.

द्रवार्द्रयोः कोऽर्थः? मधुतैलघृतादेः। उक्तं च॥८५॥
शुष्कद्रव्येष्विदं मानमेवमादि प्रकीर्तितम् ।
द्विगुणं तद् द्रवेष्विष्टं मधुतैलघृतादिषु ॥८६॥

What is the meaning of the term *dravārdra*? The term *dravārdra* (lit. liquid and wet) refers to honey, oil, ghee, etc. It is said; "The quantity described in a recipe refers to dry drugs and in the case of liquids like honey, oil, ghee, etc., the quantity should be doubled"

हारीतः
आर्द्रद्रव्यैः द्रवद्रव्यैः पलैरष्टभिरेव च ।
शुष्कद्रव्यचतुष्केण कुडवः समुदाहृतः ।।८७।।

According to Hārīta

Eight *pala-s* of wet-drugs and liquid drugs constitute one *kuḍava*. But, in the case of dry-drugs, four *pala-s* constitute one *kuḍava*.

पुष्कलावतः[६३]
आर्द्रस्याष्टपला मात्रा कुडवस्य प्रमाणतः ।
मधुतैलघृतादेश्च शुष्कद्रव्ये चतुष्पले ।।८८।।

According to Puṣkalāvata

Eight *pala-s* of wet-drugs and liquid drugs like honey, oil, ghee, etc., constitute one *kuḍava*. On the other hand, four *pala-s* of dry-drugs constitute one *kuḍava*.

विश्वामित्रः
गुडगुग्गुलुबाह्लीकैस्त्रिफलारिष्टनागरैः ।
कूष्माण्डार्द्रकनिंबानां कुडवश्चाष्टभिर्पलैः ।।८९।।
अरिष्टं रसोनः ।।९०।।

According to Viśvāmitra

Guḍa, *guggulu*, *bāhlīka*, *triphalā*, *ariṣṭa* (*rasona*), *nāgara*, *kūṣmāṇḍa*, *ārdraka* and *nimba* — eight *pala-s* of these drugs constitute one *kuḍava*.

रसदर्पणात्
लाजापायसनारिकेलसलिलैर्मूत्रैस्तथाकाञ्जिकैः;
मत्स्यांडी-मधु-तक्र-मस्तु-मदिरादीनां भवेत् द्विगुणः।
वासानिम्बपटोलकेतकिबलाकूष्माण्डकेन्दीवरी।।९१।।

वर्षाभूकुटजाश्वमारसहिताः व्योषाश्वगन्धामृताः ।
मांसी नागबलासहचरपुरं हिंग्वार्द्रकंनित्यशोः[६४] ।
ग्राह्यास्तत्क्षणमेव[६५] न द्विगुणिता ये चेक्षुजातास्तथा ।।९२ ।।

According to Rasa-darpaṇa

Lājā, *pāyasa*, coconut water, urine, *kāñjika* (vinegar), *matsyāṇḍī*, honey, butter-milk, *mastu* (whey) and alcohol — these drugs are to be taken in double the quantity.

Vāsā, *nimba*, *paṭola*, *ketaki*, *balā*, *kūṣmāṇḍa*, *indīvarī*, *varṣābhū*, *kuṭaja*, *aśvamāra*, *vyoṣa*, *aśvagandhā*, *amṛtā*, *māṃsī*, *nāgabalā*, *sahacara*, *pura*, *hiṅgu*, *ārdraka* and products of sugar-cane should be used only in the prescribed quantity. [Though these are wet-drugs, the quantity should not be doubled.]

तथा च भेलः[६६]
गुडरामठशुण्ठीनां मांसकूष्माण्डयोरपि ।
गुडूच्या गुग्गुलोश्चैव प्रस्थः षोडशभिः पलैः ।।९३ ।।

According to Bhela

In respect of drugs, viz., *guḍa*, *rāmaṭha*, *śuṇṭhī*, *māṃsa* (meat), *kūṣmāṇḍa*, *guḍūcī* and *guggulu*, sixteen *pala-s* constitute one *prastha*.

भोजः
यच्चूर्णं गुटिका या च कर्त्तव्या गुल्मरोगिणाम् ।
क्षारहिङ्ग्वजमोदाम्लवेतसैस्तान्न[६७] केवलाः ।।९४ ।।
क्रोष्टुशीर्षादिरोगेषु जटायूर्द्विगुणो मतः ।
प्रमेहादिषु रोगेषु मात्रातोऽर्धः प्रशस्यते ।।९५ ।।

According to Bhoja

Kṣāra, *hiṅgu*, *ajamodā* and *amla-vetasa* should be used only in the prescribed quantities in the case of recipes in the form of powders or pills for the treatment of *gulma* (phantom tumour). If *jaṭāyu* (*guggulu*) is to be used in a recipe for the treatment of *kroṣṭukaśīrṣa* (a type of arthritis) etc., then it should be taken in double the prescribed quantity. If, however, *guggulu* is to be used in a recipe for the treatment of *prameha* (obstinate urinary disorders including diabetes), then it is to be taken in half of the prescribed quantity.

औषध परिभाषा

[USAGE OF DRUGS]

सुश्रुतः

योऽल्पौषधकृतो योगो बहुग्रन्थभयान्मया ।

[सुश्रुत : चिकित्सा १:१३५]

द्रव्याणां तत्समानानां तत्रावापो न दुष्यति ।।९६।।

समस्तवर्गमर्धं च यथालाभमथाऽपि वा ।

प्रयुञ्जीत भिषक्प्राज्ञः कालावस्थादि[१८]भागवित् ।।९७।।

According to Suśruta

In the recipes described by me (Suśruta) only a few essential ingredients are included. This is done to avoid details. If a physician adds appropriate and similar drugs into these recipes, then no mistake is commited. A wise physician, aquainted with the differences in the nature of the time of administration and the variations in the states of diseases, can use all or half of ingredients or only those which are readily available from amongst the group of prescribed drugs.

प्रसङ्गाभिहितो वा यो बहुदुर्बलभेषजः ।

यथोपपत्तिस्तत्रापि कार्यं[१९] सर्वं चिकित्सितम् ।।९८।।

Change of Ingredients in Recipes

In a recipe, because of the context, several medicines are described which are therapeutically not so potent, one may appropriately use (omit) them while preparing the recipe for the treatment of diseases.

क्षीणानां दुर्बलाग्नीनां भेषजद्वेषिणां तथा ।

बालकानां गर्भिणीनां वृद्धानां सम्प्रदायवित् ।

मृद्वल्पौषधयोगेन भिषक् सम्यगुपाचरेत् ।।९९।।

Small Dose

The physician, aquainted with tradition, should administer *mṛdu* (less potent) medicines in smaller doses to the following categories of patients :

(1) Those who are emaciated;
(2) Those who have less power of digestion;
(3) Those who despise (do not like taking) medicines;
(4) Young children;
(5) Pregnant women; and
(6) Old people.

बलिनां बहुदोषाणां कारयेद्धि[70] विपर्ययम् ।।१००।।

Large Dose

To strong persons having more of aggravated *doṣa-s*, the physician should administer strong medicines in a large dose.

उक्तानुक्तग्रहणम्

अङ्गेप्यनुक्ते विहितं तु मूलं पानेऽप्यनुक्ते जलमाशु देयम् ।
भागेऽप्यनुक्ते समता विधेया कालेऽप्यनुक्ते दिवसस्य पूर्वम् ।।१०१।।
अनिर्दिष्ट-प्रसिद्धेषु मूलं ग्राह्यं त्वगाद्यपि ।
महान्ति यानि मूलानि काष्ठगर्भाणि यानि च ।
तेषां तु वल्कलं ग्राह्यं ह्रस्वमूलानि कृत्स्नशः[71] ।।१०२।।
अन्तःसंमार्जने मोदा'स्थाने[72] योज्या यवानिका ।
बहिःसंमार्जने मोदा'अजमोदैव गृह्यते ।।१०३।।
अंतःसंमार्जने[73] योज्यं वचास्थाने कुलिंजनम् ।
बहिःसंमार्जने सैव प्रयोक्तव्या मनीषिभिः ।।१०४।।
कृष्णजीरकयोगेन कर्त्तव्यो भक्षभेषजे ।
तस्य स्थाने विधातव्यो जीरकः कुशलो भिषक् ।।१०५।।

Unspecified Part, etc.

(1) If in a recipe, the part of the plant to be used is not specified, then the root of the herb is to be used.
(2) If the post-prandial drink is not specified, then water should be used.

(3) If the proportion in which the ingredients of a recipe is to be taken is not specified, then such ingredients are to be used in equal quantities.
(4) If the time of administering a drug is not specified, then it should be given in the morning.
(5) If in a recipe, the part of a well known plant to be used is not specified, then along with root, its bark, etc., may also be used.
(6) If it is a big tree with wood inside, then the bark of such trees should be used in medicine.
(7) If the ingredient has small root, then the entire herb is to be used in medicine.
(8) In the recipes for internal cleansing, *yavānikā* should be used in the place of *modā (ajamodā).*
(9) In the recipes for external cleansing, in the place of *modajamodā* is to be used.
(10) In the recipes for internal cleansing, *kuliñjana* should be used in the place of *vacā*.
(11) In the recipes for external cleansing, *vacā* as such should be used.
(12) If the recipe is to be used internally, then in the place of *kṛṣṇa jīraka* (black variety of *jīraka)* [*śveta*]) *jīraka* (white variety of *jīraka*) is to be used. [Ref. : Verses 35-36 of this chapter]

भद्रसौनकः[७४]
सारश्च खदिरादीनां निम्बादीनां त्वक् स्मृताः ।
फलं तु दाडिमादीनां पटोलादेश्छदस्तथा ।।१०६।

According to Bhadra-Śaunaka

(1) In the case of *khadira*, etc., the heart-wood is to be used in recipes.
(2) In the case of *nimba,* etc., the bark is to be used.
(3) Of *dāḍima*, etc., fruit is to be used.
(4) Of *paṭola,* etc., leaves are to be used.

'भद्रशौनकादपि[७५] गोरक्षमतात्'
क्वचित्पत्रं क्वचिन्मूलं क्वचित्पुष्पं क्वचित्फलम् ।
क्वचिद्बीजं क्वचिद्वल्कं क्वचित्काष्ठं क्वचिज्जलम् ।।१०७।।
क्वचिन्नालं योजनीयं क्षीरं क्षारं क्वचित्क्वचित् ।
एकैकस्यौषधस्यैवं 'यथायोगं[७६] प्रयोजयेत् ।।१०८।।

According to Bhadra-śaunaka and Gorakṣa

Depending upon their appropriateness, at times the leaves, roots, flowers, fruits, seeds, barks, woods, aqueous exudates (*jala*), tender branches (*nāla*), milky latex and at times *kṣāra* (alkali preparations) of individual ingredients are to be used in recipes.

गणोक्तमपि यद्द्रव्यं' भवेद् व्याधौ न यौगिकम् ।
तदुद्धरेद्यौगिकं हि प्रक्षिपेदप्यकीर्तितम्[७७] ॥१०९॥

Change in Gaṇa-s (Groups of Drugs)

If some ingredients mentioned in a recipe are not useful for the disease, then such ingredients should be excluded, and if some ingredients which are useful for curing the disease are not mentioned in a recipe, then such ingredients should be added to the recipe while preparing them.

नवानि सर्वद्रव्याणि प्रशस्तानि क्रियाविधौ ।
'सर्पिः[७८] कृष्णागुडक्षौद्रविडंगायससंज्ञकाः ॥११०॥
कृता ता आसवाद्यश्च न रसाश्च कदाचन ।
सदा ह्येताः पुराणानि ग्रहीतव्या विजानता[७९]' ॥
ताम्बूलं च पुराणं स्याद्धान्यं काञ्जिकमेव च ॥१११॥

Fresh and Old Ingredients

Generally, in a recipe, freshly collected ingredients are to be used. But ghee, *pippalī*, jaggery, honey, *viḍaṅga*, iron and *āsava-s* (alcoholic preparations) do not lose their potency when these are old or kept preserved for a long time. Infact, such ingredients should be used when these are old, in a recipe. Similarly, *tāmbūla*, *dhānya* (corns and cereals) and *kāñjika* (vinegar) which are old should be used in the preparation of a recipe.

सुश्रुतः
फलेषु परिपक्वं यद्गुणवत्तदुदाहृतम् ।
बिल्वादन्यत्र विज्ञेयमामं तद्धि गुणोत्तरम् ॥११२॥
[सुश्रुतः सूत्र : ४६ : २०९]

Ripe and Unripe Fruits
According to Suśruta

Among the fruits, generally the ripe-ones are therapeutically more useful. *Bilva* fruit is an exception to this rule inasmuch as the unripe fruit of it is more useful therapeutically.

वृद्धवाहडः
विरुद्धैरपराजुष्टं गन्धवर्णरसादिभिः ।
नवं द्रव्यं पुराणं वा ग्राह्यमेवं विनिर्दिशेत् ॥११३॥

According to Vṛddha-vāhaḍa
(A) ***Selection of a Drug***

A drug, whether freshly collected or old should be used in a medicine if it is not afflicted by contrary smell, colour, taste, etc. By implication, a drug which has its natural smell, colour, taste, etc., should be used in medicine.

घृते तैले च योगे च यद् द्रव्यं पुनरुच्यते ।
तत्र तद् द्रव्यमेकेन भागतो द्विगुणं भवेत् ॥११४॥

(B) ***Duplication of Ingredients***

In a recipe of medicated ghee, medicated oil or any other preparation, if a drug (ingredient) is mentioned again (for the second time), then such drug (ingredient) should be used in double the quantity.

मात्रायाः नास्त्यवस्थानं दोषमग्निं बलं वयः ।
व्याधिं द्रव्यं च कोष्ठं च वीक्ष्य मात्रां प्रयोजयेत्[८०] ॥११५॥

(C) ***Dosage of Medicines***

Regarding the dosage of medicine, there is no fixed quantity. The physician should administer medicines in appropriate dosage depnding upon the *doṣa-s* (aggravated to cause diseases), *agni* (power of digestion), strength, age, [nature of the] disease, [potency of the] medicine and [nature of the] *koṣṭha* (bowels)..

जंगमस्य वयस्थस्य रक्तलोमनखादिकम् ।
क्षीरं मूत्रं पुरीषं च जीर्णाहारे तु संहरेत् ॥११६॥

(D) *Animal Products for Therapeutic Purpose*

Young animals should be selected for the collection of blood, hair, nails, etc. Milk, urine and stool of an animal should be collected only after the digestion of its food.

कल्पना परिभाषा
[PHARMACEUTICAL PROCESSES]

चन्द्रनन्दनः
निर्यास-कल्क-निर्यूह-शीत-फाण्ट-रसक्रियाः ।
संधानगुटिकाचूर्णस्नेहाः कल्पादयः स्मृताः ।।११७।।

Different Pharmaceutical Processes According to Candra-nandana

Different pharmaceutical processes are *niryāsa* (juice), *kalka* (paste), *niryūha* (decoction), *śīta* (cold infusion), *phāṇṭa* (hot infusion), *rasa kriyā* (solid extract), *sandhāna* (alcoholic preparation), *guṭikā* (pills or tablets), *cūrṇa* (powders), *sneha* (medicated ghee or oil), *kalpa* (use of a drug with specific mode of administration for the purpose of rejuvenation), etc.

लभ्यते स्वरसो येषां तेषां क्वाथं न निक्षिपेत् ।
त्रिफलाव्यतिरेकेण मतमेतत्पतञ्जलेः ।।११८।।

(A) Juice or Decoction

If the juice of a drug can be obtained, then its decoction should not be added to a recipe. *Triphalā* is an exception to this rule. By implication, *triphalā* should always be used in a decoction form. This is the opinion of Patañjali.

सद्यः समुद्धृतात्क्षुण्णात्पटनिष्पीडितो तु यः ।
द्रव्याद्रसो विनिर्याति स रसः स्वरसश्च सः ।।११९।।

(B) *Definition of Juice*

Freshly collected drug should be crushed and strained through a cloth. The juice which comes out of it is called *rasa* or *svarasa*.

शुष्कद्रव्यमुपादाय स्वरसानामसंभवे ।
वारिण्यष्टगुणे साध्यं ग्राह्यं[८१] पादावशेषितम् ॥१२०॥
पादावशेषितं अष्टभागावशिष्टम् ॥१२१॥

(B) ***Decoction***

If it is not possible to extract juice from a drug, then such dried drugs should be boiled by adding eight times of water till one fourth of water remains. The drug should, thereafter, be strained out and the decoction is collected.

The term *pāda* used in the above verse generally means one fourth. But according to some scholars, in the present context, the term *pāda* means one-eighth.

अथ वृद्धवाहडः[८२]
परिशुष्काणां चूर्णीकृतानां आढके त्वाढकमुदकस्य ।
चाहोरात्रं स्थितं विमर्दितम् स्वरसवत्प्रयोज्यं पेयादौ ॥१२२॥

According to Vṛddha Vāhaḍa

A dried drug should be made to a powder. One *āḍhaka* of this powder should be added with one *āḍhaka* of water and kept for one day and night (24 hours). Then it should be kneaded by hand and the liquid part of it should be strained out by squeezing. This liquid may be used in the place of juice *(svarasa)* for the preparation of *peyā* (thin medicated gruel), etc.

तदाह शौनकः
द्रव्याणां परिशुष्काणामाढकः सलिलाढके ।
अहोरात्रं स्थितं वाढं मृदितं स्वरसं हितम् ॥
ग्राहयेत्साधयेत्तेन पेयायूषखडादिकम् ॥१२३॥

According to Śaunaka

One *āḍhaka* of the dried drug should be added with one *āḍhaka* of water and kept for 24 hours. Then it should be kneaded and the liquid portion of it should be strained out by squeezing. With the help of this liquid (juice), *peyā* (thin medicated gruel), *yūṣa* (vegetable soup), *khaḍa* (sour medicated drink), etc., should be prepared.

अथ पानार्थं कृष्णात्रेयः
कुडवं चूर्णितं द्रव्यं प्रक्षिप्तं द्विगुणे जले ।
अहोरात्रं स्थितं तस्माद्भवेत्स्वरस उत्तमः ॥१२४॥

According to Kṛṣṇātreya

For the preparation of a drink [from out of a dried drug], its powder should be mixed with double the quantity of water and kept for 24 hours. The juice should then be squeezed out which is excellent therapeutically.

स्वरसस्य गुरुत्वेन शुक्तिमात्रं प्रदापयेत् ।
वह्निसिद्धं रसं चैव पलमात्रं प्रदापयेत् ॥१२५॥
मधुश्वेता गुडं क्षीरं जीरकं लवणं तथा ।
घृतं तैलं च चूर्णं च कोलमात्रं रसे न्यसेत् ॥१२६॥

॥ इति स्वरसविचारः[८३] ॥

Dosage

Svarasa (juice) is heavy for digestion; hence it should be given in the dose of one *śukti*. The decoction which is prepared by boiling over fire should be given in the dose of one *pala*. In the juice, honey, sugar, jaggery, milk, *jīraka* (cumin seed powder), salt, ghee, oil and powdered drugs should be added in the dose of one *kola*.

Thus, ends the discussion on juice.

यः पिण्डश्चार्द्रपिष्टानां स कल्क इति कीर्तितः ।
वृद्धवैद्यवचः साक्षात् कल्को दृषदि पेषितः ॥१२७॥
मात्रा पिचुमिता तत्र द्विगुणं माक्षिकादिकम् ।
सितां गुडं समं दद्याद् द्रवाः देयाश्चतुर्गुणम् ॥१२८॥
आदिशब्देन तैलघृतादयः ।

॥ इति कल्कविधिः ॥

Kalka or Paste

If a wet-substance is made to a paste which could be made to a bolus-form, it is called *kalka*. According to senior physicians, such trituration should be done over a flat piece of stone and a pestle. It should be given in the dose of one *picu* and to this paste honey, oil, ghee, etc., should be added in double the quantity. Sugar and jaggery should be added to the paste in equal quantities and liquids should be added four times in quantity.

Thus, ends the description of paste.

द्रव्यादापोत्थितात्तोये प्रतप्ते निशि संस्थितात् ।
कषायो योऽभिनिर्याति स शीतः समुदाहृतः ।
आपोत्थितं निशायां तु तोयस्थं शीतमुच्यते ।।१२९।।

Cold Infusion (Śīta-Kaṣāya)

When the coarse powder of a drug is kept in hot water for one night and then strained out, the liquid, thus obtained, is called *śīta kaṣāya* or cold-infusion.

[According to some other physicians, putting the coarse powder of the drug in hot water is not essential.] It can be mixed with ordinary water, kept over-night and the liquid strained out in the next morning is called *śīta kaṣāya*.

अन्यच्च
द्रव्यात्पूतात्पलं क्षुण्णं षड्भिस्तोयपलः प्लुतम् ।
निशोषितं स विज्ञेयो हिमः शीतकषायकः ।।१३०।।

According to other physicians, one *pala* of the cleaned drug should be made to a coarse powder and soaked in six *pala-s* of water. It should be kept for one night (12 hours) and then strained out. The liquid, thus obtained, is called *hima* or *śīta-kaṣāya* (cold-infusion).

रक्तोत्पलं घृतं तैलं पुरं वज्रोदकं तथा ।
गद्याणकं प्रयोक्तव्यं कषाये हिमसंज्ञके ।।१३१।।

Drugs like *raktotpala*, ghee, oil, *guggulu* and *vajrodaka* should be added to this cold-infusion in the dose of one *gadyāṇaka* each.

चन्द्रटः
वयो रोगादिकेमध्ये क्वाथः पेयश्चतुष्पलः[८४] ।
शीतस्वरसयोरेव विधिर्ज्ञेयः कषाययोः ॥१३२॥

॥ इति शीतकषायः॥

According to Candraṭa

If the patient is of middle-age and if the disease is of moderate nature, the decoction should be taken in the dose of four *pala-s*.

The same rule [regarding dosage] is applicable to cold-infusion and juice (*svarasa*) of a drug.

Thus, ends the description of cold-infusion (*śīta-kaṣāya*).

चूर्णमुष्णेन संपृक्तं तत्फाण्टमभिधीयते ॥१३३॥

Phāṇṭa (Hot-Infusion)

If the powder of a drug is soaked in hot water and then strained [immediately], the liquid, thus obtained, is called *phāṇṭa* (hot-infusion).

शीतफाण्टयोर्भेदमाह आत्रेयः
द्रव्यं क्षुण्णमष्टगुणेम्भसि निशि स्थितः शीतः ।
फाण्टः सद्यो धृतो ज्ञेयः स्वल्पदोषबलाग्निषु ॥१३४॥
अष्टावशेषितेऽत्युष्णजले क्वाथपलं क्षिपेत् ।
विमृद्य पटपूतं तज्जलं फाण्टमिति स्मृतम् ॥१३५॥
कुडवं च जलं प्रोक्तं क्वथितं वह्निसंभवम्[८५] ।
मधुश्वेतागुडादीनां क्वाथवच्चात्र मेलनम् ॥१३६॥

॥ फाण्टः॥

Difference Between Śīta and Phāṇṭa : According to Ātreya

If the coarse powder of a drug is soaked in eight times of water, kept over-night and then strained, the liquid, thus obtained, is called *śīta* (cold-infusion). *Phāṇṭa* (hot-infusion), on the other hand, is strained out immediately. It is useful if the *doṣa-s* are mildly aggravated and if the patient has less of strength and less power of digestion (*agni*). For the Preparation of *Phāṇṭa*, water boiled and reduced to 1/8th part is used. To this hot water, one *pala* of the coarse powder of a drug is added and kneaded by hand. Then it is filtered through a cloth by squeezing. The liquid, thus obtained, is called *phāṇṭa* or hot-infusion. Generally, one *kuḍava* of boiled water is used for this purpose. Like a decoction, honey, sugar etc., are mixed with this *phāṇṭa* (hot-infusion) before giving it to a patient.

Thus, ends the description of *phāṇṭa* (hot-infusion).

चतुष्पले वारिशीते क्षुण्णं द्रव्यपलं क्षिपेत् ।
'मृत्पात्रे[८६] मंथयेत्सम्यक्तस्माच्च द्विपलं पिबेत्' ।
मधुश्वेतागुडादीनि[८७] फाण्टवन्निक्षिपेद् बुधः ।।१३७।।

।। मन्थः ।।

Mantha

One *pala* of the powder of a drug should be mixed with four *pala-s* of water, kept in an earthen vessel and properly stirred. This is called *mantha* (which is prepared by stirring) and it should be taken in a dose of two *pala-s*. Like *phāṇṭa* (hot-infusion), honey, sugar, jaggery, etc., should be mixed with this *mantha* and taken by the patient.

Thus, ends the description of *mantha*.

प्रमथ्या प्रोच्यते द्रव्यं पलमात्रं सुकल्कितम् ।
किञ्चिदन्नेन संयुक्तमथवान्नविवर्जितम् ।
'तोये[८८] चाष्टगुणे साध्यं पानमाहुः पलद्वयम्' ।।१३८।।
शेषं मन्थवत् ।।१३९।।

।। प्रमथ्या ।।

Pramathyā

One *pala* of the drug should be made to a fine paste. To this, a small amount of boiled cereals should be added. It can also be prepared without any cereal. Then it should be cooked by adding eight times of water. This is called *pramathyā*, and it should be taken in the dose of two *pala-s*. Honey, etc., should be added on the line suggested for *mantha*.

Thus, ends the description of *pramathyā*.

अथ क्वाथक्वाथ्यमात्रादिविचारः

चरकः

जघन्या द्विपला मात्रा मध्यमा च चतुष्पला ।

उत्तमा षट्पला प्रोक्ता स्नेहक्वाथौषधस्य[१०] च ।।१४०।

Dosage of Decoction, etc., : According to Caraka

Giving medicated ghee, decoction or drugs in a dose of two *pala-s* is inferior; four *pala-s* of these medicaments constitute moderate dose; and six *pala-s* of these constitute an excellent dose.

अग्निवेशः

उत्तमा स्यात्पलं मात्रा त्रिभिश्चाक्षैश्च मध्यमा ।

जघन्या च पलार्द्धेन स्नेहक्वाथौषधेषु च ।

अथौषधेषुगुडादिषु ।।१४१ ।।

According to Agniveśa

One *pala* of medicated ghee, decoction or drug constitute an excellent dose; three *akṣa-s* constitute moderate dose; and half *pala* of these drugs constitute an inferior dose.

The term 'drug' in the above statement includes jaggery and preparations of jaggery.

षट्चतुर्द्विपला मात्रा स्नेहनार्थे च योजयेत् ।

कुष्ठोदरादिषु पलं स्नेहं पक्वं च दापयेत् ।।१४२।।

Dose of Medicated Ghee

For the purpose of oleation, medicated ghee should be administered in the dose of either six, four or two *pala-s*. For the treatment of *kuṣṭha* (obstinate skin diseases including leprosy), *udara* (obstinate abdominal diseases including ascites), etc., cooked medicated ghee should be administered in the dose of one *pala*.

चरकः

मन्दबुद्धिनिरासार्थं नियतं मानमुच्यते ।

उक्तं तन्मूलमानस्य हीनमध्याधिकं बहुः ।
तत्रापि रोगद्रव्याग्निदेहं वीक्ष्य प्रयोजयेत् ।।१४३।।

According to Caraka

To assist physicians with low intellect, the limit of dosage is explained. The basic dose may vary differently, viz., inferior, medium and excess. This is to be determined on the basis of the nature of the disease, drug, digestive power and physique of the patient.

वराहमिहिरः

माषकादिपलं यावद् दद्यात् षोडशकं जलम् ।
तदूर्द्ध्वं कुडवं यावत्तोयमष्टगुणं भवेत् ।।१४४।
प्रस्थादेः कुडवादूर्ध्वं सलिलं च चतुर्गुणम् ।
प्रस्थादितः क्षिपेन्नीरं खारी यावच्चतुर्गुणम् ।।१४५।।

According to Varāha-mihira

If the quantity of the drug is from one *māṣa* to one *pala*, then sixteen times of water should be added to it and boiled for preparing the decoction. If the quantity is above one *pala* upto one *kuḍava*, then eight times of water should be added for preparing the decoction. If the quantity is above one *kuḍava* upto one *prastha*, then four times of water should be added. If the quantity is above one *prastha* upto one *khārī*, then [also] four times of water should be added to it and boiled for preparing the decoction.

क्षारपाणिः

मृदौ चतुर्गुणं देयं कठिनेऽष्टगुणं जलम् ।
कठिनात्कठिने देयं बुधैः षोडशिकं जलम् ।।१४६।।
मृद्वादिक्वाथसंघातैर्मानानुक्ते चिकित्सकः ।
मध्यस्योभयगामित्वादिच्छन्त्यष्टगुणं जलम् ।।१४७।।

According to Kṣārapāṇi

If the drug used for decoction is soft, then four times of water should be added and boiled; if it is hard then eight times of water should be added; and if it is very hard then 16 times of water should be added and boiled for preparing the decoction. If the recipe is a mixture of soft, hard and very hard drugs and the quantity of water to be added is not specified, then it should be treated as a medium type of recipe (which is applicable to both soft and hard drugs) and eight times of water should be added to this recipe for preparing the decoction.

क्वाथ्यद्रव्यपले वारिद्विरष्टगुणमिष्यते ।
चतुर्भागावशेषं[११] तु पेयं पलचतुष्टयम् ॥१४८॥
दीप्तानलं महाकायं पाययेत्तं जलाञ्जलिम् ।
अन्येश्चार्द्धं परित्यज्य प्रवदन्ति चिकित्सकाः ॥१४९॥

To one *pala* of the drug, sixteen *pala-s* of water should be added to prepare the decoction. After boiling, four *pala-s* of water should be remained. [This should then be filtered]. This decoction (one *añjali* in quantity) should be administered to a patient having strong power of digestion and having a robust physique.

According to other physicians, only half of this quantity should be administered to the patient and the other half should be rejected.

भेलः[१३]
क्वाथत्यागमनिच्छन्तस्त्वष्टभागावशेषितम् ।
पारंपर्योपदेशेन वृद्धवैद्याः पलं द्वयम् ॥१५०॥

According to Bhela

Some physicians do not like to reject half of the decoction (mentioned above). Therefore, according to tradition and on the advice of senior physicians, they add 16 *pala-s* of water to one *pala* of the drug and boil till 1/8th of the water remains. This decoction which is two *pala-s* in quantity is administered to the patient.

चूर्णं कषायः शिशिरः शृतश्च
फाण्टः सकल्कस्वरसस्तथैव ।
पञ्चैव कल्काः खलु भेषजानां
यथोत्तरं ते गुरवः प्रदिष्टाः[१४] ॥१५१॥

(1) *Cūrṇa* (powder), (2) *kaṣāya* (decoction), (3) *phāṇṭa* : both *śiśira* (cold-infusion) and *śṛta* (hot-infusion), (4) *kalka* (paste), and (5) *svarasa* (juice) - these are five types of pharmaceutical preparations of drugs. Of these, the succeeding ones are heavier than the preceding ones. [These five pharmaceutical processes are called here as *kalka* (lit. meaning paste). This seems to be a calligraphic error. Generally, Ayurvedic texts describe them as five types of *kaṣāya-s*.]

अथ क्वाथकल्पना

वह्नौ तु क्वथितं द्रव्यं शृतमाहुश्चिकित्सकाः ।
क्वाथः क्वाथ्यसमो ग्राह्य इति वैद्यपरम्परा ॥१५२॥

Preparation of Decoctions

If a drug is boiled [with water] over the fire, then the product, according to physicians, is called *śṛta* or decoction. The quantity of decoction should be the same as the quantity of the drug used for preparing the decoction. [By implication, if one *pala* of the drug is used then 16, 8 or 4 times of water should be added to it, boiled and reduced to 1/16th, 1/8th or 1/4th respectively. After straining, this decoction should be administered to the patient.] This [according to the another] is the traditional practice of ayurvedic physicians.

आत्रेयः

पाचनो दीपनो यश्च शोधनः शमनस्तथा ।
तर्पणः क्लेदनः शोषणः क्वाथः सप्तविधो मतः ॥१५३॥

According to Ātreya

(A) Varieties of Decoction

Decoction is of seven types, viz., (1) *pācana* (carminative), (2) *dīpana* (which stimulates the power of digestion), (3) *śodhana* (which cleanses the body), (4) *śamana* (which alleviates the aggravated *doṣa-s*), (5) *tarpana* (which refreshes), (6) *kledana* (which helps in producing stickiness), and (7) *śoṣaṇa* (which dries up the tissues).

पाचनः पचते दोषान्दीपनोद्दीप्यतेऽनलम् ।
शोधनो मलशोधी स्याच्छमनः शमते गदान् ॥१५४॥
तर्पणस्तर्प्यते धातून्क्लेदी हृत्क्लेदकारकः ।
विशोषी शोषमादत्ते तस्मात्क्वाथान्परीक्षयेत् ॥१५५॥

(B) Effects of Different Types of Decoction

Pācana type of decoction helps in the metabolic transformation of tissue elements. *Dīpana* type of decoction stimulates the power of digestion. *Śodhana* type of decoction eliminates waste products from the body. *Śamana* type of decoction alleviates diseases. *Tarpaṇa* type of decoction provides nourishment to tissues. *Kledana* type of decoction produces stickiness of the heart. *Śoṣaṇa* type of decoction causes dryness of the body. Therefore, the physician should examine the decoctions carefully.

विशोषीं क्लेदिं[१५] विज्ञाय वमनं कारयेद् बुधः ।।१५६।।

(C) To Counter-act Adverse Effects

If a patient has taken *viśoṣī* or *kledi* type of decoction, then [to counter-act their adverse effects on the body], a wise physician should administer emetic therapy.

पाचनोऽर्धावशेषी स्यात् शोधनोऽर्द्धरसांशकः ।
क्लेदनश्चतुरांशश्च शमनोऽष्टावशेषितः ।।१५७।।
दीपनीयो दशांशस्तु तर्पणश्च षडंशकः ।
विशोषी षोडशांशश्च क्वाथभेदाः प्रकीर्तिताः ।।१५८।।

(D) Extent of Boiling

In *pācana* type of decoction, boiling should be done till half of the water remains. Similarly, *śodhana* type of decoction should be boiled till half of the water remains. *Kledana* type of decoction should be boiled till one-fourth of water remains. *Śamana* type of decoction should be boiled till one eighth of water remains. *Dīpana* type of decoction should be boiled till one tenth of water remains. *Tarpaṇa* type of decoction should be boiled till one sixth of water remains. *Viśoṣī* type of decoction should be boiled till one sixteenth part of the water remains. These are the different varieties of decoction.

पाययेदातुरं सामं[१६] पाचनं सप्तमेऽहनि ।
शमनेनाथवा दृष्ट्वा निरामं समुपाचरेत् ।।१५९।।

निशासु पाचनो देयो ज्ञात्वा दोषबलाबलम् ।
तत्तु नवज्वरे पीतं दोषकृन्न च दोषहृत् ।
पूर्वाह्णे शमनो देयोऽपराह्णे दीपनस्तथा ॥१६०॥
तर्पणश्चोत्क्लेदनश्च कल्प्यं[१७] पानाय दापयेत् ।
निशीथे शोषणो देयः श्लैष्मिके प्रथमेऽहनि ।
दद्यात्सूर्योदयात्पूर्वं शोधनीयं भिषक्तमः ॥१६१॥

(E) Time of Administration

The patient having *āma-doṣa* (product of defective digestion and metabolism), should be administered *pācana* type of decoction on the seventh day. If the patient is free from this *āma-doṣa*, then *śamana* type of decoction should be administered. *Pācana* type of decoction should be administered at night after examining the strength or weakness of *doṣa-s*. If decoction is administered to a patient having freshly occured fever, then it aggravates the *doṣa-s* and does not alleviate them. *Śamana* type of decoction should be administered in the morning. *Dīpana* type of decoction should be administered in the afternoon.*Tarpaṇa* and *kledana* types of decoction should be administered only after the patient has become free from the disease. *Śoṣaṇa* type of decoction should be administered at night. If *kapha* is aggravated then it should be administered during the first part of the night. *Śodhana* type of decoction should be administered before sun-rise.

वरमाशीविषं नैव क्वथितं ताम्रभाजने ।
पीतमत्यग्निसंतप्ता भक्षिता[१८] वाप्ययोगुडा ॥१६२॥
वमनार्थं ताम्रपात्रं प्रसिद्धम् ॥१६३॥

(F) Vessel for Boiling

A copper vessel should never be used for boiling a decoction: The decoction, thus prepared, is worse than a strong poison. Taking such decoction is like taking an excessively hot iron-ball. Of course, for preparing a recipe of emetic therapy, copper vessel is popularly used.

प्रक्वाथ्य शीतो निर्यूहः पुनस्तप्तो भवेद् यदा[१९] ।
पानीयं वा पुनस्तप्तं विषवद्धन्ति मानवम् ॥१६४॥

घृतं तैलं च पानीयं कषायं वाञ्जनादिकम् ।
पक्त्वा शीतं पुनस्तप्तं तत्सर्वं स्याद्विषोपमम् ।।१६५।।

(G) Repeated Boiling

If a boiled and cooled decoction or simple water is boiled again and taken, then it kills a person (who takes it) like a poison. In addition to decoction and water described above, if the boiled and cooled ghee or oil or *añjana* (collyrium) is again heated and used, then they work like poisons.

घृतं क्षौद्रं जलं तैलं धान्यं ताम्बूलमौषधम् ।
नवं पुराणसंमिश्रं न सेव्यं सुखवाञ्छता ।।१६६।।

(H) Mixture of Fresh and Old

A person desirous of good health should not mix freshly collected and old (preserved) ghee, honey, water, oil, cereals, betel-leaf and medicines, and use them.

विदीर्यते च स्फुटते पतते[100] क्वाथभाजनः ।
गन्धवर्णरसैर्युक्तः क्वाथश्च सुखदायकः ।।१६७।।

(I) Auspicious Decoction

If while preparing a decoction, the vessel breaks, gets cracked or falls down; and if the decoction is endowed with appropriate smell, colour and taste, then such a decoction is useful for the patient.

आत्रेयात्
क्वाथपाने क्लमो मूर्च्छा वैक्लव्यं च शिरोव्यथा ।
यदा संजायते चाशु वामयेद्रोगिणं तदा ।।१६८।।

According to Ātreya

(A) *Adverse Effects and Their Treatment*

If a patient, after taking the decoction, gets mental fatigue, fainting, uneasiness and headache, then he should be given emetic therapy immediately.

षोडशाष्टचतुर्भागं वातपित्तकफार्तिषु ।
क्षौद्रं कषाये दातव्यं विपरीतात्र शर्करा ।।१६९।।

(B) Addition of Honey and Sugar

In the decoctions for patients suffering from diseases caused by *vāyu*, *pitta* and *kapha*, honey should be added in quantity of 1/16th, 1/8th and 1/4th respectively. In such decoctions, sugar should be added in the quantity of 1/4th, 1/8th and 1/16th respectively.

काश्यपः

जरणोषणशुण्ठ्यादिः शाणिकंहिंगुमाषिकम्[१०१] ।
गुडक्षीरसितादीनां कर्षं क्वाथे विनिक्षिपेत् ।।१७०।।
नस्येषु च प्रयोक्तव्यं माषकं[१०२] हिंगुसैन्धवम् ।।१७१।।

According to Kāśyapa

In the decoctions, *jaraṇa*, *ūṣaṇa*, *śuṇṭhī*, etc., should be added in the dose of one *śāṇa*; *hiṅgu* should be added in the dose of one *māṣa;* and jaggery, milk, sugar, etc., should be added in the dose of one *karṣa*. To a recipe for inhalation therapy, *hiṅgu* and *saindhava* should be added in the dose of one *māṣa*.

सुश्रुतात्

व्योषं शिलाजतुक्षारं लवणं हिंगुजीरकम् ।
क्षिपेत् टंकमितं क्वाथे तैलं क्षीरं घृतं गुडम् ।।१७२।।

According to Suśruta

In a decoction, *vyoṣa* (*trikaṭu*), *śilājatu*, *kṣāra* (alkali preparation), salt, *hiṅgu*, *jīraka*, oil, milk, ghee and jaggery should be added in the quantity of one *ṭaṅka* each.

चरकः

क्षीरं घृतं गुडं तैलं मूत्रं चान्यद् द्रवं तथा ।
कल्कं चूर्णं गुग्गुलुं च क्वाथे कर्षसमं क्षिपेत् ।।१७३।।

According to Caraka

In a decoction, milk, ghee, jaggery, oil, cow's urine, other types of liquid, paste, powder and *guggulu* should be added in the quantity of one *karṣa* each.

क्वाथेन चूर्णपानं यत्तत्र क्वाथप्रधानता ।
प्रवर्तते न तेनात्र चूर्णापेक्षी चतुर्द्रवः ।।१७४।।

If a powdered recipe is required to be taken along with a decoction, then the rule of taking a liquid in the dose of four times of the powder is not applicable.

'आर्येन[१०३] क्वाथे व्योषादीनां टंकमात्रा प्रयोगः प्रोक्तः ।।१७५।।
चरकेन कर्षमात्राः आवापस्य प्रोक्ता ।।१७६।।
अत्र कर्तव्यमाह' ।।१७७।।

According to the preceptor (Suśruta), *vyoṣa*, etc., are to be added in the dose of one *ṭaṅka*. Caraka, however, describes one *karṣa* of these drugs to be added. [In view of this controversy], the duty of the physician is described as follows [by Kṛṣṇātreya].

कृष्णात्रेयः
क्वाथे द्रव्यान्तराक्षेपो चूर्णाद्यैः क्रियते हि यः ।
आवापापोदनं प्रोक्तं कर्षमात्रं क्षिपेद् बुधः ।।१७८।।

According to Kṛṣṇātreya

Addition of other substances like powder, etc., in a decoction is called *āvāpa*. Such drugs should be added in the dose of one *karṣa*.

प्रक्षिप्ते आवापे पुनरपि द्रव्यान्तराक्षेपः क्रियते।
यत्तदृषिभिःसंज्ञा कथिता प्रतीवापः ।।१७९।।
प्रतीवापस्य मात्रा तु शाणतुल्या प्रकीर्तिता ।।१८०।।

Pratīvāpa

Adding a drug to a decoction etc., is called *āvāpa*. If, however, another drug is added to the recipe thereafter, then it is called *pratīvāpa*. Such drugs as *pratīvāpa* should be added in the quantity of one *śāṇa*.

रसार्णवात्

आवर्तितेषु लोहादौ प्रतीवापं प्रचक्ष्महे ।
प्रतीवापो निषेकश्च अभिषेकस्तथैव च ॥१८१॥
प्रतिवापः पुनः योज्यो निषेकस्तदनन्तरम् ।
छादनं तु प्रतीवापो निषेकं मज्जनं विदुः ॥१८२॥
अभिषेकं तदिच्छन्ति स्रपनं[104] क्रियते तु यः ।
उष्णेनैव हि काङ्क्षन्ति न[105] शीतेन कदाचन ॥१८३॥

According to Rasārṇava

After melting iron (metals), etc., *pratīvāpa* should be added which will be described now. *Pratīvāpa*, *niṣeka* and *abhiṣeka*, these are the three different pharmaceutical processes. First of all, *pratīvāpa* should be added and *niṣeka* should be added thereafter. A substance for *pratīvāpa* is sprinkled over the surface of the melted iron. The substance which is added to melted iron, etc., for further liquefaction is called *abhiṣeka*. Such drugs for *pratīvāpa*, *niṣeka* and *abhiṣeka* are added only to a hot-substance and never to a cold substance.

अथ वमनीयक्वाथादिमात्रा[106]ऽऽह भेलः

नवप्रस्था भवेज्ज्येष्ठा मध्यमा षट् प्रकीर्तिता ।
निःक्वाथ्यस्य त्रयः पञ्च मागधा तु कनीयसी ॥१८४॥
मागधा मगधप्रस्थेनेत्यर्थः ॥१८५॥

According to Bhela
Dose of Emetic Decoctions, etc.

For the purpose of emesis, administration of decoction in the dose of nine *prastha-s* is excellent; in the dose of six *prastha-s* is medium; and in the dose of three *prastha-s* it is small. Similarly, five *prastha-s* according to *Māgadha* type of measurement is the small dose.

अथ सिद्धसारः

त्रिपलं श्रेष्ठमाख्यातं द्विपलं मध्यमं भवेत् ।

क्नीयस्तु पलं विद्यादिति मे निश्चिता मतिः ।
कल्कचूर्णादिषु सदा[१०७] यथासंख्यं विनिर्दिशेत् ।।१८६।।

According to Siddhasāra

The excellent dose of pastes and powders is three *pala-s,* the medium dose is two *pala-s,* and the small dose is one *pala*. [This according to *Siddhasāra* is most appropriate].

पित्तेन स्यान्मृदुकोष्ठः क्रूरो वातकफाश्रयात् ।
मध्यश्च समदोषत्वात् मात्रा योज्यानुपूर्विकी ।।१८७।।
सा च मात्राभेदेनोक्ता ।।१८८।।

Aggravated *pitta* causes soft bowel movement and aggravated *vāta* and *kapha* cause costive bowel. If these *doṣa-s* are in equilibrium, the bowel is of moderate type. Therefore, the dosage of drugs should be selected approximately.

द्विपलं श्रेष्ठमाख्यातं मध्यमं तु पलं भवेत् ।
पलार्द्धमुपयुञ्जीत[१०९] क्नीयस्तु विरेचने ।।१८९।।

।। इति विरेचनमात्रा ।।

Dosage of Purgatives

For the purpose of purgation, a drug should be administered in the dose of two *pala-s* which is excellent, or in the dose of one *pala* which is medium or in the dose of half *pala* which is small.

अथ हारीतः
स्नेहो गुडो मांसरसाः पयांसि
साम्लानि मूत्रं मधु सैन्धवं च ।
एतान्यनुक्तान्यपि दापयेत्तु
युक्त्या निरूहे मदनात्फलं च ।।१९०।।

According to Hārīta

In a recipe for *nirūha* (a type of enema), the physician should always add *sneha* (ghee, oil, etc.), jaggery, meat-soup, milk, sour preparations (like vinegar), cow's urine, honey, rock-salt and fruits of *madana*, even if these are not specified in the formula.

अथ पाराशरः
निरूहस्य प्रमाणं तु प्रस्थं पादोत्तरं परम् ।
मध्यमं प्रस्थमुद्दिष्टं हीनं तु कुडवास्त्रयः ।।१९१।।

According to Pārāśara

The best dose of *nirūha* is one and one fourth of *prastha*, the medium dose is one *prastha*, and the inferior dose is three *kuḍava-s*.

अथ खरनादः
सर्वेष्वेव निरूहेषु मदनं[११] सम्प्रयोजयेत् ।
स्नेहं गुडं माक्षिकं च लवणं चापि युक्तितः ।।१९२।।
मधुशुक्त्या गुडपलं कर्षार्द्धं लवणस्य च ।
निरूहे स्नेहभागः स्यात् षष्ठः पित्ते कफेऽष्टमः ।
वाताधिके[१२] चतुर्भागः प्रकृतिस्थे च पित्तवत् ।।१९३।।

According to Kharanāda

In all the recipes of *nirūha*, *madana* should be used; in addition, oil, ghee, jaggery, honey and salt should be used appropriately. Honey should be added to the recipe in the dose of one *śukti*, jaggery in one *pala*, and salt in the dose of half *karṣa*. In a recipe of *nirūha*, oil and ghee should be added in 1/6th quantity if *pitta* is aggravated , in 1/8th quantity if *kapha* is aggravated, and in 1/4th quantity if *vāyu* is aggravated. If all the three *doṣa-s* are in a state of equilibrium, the quantity of oil or ghee should be 1/6th in quantity (like aggravated *pitta*).

दधिक्षीरं पयो मूत्रं[१३] कांजिकं मदिरादयः ।
यस्मिन्निरूहे निर्दिष्टाः प्रमाणं न च कीर्तितम् ।
तस्मिन्दोषादिकं[१४] बुद्ध्वा युक्त्या संविभजेदधः ।।१९४।।

If in a recipe of *nirūha* (a type of medicated enema), curd, milk, water, cow's urine, *kāñjī* (a type of vinegar), wine, etc., are mentioned to be added but their quantities are not described, then their quantities are to be determined by the physician on the basis of the *doṣa*, etc., involved in the causation of the disease.

वाते पित्ते कफे क्षौद्रं स्नेहकल्कगुडादयः ।
क्वाथादपि पृथग्बस्तिश्चतुर्विंशतिभिः[११५] पलैः ।।१९५।।

In *vātika*, *paittika* and *kaphaja* types of diseases, honey, oil, ghee, pastes of drugs, jaggery, etc., should be added in the quantity of 24 *pala-s* to the decoction. [The meaning of this verse is not clear].

वाते गुडं सिता पित्ते कफे सिद्धार्थकादयः ।
कल्कः क्वाथ-रसक्षीरं-मूत्रं प्रायं द्रवं क्षिपेत् ।।१९६।।

To a recipe of *nirūha* (a type of medicated enema), jaggery should be added if *vāyu* is aggravated, sugar should be added if *pitta* is aggravated, and mustard, etc., should be added if *kapha* is aggravated. In addition, pastes, decoctions, juice, milk, cow's urine and other liquids should be added to such recipes.

त्रिंशन्मात्रास्थिते बस्तौ ततश्च क्षुद्रको भवेत् ।।१९७।।

।। इति निरूहबस्तिपरिभाषा ।।

[The meaning of this line is not clear].

Thus, ends the description of *nirūha basti*.

सुश्रुतश्च
मया चात्र निरूहाणां या मात्रा परिकीर्तिता ।
पादावशिष्टास्ताः कार्याः स्नेहबस्तिषु देहिनाम् ।।१९८।।

।। इत्यनुवासनम् ।।

According to Suśruta

Whatever quantity has been described by me (by Suśruta) for the preparation of the recipe for *nirūha* (a type of medicated enema) should be used for *anuvāsana* (another type of medicated enema) in one fourth quantity.

Thus, ends the description of *anuvāsana*.

अथ मंडादिकल्पना

शिंबीधान्यकृतं[११६] तोयं निर्यूह इति संज्ञितः ।

तण्डुलैश्च कृतो मण्डः साधनं तस्य कथ्यते ॥१९९॥

Preparation of Maṇḍa, etc.

The decoction prepared by boiling *śiṃbī-dhānya* (pulses and legumes) in water is called *niryūha*. The gruel prepared of rice is called *maṇḍa*. Its method of preparation will be described hence forth.

वृद्धसुश्रुतः

सिक्थैर्विरहितो मण्डः पेया सिक्थसमन्विता ।

विलेपी बहुसिक्था स्याद्यवागूर्विरलद्रवा ॥२००॥

[सुश्रुत : सूत्र : ४६:३४४-३४५]

According to Vṛddha Suśruta

Maṇḍa is free from sticky material whereas *peyā* is sticky. *Vilepī* is very sticky and *yavāgū* contains very little quantity of liquid i.e. it is semi-solid in consistency.

अन्नं पञ्चगुणे साध्यं विलेपी च चतुर्गुणे ।

चतुर्दशगुणे मण्डो यवागूः षड्गुणेम्भसि ॥२०१॥

स्याद्धितः साधितो यूषस्त्वष्टादशगुणे जले ॥२०२॥

Quantity of Water

Anna (cooked rice) is prepared by boiling with five times of water. *Vilepī* is prepared by boiling with four times of water. *Maṇḍa* is prepared by adding fourteen times of water. *Yavāgū* is prepared by boiling with six times of water. *Yūṣa* (vegetable soup) is prepared by boiling with eighteen times of water.

अग्निवेशः

यदप्सु शृतशीतं तं षडङ्गादि प्रयुज्यते ।
कर्षमात्रं ततो द्रव्यं साधयेत्प्रास्थिकेऽम्भसि ।।२०३।।
अर्द्धशृतं[117] प्रयोक्तव्यं पानपेयादिसंविधौ ।
कर्षार्द्धं वा कणाशुण्ठ्योः कल्कद्रव्यस्य वा पलम् ।।२०४।।
विनीय पाचयेद्युक्त्या वारिप्रस्थेन चापरान् ।
यूषांश्चैव रसांश्चैव कल्पनानेन साधयेत् ।।२०५।।

According to Agniveśa

In *Ṣaḍaṅga kaṣāya*, etc., which are prepared by boiling with water and then by cooling, drugs should be added in the quantity of one *karṣa* and it should be boiled by adding one *prastha* of water. After it is reduced to half, the drug should be filtered out and the liquid should be administered for drinking or for the preparation of *peyā* (thin gruel), etc. Alternatively, half *karṣa* of each of *pippalī* and *śuṇṭhī* or one *pala* of the paste of other drugs should be appropriately cooked in one *prastha* of water. With the help of this decoction, vegetable-soups (*yūṣa-s*) and meat-soups (*rasa*-s) should be prepared.

'अत्र'[118] कर्षः एव कर्षार्द्धं न तु कर्षार्द्धं कर्षस्यार्द्धम् ।
तेन तीक्ष्णत्वेन कणाशुण्ठ्योः समानगुणत्वात्कर्षः' ।
तदतिरिक्तं मरिचचित्रकादीनां कर्षः रसप्रधानमांसादि-
द्रव्यस्य पलं सर्वत्र वारिप्रस्थे इति सम्बन्धः ।।२०६।।

The term *karṣārdha* used in the above verse means one *karṣa* i.e. the total quantity of *pippalī* and *śuṇṭhī* should be one *karṣa* and not half *karṣa*. This [small] quantity of one *karṣa* is mentioned here because both *pippalī* and *śuṇṭhī* are sharp (*tīkṣṇa*) in their attribute. Similarly, drugs like *marica*, *citraka* etc. should be used in the quantity of one *karṣa*. Ingredients dominated by *rasa* (taste) like meat are to be used in the quantity of one *pala*. In all such cases, the quantity of water should be one *prastha*.

नलः
प्रस्थेऽम्भसि पलं साध्यं मांसं पादस्थिते रसः।
कंसाप्सु कुडवं मांसं पक्त्वा पादावशेषितम्।
तेन क्वाथेन विपचेद्यवागूं प्रोक्तकर्मसु ।।२०७।।

According to Nala
Preparation of Meat-soup

One *pala* of meat should be cooked in *prastha* of water and reduced to one fourth for the preparation of meat-soup. If the quantity of meat is one *kuḍava*, then it should be cooked in one *kaṃsa* of water and reduced to one fourth for the preparation of meat-soup. With this decoction (meat-soup), *yavāgū* (thick gruel) should be prepared and used in therapies.

अस्नेहलवणं सर्वमकृतं कटुकैर्विना ।
विज्ञेयं लवणस्नेहकटुकैः संयुतं कृतम् ।।२०८।।

Kṛta and Akṛta

Soups prepared without the addition of fat (oil, ghee etc.,), salt and pungent ingredients are called *akṛta*. On the other hand, soups prepared by adding salt, fat and pungent [spices] are called *kṛta*.

अथ यूषलक्षणमाह नलः[119]
भृष्टमुद्गदलानां तु पलैकेन विपाचितः ।
पूतापनीतविदलस्तनुर्यूषः कृताकृतः[120] ।।२०९।।

Vegetable Soup
According to Nala

One *pala* of the seeds of *mudga* should be roasted. Then the husk of these seeds should be removed and boiled with water. The thin liquid, thus prepared, is called *yūṣa* (vegetable soup). Thereafter, it can be sizzled with fat, salt and pungent spices which is called *kṛta yūṣa*. If such ingredients are not added then it is called *akṛta yūṣa*.

वृद्धवैद्याः पलं द्रव्यं ग्राहयन्ति जलाढके ।
भेषजस्यातिबाहुल्यात्क्वाचिदरुचिर्भवेत् ।।२१०।।

पेया मण्डादियोगेषु भेषजं यत्प्रकीर्तितम् ।
तत्तथैव प्रयोक्तव्यमरुचिर्न भवेद्यथा ।।२११।।

।। इति सर्वत्र ।।

According to Experienced Physicians (Vṛddha Vaidya)

Experienced or senior physicians use one *pala* of the drug and boil it in one *āḍhaka* of water to prepare soup. If the ingredients are more in quantity, they at times cause *aruci* (anorexia), i.e. the patient may not like to take such soups.

Similarly, medicinal ingredients mentioned for the preparation of *peyā* (thin gruel) and *maṇḍa* (another type of thin gruel) should be added appropriately (in small quantity) so that the recipe becomes delicious for the patient. This is a general rule.

अथ चूर्णाः च

अत्यन्तशुष्कं यद्द्रव्यं कुट्टितं वस्त्रगालितम् ।
चूर्णं स्यात्क्षोदको रेणु रजो मात्रास्य तिन्दुकम् ।।२१२।।

Powders

If an excessively dry drug is pounded and strained through a cloth, then it is called *cūrṇa* (powder). Its synonyms are *kṣodaka*, *reṇu* and *rajas*. It is administered in the dose of one *tinduka*.

चूर्णेषु चूर्णद्विगुणा सिता[२१] चूर्णसमो गुडः ।
चतुर्गुणा च भवति सिता दोषं बलं प्रति ।।२१३।।

In a recipe of powders, sugar should be added in double the quantity of the powder of drugs and the quantity of jaggery should be equal to that of the drugs. Depending upon the nature of the aggravated *doṣa-s* and strength of the patient, four times of sugar may also be added to a recipe of powder.

लिहेच्चूर्णं द्रवैः सर्वैर्घृताद्यैर्द्विगुणैर्ध्रुवम् ।
पिबेच्चतुर्गुणैरेवं गुडश्चूर्णसमो मतः ।।२१४।।

Anupāna for Powders

A powdered recipe should be made to a linctus by adding double the quantity of liquids like ghee, etc., and administered. If it is to be taken with water or decoction, the latter should be four times in quantity. If a powdered recipe is to be taken along with jaggery, then the latter should be taken in equal quantity.

वसिष्ठः
चूर्णस्तु द्विविधो ज्ञेयो एकान्तश्च सितायुतः।
एकान्तः कर्षमात्रः स्यादपरः शुक्तिमात्रकः ।।२१५।।

Varieties of Powder
According to Vasiṣṭha

Powdered-recipes are of two types, viz.,

(1) those prepared exclusively of drugs, and
(2) those containing drugs and added with sugar.

The former type is administered in the dose of one *karṣa* and the latter in the dose of one *śukti*.

अथ गुटिकादयः
गुडादिवर्तितश्चूर्णो वर्तिः स्याद्गुटिका गुडः।
मोदको वटकः पिण्डी तन्मात्रं चूर्णवन्मतम् ।।२१६।।

Pills

If the powder of drugs is mixed (triturated) with jaggery, etc., and rolled into pills, then it is called *varti, guṭikā, guḍa, modaka, vaṭaka* and *piṇḍī*. The dose of these pills is similar to that of powders.

मोदकेषु द्विगुणितो गुडः सिता चतुर्गुणा।
पक्वेन वटकाः कार्याः गुडेन सितयाऽथवा।
परं हि वह्निसंपर्काल्लघिमानं भजन्ति ते।।२१७।।

Modaka (Large Pills)

Modaka-s (large pills) are prepared by double the quantity of jaggery or four times in quantity of sugar. Both the jaggery and sugar are to be cooked (by adding water and made to a syrup) for preparing *vaṭaka-s* (large size pills). Because of cooking over fire, these preparations become lighter for digestion.

चूर्णावलेह - गुटिका - कल्कानामनुपानकम् ।
वातपित्तकफातंके द्वित्र्येकपलमाहरेत् ।।२१८।।

Anupāna (Vehicle)

The vehicle *(anupāna)* for powders, linctus, pills and pastes for the diseases caused by *vāyu*, *pitta* and *kapha* should be two, three and one *pala-s* respectively.

गोपुरः
सितागुडादिसंयोगाद् गुटिका या प्रजायते ।
शुक्तिमात्रा मता तस्याः शेषाः कर्षसमा मताः ।।२१९।।

।। इति गुटिका ।।

According to Gopura

Guṭikā (pill) which is prepared by adding sugar, jaggery, etc., should be administered in the dose of one *śukti*. The dose of the remaining medicines is one *karṣa*.

Thus, ends the description of pills.

क्वाथादीनां पुनः पाकाद्घनभावो रसक्रिया ।
मात्रा रसक्रियायाश्च विद्यात्पाणितलं बुधः ।।२२०।।

।। रसक्रिया ।।

Rasakriyā (Solid Extract)

When decoctions etc., are cooked again to make them semi-solid, it is called *rasa kriyā*. Its dose is one *pāṇitala*.

Thus, ends the description of *rasa kriyā*.

लेहे यत्रास्ति यो भागोऽनिर्दिष्टो द्रवकल्कयोः ।
तत्रापि पादिकः कल्को द्रवात्कार्यो विजानता ।।२२१।।

Leha (Linctus)

If the ratio of liquids and pastes of drugs in a recipe of linctus is not specified, then the latter (paste) should be taken one fourth in quantity of the former (liquid).

तुला द्रव्यं जले द्रोणे द्रोणे द्रव्यं तुला मता ।
देयो गुडः सिता वापि इति सर्वत्र निश्चितम् ।
अवलेहश्च लेहश्च तस्य मानं पलद्वयम् ।।२२२।।

If for the preparation of a linctus one *tulā* of drug is prescribed to be used, then this drug should be boiled in one *droṇa* of water. Similarly, if the quantity of drug is not specified, in the recipe, then one *tulā* of the drug should be taken and boiled in one *droṇa* of water. To this decoction, jaggery and sugar should be appropriately added and the linctus should be prepared. This type of preparation is called *avaleha* or *leha* and it should be administered in the quantity of two *pala-s*. [There appears to be some mistakes in the text.]

वाग्भटः

सुखमर्द्यः सुखस्पर्शो गन्धवर्णरसान्वितः ।
पीडितो भजते मुद्रां गुडपाकमुपागतः[१२२] ।।२२३।।
यदा दर्वीप्रलेपः स्याद्यावद्धा तन्तुली भवेत् ।
तोयपूर्णे यदा पात्रे क्षिप्तो न प्लवते गुडः ।।२२४।।
क्षिप्तस्तु निश्चलं तिष्ठेत्पतितस्तु न शीर्यति ।
एषः पाके गुडादीनां सर्वेषां परिकीर्तिता ।।२२५।।

According to Vāgbhaṭa

Signs of proper *guḍa-pāka* (proper cooking of linctus) are as follows :

(1) The paste should be soft in rubbing.
(2) The paste should be soft in touch.
(3) The paste should possess appropriate smell, colour and taste.
(4) If the paste is pressed between two fingers then finger prints should be appeared over the paste.
(5) The paste should stick to the stirring-spoon.
(6) Threads should appear when a small portion of the paste is lifted out of the vessel.
(7) If a small portion of the linctus is placed on a cup filled with water, it should not float over it, it should remain stable in the

water and it should not get dissolved in water.

The above criteria indicates proper cooking of all types of linctus.

भेलः[१२३]

रसक्रियाद्या ये लेहाः गुडाश्चैव प्रकीर्तिताः ।
तेषां विन्दुर्जले न्यस्तो न शीर्येत्पक्वलक्षणम् ॥२२६॥

॥अवलेहः[१२४]॥

According to Bhela

If a drop of *rasa kriyā* (solid extract), *leha* (linctus) or *guḍa* (linctus prepared with jaggery) is put in water and it does not get dissolved, then it is the sign of proper cooking of these preparations.

Thus, ends the description of linctus.

परासरः[१२५]

पुटेन पच्यते यस्मात्पुटपाकस्ततो मतः ।
सुपिष्टं कुडवं द्रव्यं वारिणा काञ्जिकेन वा ॥२२७॥
पुटकान्तरगतं बद्धं सान्द्रपंकेन लेपितम् ।
अङ्गुष्ठमानतः पश्चादूगोमयेनाग्निना बुधः ॥२२८॥
सिन्दूरवर्णतां प्राप्तं ग्राहयेत्तद्रसं शुभम् ।
शीतलेन रसावाप्तिर्भवेदिति[१२६] विनिश्चितम् ।
पुटपाकस्य पाकोऽयं बहिरारक्तवर्णता ॥२२९॥
पलमात्रो रसो ग्राह्यः कर्षमात्रं मधु क्षिपेत् ।
कल्क-चूर्ण-द्रवाद्याश्च देया स्वरसवदूबुधैः ॥२३०॥

॥ पुटपाक ॥

Puṭapāka : According to Parāsara

If a drug is made to a bolus form, wrapped with cloth, leaf, grass etc., and cooked (roasted) over fire, then it is called *puṭapāka*.

One *kuḍava* of the drug should be made to a fine paste by triturating with water or vinegar, made to a bolus-form, wrapped with leaves, grass, etc., smeared with mud and cooked with cow-dung cakes of half-inch thickness. When the bolus becomes red hot, it should be taken out of fire, allowed to cool down, wrapped material should be scrapped out and the juice of the drug should be squeezed out after it becomes cool. This is called *puṭa-pāka*. It should be ensured that the bolus containing the drug becomes red-hot while cooking (roasting) over the fire. One *pala* of this juice should be added with one *karṣa* of honey. To this, paste, powder, liquids, etc. should be added as per the quantities prescribed for ordinary juice (*svarasa*).

Thus, ends the description of *puṭa-pāka*.

द्रवेण यावता द्रव्यमेकीभूयार्द्रतां व्रजेत् ।
तावत्प्रमाणं निर्दिष्टं भिषग्भिर्भावनाविधौ ।।२३१।।
भाव्यद्रव्यसमं क्वाथं क्वाथोऽष्टांशस्तु तेन हि ।
आर्द्रं यावद्धि तद्भाव्यं सप्ताहं भावनाविधौ ।।२३२।।

Bhāvanā (Impregnation)

To a drug, liquids should be added in such quantities by which the drug gets fully mixed up with the liquid and becomes wet. This is quantity of a liquid used for *bhāvanā* (impregnation).

For *bhāvanā* (impregnation), a drug should be boiled by adding eight times of water and reduced to one fourth. This decoction should be added to equal quantity of another drug which is to be impregnated till the drug becomes fully wet (soaked with the decoction). This process should be repeated for seven days. This pharmaceutical process is called *bhāvanā*.

चरकः

"अकालेऽल्पातिमात्रं वा पुराणमवभावितम्[१२७] ।
असम्यक्संस्कृतं चैव व्यापदौषधमुच्यते[१२८]" ।।२३३।।

[चरक: सिद्धि : ६:२८]

According to Caraka

The following are the faults of a medicine :

(1) If a medicine (herb) is collected in improper time;
(2) If a medicine is administered in less or more in quantity;
(3) If the ingredients of the recipe are old (not fresh);
(4) If the ingredients are not properly impregnated; and
(5) If the ingredients are not properly processed or purified.

अथ शिलाजतु
"ग्रीष्मेऽर्कतप्ताः गिरयो जतुतुल्यं वमन्ति यत्।
हेमादिषड्धातुरसं प्रोच्यते तच्छिलाजतु[१२१]" ।।२३४।।
[अष्टाङ्गहृदय : उत्तरस्थान : ३९ : १३१]

Śilājatu (Mineral pitch)

When the stones in the mountain become excessively hot because of sun-rays during summer season, wax-like exudate comes out of them. This exudate contains the essence of six types of metals like gold, etc., and it is called *śilājatu*.

क्षिप्तमग्नौ न दह्येत लिङ्गाकारमथापि च ।
जले जटिलतां याति तच्च श्रेष्ठं शिलाजतु ।।२३५।।

Test of Śilājatu

A small quantity of *śilājatu* should be placed over a red hot charcoal. It should not be get burnt but should take the shape of a *śiva-liṅga* (cylinder). When *śilājatu* is placed in a cup of water, it should be knotty in appearance. *Śilālatu*, having these characteristic features is excellent in quality.

"गोमूत्रगन्धि कृष्णं गुग्गुल्वाभं विशर्करं मृत्स्नम् ।
स्निग्धमनम्लकषायं मृदु गुरु च शिलाजतु श्रेष्ठम्" ।।२३६।।
[अष्टाङ्गहृदय : उत्तरस्थान : ३९ : १३३]

Characteristics of Śilājatu

Excellent type of *śilājatu* has the following characteristic features:

(1) It should smell like cow's urine;
(2) It is black in colour;
(3) It looks like *guggulu* (gum-resin of *Commiphora mukul*);
(4) It should be free from sand particles;
(5) It should be free from sliminess;
(6) It should be unctuous;
(7) It should not be sour but astringent in taste; and
(8) It should be soft and heavy.

वसिष्टः

तदेतदीदृशमपि धूपितशोधितभावितमेव योज्यमिति वृद्धाः ।
धूपादि[३०]कल्पना ग्रंथांतरादवगन्तव्या ।।२३७।।

According to Vasiṣṭha

Śilājatu having the above mentioned characteristic features should be fumigated, purified and impregnated before using in medicines. The methods of fumigation, etc., should be determined on the basis of other texts on this subject.

लोहाढकी-निम्ब-गुडूचि-सर्पिर्यवैर्यथावत्परिधूपयेच्च ।
संतानिका कीट-पतंगदंशदुष्टौषधीदोषनिर्बहणाय ।।२३८।।

।।शिलाजतुधूपनम्।।

Fumigation of Śilājatu

Śilājatu should be appropriately fumigated with the help of *guggulu*, *āḍhakī*, *nimba*, *guḍūcī*, ghee and barley. Such fumigation helps to remove *santānikā* (formation of scum), affliction by parasites and insects, and adulteration by poisonous drugs.

Thus, ends the description of *śilājatu* fumigation.

उष्णो[३१] तु काले रवितापयुक्ते शुभ्रे निवाते समभूमिभागे ।
चत्वारि पात्राण्यसितायसानि न्यस्तातपे दत्तमनोवधानः ।।२३९।।
शिलाजतुश्रेष्ठमवाप्य पात्रे प्रक्षिप्य तस्माद्द्विगुणं च तोयम् ।
उष्णं तदुष्णोदकमन्तर्दत्वा विशोषयेत्तन्मृदितं यथावत् ।।२४०।।
ततश्च यत्कृष्णमुपैति चोदूर्ध्वं पात्रे तदन्यत्र ततो निधाय ।
ततश्च पात्रादपरे च पात्रे तस्माच्च पात्रादपरत्र[३२] भूयः ।।२४१।।
पुनस्ततोऽन्यत्र निधाय कृष्णं यत्संहतं तत्पुनराहरेच्च ।
यदा विशुद्धं जलमच्छमूर्ध्वं प्रसन्नभावान्मलमेत्यधस्तात्[३३] ।
तदा त्यजेत्तत्सलिलं मलं[३४] च शिलाजतु स्याज्जलशुद्धमेवम् ।।२४२।।

Purification of Śilājatu

In summer season when the sun rays are hot, when the sky is clear, when there is no strong current of wind and in a levelled ground, four vessels made of black iron should be carefully kept. In one of these vessels, *śilājatu* of good quality should be placed. Into this vessel, double the quantity of warm water should be added and gently squeezed with the help of hands. This should then be allowed to remain exposed to the sun. A black-coloured scum will then appear over the surface of water. This should be collected and kept in the second vessel and warm water should be added to it. After some time, scum will again appear over it which should be collected and transferred to the third vessel. Similarly, the scum of the third vessel should be transferred to the fourth vessel. At the end, the water will remain clean and the dirt in *śilājatu* will settle down at the bottom of the vessel. Thereafter, the dirt settled at the bottom is thrown out and the water is decanted. This is the method of purifying *śilājatu* with the help of water.

विशोधयेत्पित्तहरैश्च पित्ते कफे कफघ्नैश्च कषाययोगैः ।
वातेऽनिलघ्नैर्दशमूलयुक्तैः स्वयोनिनिघ्नैश्च चतुर्थभागे[३५] ॥२४३॥

Processing of Śilājatu for Different Doṣa-s

For the treatment of *paittika* diseases, *śilājatu* should be processed with the decoction of *pitta*-alleviating drugs. For *kaphaja*-diseases, *śilājatu* should be processed with the decoction of *kapha*-alleviating drugs. Similarly, for *vātika*-diseases, it should be processed with *vāyu*-alleviating drugs along with *daśa-mūla*. For this purpose, the decoctions should be prepared by [boiling drugs with eight times of water and reducing to] one fourth.

पथ्या-गुडूची-जल-निम्ब-धात्री-बिभीतकैश्चैव महाकषायैः ।
चतुर्थशेषेण जलेन तेन तद्भावयेन्नैकश एव विद्वान् ॥२४४॥

Special Decoction for Processing Śilājatu

Pathyā, *guḍūcī*, *mustā*, *nimba*, *dhātrī* and *bibhītaka* should be boiled by adding eight times of water and reduced to one fourth. With this decoction, *śilājatu* should be impregnated for several times by a wise physician.

वृद्धसुश्रुतः
आरग्वधादिकेनापि सालसारादिकेन वा ।

शिलाजतुसमं द्रव्यं क्वाथ्यमष्टगुणे जले ।
पादावशेषितात्पूतं तस्मिन्कोष्णे विनिक्षिपेत् ।।२४५।।

According to Vṛddha Suśruta

Drugs belonging to *Āragvadhādi* group or *Sālasārādi* group should be taken in quantity equal to *śilājatu*. To these drugs, eight times of water should be added, boiled and reduced to one fourth. The decoction should then be strained out. *Śilājatu* should be added to this decoction when it is warm.

आम्नायविदः
भावना व्यतिरेकंच तन्त्रान्तरवचनमिदमवश्यमनुसरणीयम् ।
निःशर्करं[३६] च मृत्स्नं च सेवेन्नित्यं गतभ्रममिति ।।२४६ ।।

According to Wise Physicians

If *śilājatu* is to be used without impregnation, then one should follow the instructions provided in another text according to which *śilājatu* should be free from sand particles, homogenous and free from adulterants.

तद्वचनं हि
समं गिरिजमष्टगुणिते निःक्वाथ्य भावनौषधं तोये ।
तन्निर्यूहेऽष्टांशे पूतोष्णे प्रक्षिपेद्गिरिजम् ।
तत्समरसतां यातं संशुष्कंप्रक्षिपेत्[३७] घर्मे भूयः ।
स्वै स्वैरेव क्वाथैर्भाव्यं वारान्भवेत्सप्ततः ।।२४७ ।।

They have also described the process of impregnation with decoctions and pastes in a different way. According to them, "The quantity of drugs for preparing decoction should be same as that of *śilājatu*. These drugs should be boiled by adding eight times of water and after boiling the water should be reduced to one eighth. To this decoction, *śilājatu* should be added and kept till it gets dried by absorbing the essence of the decoction. Thereafter, *śilājatu* should be dried in sun. In each of the decoctions, *śilājatu* should be impregnated for seven times.

वाग्भटः[138]

एकद्वित्रिषु[139] सप्ताहं कर्षमर्धपलं पलम् ।
हीनमध्यमोत्तमो योगः शिलाजस्य प्रकीर्तितः[140] ।।२४८।।

[अष्टाङ्गहृदय : उत्तरस्थान ३९ : १४०]

Dose of Śilājatu : According to Vāgbhaṭa

Śilājatu should be administered for one week in the dose of one *karṣa*, half *pala* and one *pala* which are inferior, medium and superior respectively.

चरकः

प्रयोगः सप्तसप्ताहास्त्रयश्चैकश्च सप्तकः ।
निर्दिष्टस्त्रिविधस्तस्य परो मध्योऽवरस्तथा ।।२४९।।

[चरक : चिकित्सा : १:३:५४]

According to Caraka

Śilājatu should be administered for seven weeks, three weeks or one week. These three modes of administration represent the excellent, medium and inferior dosage respectively.

मात्रा पलमर्धपलं स्यात्कर्षस्तु कनीयसी ।।२५०।।

।। इति हारीतः ।।

According to Hārīta

The dose of *śilājatu* should be either one *pala* or half *pala.* One *karṣa* is the smallest dose of *śilājatu.*

तत्संभावितदेहस्तु कपोतादीन्परित्यजेत् ।
कुलत्थं काकमाचीं च रूक्षभोज्यं तथैव च ।।२५१।।

Diet

A person taking *śilājatu* should avoid the meat of *kapota,* etc., *kulattha*, *kākamācī* and ununctuous food.

स्नेहादिकंचापि शिलाजमेव न हन्ति तद्वर्णमलं विदध्यात् ।
यदाविरूक्षे वपुषि प्रदत्तं विशोषणं[141] क्लेदनमादधाति[142] ।।२५२।।

Unctuous Food

Fats (like oil and ghee) do not impair the effects of *śilājatu*. On the other hand, they help in promoting the complexion of the patient. If it is administered to a patient having a dry (ununctuous) body, then it causes emaciation (depletion of tissue elements) and produces stickiness (*kledana*) in the body.

समत्वाच्च गुरुत्वाच्च गुग्गुलोः करणक्रमः ।।२५३।।

।। इति शिलाजतुविधानम् ।।

Guggulu and Śilājatu

Guggulu and *śilājatu* have come identical properties in asmuch as both are heavy in attribute. Therefore, the procedure prescribed for the purification (processing) of *śilājatu* should be followed for *guggulu* also.

Thus, ends the description of processing *śilājatu*.

जलमष्टगुणं दत्वा पलं खण्डिततण्डुलात् ।
भावयित्वा ततो देयं तु तण्डुलोदकक्कर्मणि ।।२५४।।

।। तण्डुलोदकम् ।।

Taṇḍulodaka

One *pala* of rice should be coarsely pounded. To this, eight times of water should be added for impregnation. The liquid, thus obtained, is called *taṇḍulodaka* which is used in medicines.

उद्धृत्य मुष्टिनाच्छाद्य सुगुप्तं यन्निधापयेत् ।
तं मुष्टियोगमित्याहुर्विबुधाः भिषगीश्वराः ।।२५५।।

।। इति मुष्टियोगः ।।

Muṣṭi Yoga

Drugs which are taken out covered inside the fist and given to the patient is called *muṣṭi yoga*.

घृताभ्यक्ता गुदे क्षेप्या अङ्गुष्ठाभा सुसंहता[४३] ।
मलप्रवर्तिनी वर्तिः फलवर्तिर्मता बुधैः ।।२५६।

Phala-varti (Suppository)

A cylindrical and compact suppository of the size and shape of thumb, which is smeared with ghee and inserted into the anus for inducing bowel movement is called *phala varti.*

रक्तोत्पलं मधुरसं त्रिगुणं समुदाहृतम् ।
विमलं किञ्चिदधिकं दत्वा वर्तिं प्रकल्पयेत् ।
रक्तोत्पलं गुडं प्रोक्तं विमलं सैन्धवं मतम् ।।२५७।।

Raktotpala (jaggery) should be added with three times of honey. To this, a small quantity of *vimala* (rock-salt) should be added and from out of this paste, a *varti* (elongated pill) should be prepared. In the present context, *raktotpala* is *guḍa* (jaggery) and *vimala* is *saindhava* (rock-salt).

आत्रेयात्
गुडाच्चतुर्गुणं मूत्रं प्रदद्याद्वा स्वबुद्धितः ।।२५८।।

।। फलवर्तिः ।।

According to Ātreya

In the *varti*, four parts of cow's urine should be added to one part of jaggery by the physician according to his own judgement.

Thus, ends the description of *phala varti.*

द्रव्यादष्टगुणं क्षीरं क्षीरात्तोयं चतुर्गुणम् ।
क्षीरावशेषः कर्त्तव्यः क्षीरपाके त्वयं विधिः ।।२५९।।

।। इति क्षीरपाकविधिः ।।

Kṣīrapāka (Preparation of Medicated Milk)

For the preparation of *kṣīrapāka* (medicated milk), to one part of the drug , eight parts of milk and 32 parts of water should be added and boiled till one fourth remains.

Thus, ends the description of *kṣīrapāka* (medicated milk).

अनेनैव प्रकारेण वज्रकाञ्जिकसाधनम्[१४४] ।।२६०।।

।। इति काञ्जिकम् ।।

Vajra Kāñjika (A Type of Vinegar)

In the above mentioned manner, *vajra kāñjika* should be prepared.

Thus, ends the description of *kāñjika* (vinegar).

दोषघ्नो विषहा वर्ण्यो लेपस्त्वेवंविधो[१४५] मतः ।
द्वौ तस्य कथितौ भेदौ प्रलेपाख्यप्रदेहकौ ।।२६१।।

Lepa (Ointment)

Lepa (external application of drugs in the form of paste or ointment) cures aggravated *doṣa-s* and poisons and promotes complexion. It is of two types, viz., *pralepa* and *pradeha*.

सुश्रुतात्
कुष्ठ-वीसर्प-पिडका-व्रण-शोफामयेषु च ।
दशांगादिः कठिल्लादिः लेपाः दोषहरा मताः ।।२६२।।

According to Suśruta

In diseases like *kuṣṭha* (obstinate skin diseases including leprosy), *visarpa* (erysipelas), *piḍakā* (pimples), *vraṇa* (ulcers) and *śopha* (oedema), *Daśāṅga lepa*, *Kaṭhillādi lepa*, etc., help in the alleviation of *doṣa-s*.

आरुष्करो घटिकादिः शोफघ्नो विषहा मतः ।।२६३।।

Āruṣkara lepa, *Ghaṭikādi lepa*, etc., cure oedema and poisoning.

वली-पलित-खालित्य-नीलि-व्यङ्गादिकानपि ।
नाशयेदतिलोमं च तथा कृष्णीकरं भवेत् ।
वर्धयेच्चेन्द्रियाणां वै लेपो वर्णकरो मतः ।।२६४।।

Lepa-s [of different types] in general, cure wrinkling of skin, graying of hair, baldness, blue moles, freckles, etc. They remove excess of hair and make the [depigmented] skin black. They promote the functioning of sense organs and help in the promotion of complexion.

सुशीतो लेपसंज्ञः स्यादुष्णः[१४६] प्रोक्तः प्रदेहकः ।
प्रलेपः शीतलः प्रोक्तो रक्तपित्तहरः परः ।
प्रदेहः कफवातघ्नः पाचनः परिकीर्तितः ।।२६५।।

Varieties

Cold ointment is called *lepa* and hot ointment is called *pradehaka*. *Pralepa* type of ointment is cold and it cures *rakta pitta* (a disease characterised by bleeding from different parts of the body). *Pradeha* alleviates *vāyu* and *kapha* and it causes *pācana* (suppuration of abscesses).

यदार्द्रं माहिषं चर्म तस्योत्सेधेन[१४७] लेपनम् ।
लोमाभिमुखमादेयौ प्रलेपाख्यप्रदेहकौ ।।२६६।।

Mode of Application

Both the *pralepa* and *pradeha* types of ointment should be applied in thickness like that of a wet buffalo leather. The application of these ointments should be from the centre to the perifery on the line of hair growth (*anuloma*).

अंगुष्ठस्य चतुर्भागो मुखलेपो विधीयते ।।२६७।।

In the face, ointment should be applied in the thickness of one fourth of one *aṅguṣṭha* (thumb breadth).

न रात्रौ लेपनं दद्याद् दत्तनिपतितं[१४८] तथा ।
न च पर्युषितं चापि शु[ष्य]मानं[१४९] न धारयेत् ।
न चापि मुखमालिंपेत्तेन दोषः प्रसिच्यते ।।२६८।।

Time of Application

Ointment should not be applied at night. After the ointment is removed, it should not be used again. Stale ointment should not be used. Similarly, prepared ointment which is dried up should not be used. The dried ointment should not be used even over the face because it aggravates *doṣa-s*.

डल्हणः
तमसाऽपिहितो ह्यूष्मा रोमकूपेषु संस्थितः ।
विना लेपेन निर्याति रात्रौ नालेपयेदतः ।।२६९।।

According to Ḍalhaṇa

Heat, located in the hair-roots, is slightly prevented from coming out because of the effect of the darkness at night. If ointment is applied at night, it completely inhibits such emission of heat. On the other hand, if ointment is not applied, then such heat-emission does take place (though in less quantity). Therefore, ointment should not be applied at night.

सुश्रुतः[१५०]
अपाकिशोफविषमे गम्भीरे कफवायुना ।
संयुक्तरक्ते विहितो रात्रौ लेपश्च निश्चितम् ।
शुष्कमानमुपेक्षेत प्रदेहं पीडनं प्रति ।।२७० ।।

According to Suśruta

If the oedema caused by *kapha* and *vāyu* is not suppurated, if it is irregular (uneven), if it is deep-seated, and if it is associated with vitiated blood, then ointment should certainly be applied at night. The ointment which is in the process of getting dried up should not be used because it may cause contraction of the tissues.

तथा हि शुष्को ह्यपार्थको[१५१] रुक् चान्यत्रावपीडयितव्यात् ।
अपार्थको निष्फलः । पीडयितव्यो व्रणाधिकारोक्तः यो
व्रणः पीडयितव्यो भवति तस्मादन्यत्र शुष्यमानं
नोपेक्षेत इत्यर्थः । निशि लेपः पर्युषितः कुर्य्याद्व्रणोक्त-
पिडकाचितम् । दत्तं निःपतितं चैव हीनवीर्यत्वमाप्नुयात् ।।२७१ ।।

Similarly, application of the dried ointment is useless and it gives rise to pain. This, therefore, should not be used unless the ulcer is required to be squeezed out (*piḍayitavya*). The term *apārthaka* used in the first line means useless. In the topic describing various types of ulcers, some are described to be suitable for being squeezed out (*pīḍayitavya*). For such type of ulcers, dried ointment can be used. For others, dried ointment should not be used and if required, semi dried ointment can be used for their treatment. If ointment is applied at night and if stale ointment is used [even during day time], then pimples, as described in the topic on ulcers, appear. If the ointment is already applied earlier but subsequently removed, such ointment loses its potency and should not be used.

सुश्रुतः
षड्भागं पैत्तिके स्नेहश्चतुर्भागं च वातिके ।
अष्टभागं तु कफजे स्नेहमात्राः प्रदापयेत् ।।२७२।।

According to Suśruta

In an ointment, fats (oil, ghee, etc.,) should be added one sixth, one fourth and one eighth in quantities for the treatment of *paittika*, *vātika* and *kaphaja* types of ailments respectively.

कृष्णात्रेयः
षोडशांशं षडंशं च चतुर्थांशं प्रदापयेत् ।
लेपप्रदेहयोः क्षौद्रं विपरीतं क्षिपेत्तिलम् ।
विकारतत्त्व-प्रकृति-प्रमाणं सैन्धवादिके ।।२७३।।

According to Kṛṣṇātreya

In the recipes of *lepa* (cold ointment) and *pradeha* (hot ointment), honey should be added in the quantities of 1/16th, 1/6th and 1/4th [respectively for *vātika*, *paittika* and *kaphaja* ailments). The quantity of sesame seed (or oil), on the other hand, should be 1/4th, 1/6th and 1/16th of the recipe for *vātika*, *paittika* and *kaphaja* ailments respectively. In a recipe of ointment rock-salt, etc., should be added keeping in view the nature of the ailment and constitution of the patient.

उपनाहो मतः तस्माद्यस्मादुपरि बध्यते ।
स्नेहाम्ललवणं तत्र व्यक्तं कृत्वा विनिक्षिपेत् ।।२७४।।
विषदोषहरावाद्यौ तयोरर्थे विधिस्त्वयम् ।
यस्तु वर्ण्यो न तस्यैषा इति वृद्धपरंपरा ।।२७५।।

Upanāha

'*Upanāha*' is called because it is wrapped (*nāha*) with the help of a cloth over (*upa*) the skin. In such recipes fats, sour things and salt should be added liberally.

The first two ingredients (fats & sour things) are anti-poisons; hence these are described to be added in more quantity. If however, the recipe is to be given for promoting complexion, then this rule should not be followed. This is in accordance with tradition of old physicians.

रत्नाकरात्[152] शिरोलेपविधिर्लिख्यते

उक्तानुक्तेषु लेपेषु संवेष्ट्यैरण्डपत्रकैः ।
कुर्यादिरात्रौ दिवास्नानं युक्तिरेषा प्रकीर्तिता[153] ।।२७६।।

।। इति लेपविधिः ।।

Śirolepa : According to Rasaratnākara

Recipes for application over the head (*śirolepa*) are described in Ayurvedic classics. Sometimes physicians, out of their experience, use other such recipes. These two categories of recipes should be applied over the head, covered with castor-leaf and then tied with the help of a cloth. This should be done at night and in the next morning the ointment should be washed out at the times of bath. This procedure should be followed for *śirolepa*.

Thus, ends the description of ointments.

यत्र नस्तक्योः क्वाथं पातव्यमिति भाषितम् ।
पाणिशुक्तिसमा मात्रा दातव्या पारिभाषिकैः ।।२७७।।
माषिके हिंगुसिन्धूत्थे शर्कराद्याश्च शाणिकाः ।
स्नेहस्यौषधसिद्धस्य मात्रात्वष्टौ च विन्दवः ।।२७८।।
प्रत्येकशो नस्तक्योरिति सर्वत्र निश्चितम् ।
स्नेहस्य केवलस्याथ मात्रा शुक्तिसमा मता ।।२७९।।
संतर्पणस्य नस्यस्य मात्रा कर्षसमा मता ।
तीक्ष्णस्य शुक्तिपादः स्याद्गुंजा प्रधमने मता ।।२८०।।

।। भद्रशौनकत्तस्य मात्रा ।।

Inhalation Therapy : According to Bhadraśaunaka

If a decoction is described to be inhaled through the nostrils, then the dose of this docoction should be one *pāṇi śukti*. In such a recipe, *hiṅgu* and *saindhava* should be added in the dose of one *māṣa*, and sugar, etc., should be added in the quantity of one *śāṇa*. The dose of medicated oil or medicated ghee for inhalation therapy is eight drops in each nostril. Simple oil or ghee (not medicated) should be used in the dose of one *śukti* for inhalation therapy. The dose of the *santarpaṇa* (nourishing) type of inhalation therapy is one *karṣa*. Sharp type (*tīkṣṇa*) of inhalation therapy should be used in the dose of one fourth of a *śukti*. *Pradhamana* type (which is blown into the nostrils) of inhalation therapy should be administered in the dose of one *guñjā*.

आसंचारी मुखे पूर्णे गंडूषः क्वलोन्यथा[154] ।
द्रवेषु दद्याच्चूर्णं हि गण्डूषे कर्षमात्रकम् ।
पलमात्रं द्रवं सर्वं गण्डूषे दापयेद्बुधः ।।२८१ ।।
वारमेकम्[155] ।।२८२ ।।

Gaṇḍūṣa and Kavala (Gargling)

If the mouht is filled with a potion which is made to move in it (the mouth), then it is called *gaṇḍūṣa* (gargling). *Kavala*, on the other hand, is different from it inasmuch as the potion does not move in the mouth and it is just held in it.

For *gaṇḍūṣa*, drugs in powder form should be added in the quantity of one *karṣa* and quantity of all the liquids should be one *pala*. This quantity is in respect of one-time *gaṇḍūṣa* (gargling).

द्रवेण कार्यो गंडूषः कल्केन क्वलः स्मृतः ।
कल्के सकल्करूपः स्यान्न तु सूक्ष्मं प्रदापयेत् ।
एक-द्वि-त्रि-चतुः-पञ्च वारान्कुर्यादनलसः ।।२८३ ।।

For *gaṇḍūṣa*, the drug is used in liquid form and for *kavala*, it is in paste form. The paste for *kavala* should be in coarse form and not fine. *Gaṇḍūṣa* and *kavala* should be done one, two, three, four or five times without any break.

अङ्गुल्यग्रेण चूर्णादीन् नीत्वा जिह्वादिकं शनैः ।
सारणं यत्प्रकुर्वीत तस्मात्तत्प्रतिसारणम् ।।२८४ ।।
कोलास्थिमात्रं भैषज्यं प्रतिसारणकर्मणि ।।२८५ ।।

।। क्वलगण्डूषप्रतिसारणमात्रा ।।

Pratisāraṇa

Drugs in powder form should be taken with the help of the fingertip and applied over tongue, etc. Since such applications cause salivation (*sāraṇa*), the process is called *pratisāraṇa*. For *pratisāraṇa*, the quantity of drugs should be like that of the seed (stone) of a jujuba fruit.

Thus, ends the description of the dose of drugs for *gaṇḍūṣa*, *kavala* and *pratisāraṇa*.

क्षारौषधीश्चतिं कृत्वा तिलनालेन दीपयेत् ।
निःक्वाथ्य षड्गुणे तोये श्रापयेच्च कुसुम्भवत् ।।२८६।।
यावदच्छः पिच्छिलश्च रक्तश्चैव प्रजायते[१५६] ।
चतुर्गुणेन तोयेन भावनार्थं शृतं भवेत् ।
भक्तादिसाधने श्राव्यं जलेन त्रिगुणेन च ।।२८७।।

Kṣārodaka (Preparation of Alkaline Water)

Drugs to be used for the preparation of *kṣāra*, should be cut into pieces and burnt into ashes with the help of the fuel of sesame-stalk. This should then be mixed with six times of water and the supernatant fluid should be decanted. This process of adding water and decantation should be repeated till the water thus collected is transparent, slimy and red like the water from [the bark of] *kusumbha*.

For the purpose of *bhāvanā* (impregnation), this alkaline water should be further boiled by adding four times of water, and for the preparation of rice, etc., it should be boiled by adding three times of water.

क्षारश्च द्विविधो ज्ञेयः पानीयः प्रतिसारणः ।
पलमात्रं च पातव्यं क्षेप्यं गद्याणकत्रयम् ।।२८८।।
स्नेहं कर्षसमं क्षेप्यं यथादोषबलं प्रति ।।२८९।।
प्रतिसारणके मात्रा श्रेष्ठा शुक्तिसमा मता ।।२९०।।

Varieties of Kṣāra

Alkali preparations are of two types, viz., *pānīya* (meant for drinking) and *pratisāraṇa* (meant for local application).

The former type is taken in the dose of one *pala* [of water] to which the *kṣāra* is added in the dose of three *gadyāṇaka-s*. To this recipe, about one *karṣa* of fat (oil or ghee) should be added depending upon the nature of the aggravated *doṣa-s* and strength of the patient.

The excellent dose of *pratisāraṇaka* type of *kṣāra* (alkali preparation) is one *śukti*.

सुश्रुतः
सर्वावयवसाध्येषु पलाशलवणादिषु ।
व्यवस्थितो न कालोऽत्र यत्र सर्वो विधीयते ।।२९१।।
क्षारचूर्णस्य मात्रा च गद्याणत्रयसंमता[५७] ।
अथवा क्षारलवणं कारयेल्लवणं यथा ।।२९२।।
।। इति क्षारविधिः ।।

According to Suśutra

When a *kṣāra* (alkali preparation) is prepared of the entire plant like *palāśa* by adding salt etc., there is no fixed time for their use, i.e. these alkali preparations can be used at any time depending upon the requirement of the patient. The powder of *kṣāra* should be administered in the dose of three *gadyāṇa-s*. When a *kṣāra* is mixed with salt (*lavaṇa*), then it should be administered in a dose prescribed for salts.

अथ वृद्धसुश्रुतः
आसवादिषु साध्येषु द्वात्रिंशद्गुणसंमतम् ।
खदिरादेः प्रतिपलं जलमाहुश्चिकित्सकाः ।।२९३।।
अष्टावशेषितं कृत्वा गुडं क्वाथसमं क्षिपेत् ।
प्रपुराणं गुडं देयं कफश्चाग्निवधोन्यथा ।।२९४।।
।। इति ।।

According to Vṛddha Suśruta
Preparation of Āsava

In the preparation of *āsava* etc., *khadira*, etc., should be added in the quantity of one *pala*, and the water should be added in the quantity of thirty two times of it. After boiling, the water should be reduced to one eighth. The quantity of jaggery should be same as that of the decoction. In *āsava-s*, the jaggery to be added should be very old (*prapurāṇa*) because fresh jaggery aggravates *kapha* and suppresses the power of digestion (*agni*).

क्वाथ्यद्रव्यस्य बाहुल्यादुदकं स्वल्पमेव चेत् ।
सम्यक् पाकं न मुञ्चन्ति हीनवीर्यं तु[१५८] केवलम् ।।२९५।।

Water for Decoction

If in a preparation of *āsava*, several drugs are prescribed for decoction and less quantity of water is used for boiling, then all the essence of these drugs do not come into the decoction and such decoctions are deficient of therapeutic potency.

क्वाथ्यद्रव्यं घटसमं जलं दशघटं क्षिपेत् ।
निःक्वाथ्य पादशेषं तु गुडं सार्धघटं न्यसेत् ।
विमृद्य संधितं यच्च तच्चासवमितीरितम् ।
पादावशेषितं चतुर्थावशेषितमित्यर्थः ।।२९६।।

Drugs for decoction should be taken in the quantity of one *ghaṭa*, and to this, eight *ghaṭa-s* of water should be added. This should be boiled till one fourth of water remains. Thereafter, the decoction should be filtered out. To this decoction, half a *ghaṭa* of jaggery should be added and stirred with the help of hands. This should then be allowed to get fermented. This preparation is called *āsava*.

विना क्वाथेन संधानमासवः प्रोच्यते किल ।
गुडं क्वाथौषधसमं[१५९] जलं चापि चतुर्गुणम् ।।२९७।।
आसवारिष्टमद्येषु ह्यावापश्च दशांशकः ।
क्षौद्रं च गुडपादोनं प्रदातव्यं भिषक्तमैः ।।२९८।।

If an alcoholic preparation is made without adding decoction (i.e. by adding drugs and water separately without boiling and making a decoction) then it is called *āsava*. In such preparation, the quantity of jaggery should be same as that of the drugs and water should be added four times in quantity. In *āsava-s, ariṣṭa-s* and *madya-s*, the *āvāpa* (drugs which are added in powder form at the end) should be 1/10th in quantity and honey should be 3/4th in quantity of jaggery.

गोपुरः

अरिष्टेषु च सर्वेषु द्रोणे पलशतं गुडम् ।
चिरस्थायिष्वरिष्टेषु द्विगुणं गुडमावपेत् ।।२९९।।

According to Gopura

In all types of *arista*, one hundred *pala-s* of jaggery should be added to one *drona* of water. If it is intended to keep the *arista* for a long time, then double the quantity of jaggery should be added.

अनुक्तमानारिष्टेषु द्रवद्रोणे गुडं तुलाम् ।
क्षौद्रं क्षिपेद् गुडस्यार्द्धं प्रक्षेपस्तु दशांशिकः ।
तद्विधेषु च द्रष्टव्या मद्यकर्त्तव्यता[१६०] बुधैः ॥३००॥

If in a recipe of *arista*, the quantity in which drugs, etc., are to be added is not specified, then in one *drona* of liquid, one *tulā* of jaggery, half *tulā* of honey and $^1/_{10}$th *tulā* of *praksepa* (drugs in powder form added to the recipe at the end) should be added. Similar procedure should be followed for the preparation of *madya*.

आसवारिष्टयोर्यत्र न गुणं लभ्यते तदा[१६१] ।
एकद्वित्रिशृतं कृत्वा दापयेद्गुणवृद्धये ॥३०१॥

If an *āsava* or *arista* does not produce the desired therapeutic effect, then the drugs should be boiled once, twice or thrice more and the recipe should be prepared. This enhances the therapeutic efficacy of the recipe.

अत्र भद्रशौनकः
स्रावणार्थे तु[१६२] सन्धाने पुनः कंसमितं गुडम् ।
दत्वा यन्त्रे प्रदातव्यं पारम्पर्योपदेशतः ।
भक्तसंज्ञा भवेदस्य सम्यक् स्रावार्थमाचरेत् ॥३०२॥

According to Bhadraśaunaka

For the purpose of distillation, in the fermented liquid, one *kamsa* of jaggery should again be added, and thereafter, the material should be placed in the distilling apparatus for distillation. If properly distilled, the product is called *'bhakta'*.

अथ जलविचारः
यथा यथा जलं चात्र विरसं पत्तलं भवेत् ।
तथा तथा गुडं देयं ह्यधिकं सम्प्रदायतः ।

तथा तथा भवेदत्र स्रावो बहुतरः शुभः ।।३०३।।

Addition of Water & Jaggery

If the *āsava* is tasteless and thin (like ordinary water), then according to tradition, more and more of jaggery should be added to the recipe. By such addition of jaggery, the recipe produces more and more of useful distillate.

अनुक्ते दशमूलादौ बब्बूलबदरादिकम् ।
स्रावणार्थे प्रदातव्यं नासवादौ कदाचन ।।३०४।।

If *daśamūla*, etc., are not mentioned in the recipe, then *babbūla*, *badara*, etc., should be added to it for the purpose of distillation. In ordinary *āsava*, etc., such drugs (*babbūla*, etc.) should never be added.

[धातकीमहत्वम्]

अनुक्तेऽपि च प्रस्थार्धं धातकीकुसुमं क्षिपेत् ।।३०५।।

Importance of Dhātakī

In the recipes of *āsava*, etc., half a *prastha* of *dhātakī* should be added even if it is not specified in the text.

स्रावणार्थेषु[१६३] संधेयं मधुकुष्ठविवर्जितम् ।
कुष्ठेन शिरसः पीडा छर्दिः[१६४] पुष्परसाद्भवेत् ।।३०६।।

Honey and Kuṣṭha

If the recipe is intended to be distilled, then honey and *kuṣṭha* should not be added to it because *kuṣṭha* causes headache and honey causes vomiting [if added to such recipes].

अरिष्टासवयोर्मात्रा प्रोत्तमा कुडवान्विता ।
यथा यथा शृतं मद्यं मात्रा चाल्पा तथा तथा ।।३०७।।

Dosage

The dose of *āsava* and *ariṣṭa* is one *kuḍava*. The distilled preparations are to be given in smaller dose.

अथ स्वस्थे मात्रा

यावन्न चलते दृष्टिर्यावन्न क्षोभते मनः ।
पानमात्रा परा तावद्विपरीता विषोपमा ।।३०८।।

Dose for a Healthy Person

A healthy person should take these preparations in such a dose as would not cause intoxicated movement of eye-balls and perversion of mental activities. This is the limit of taking alcoholic drinks. If a person drinks more than that then it works as a poison.

द्रव्यगुणमालायाम्

धातकी सगुडो मद्यो भेदो गौडः प्रकीर्तितः ।

[शार्कर]

शर्कराधातकी-तोय-क्वथितैः शार्करो मता ।।३०९।।

According to Dravyaguṇamālā

The alcoholic prerparation made out of *dhātakī* and *guḍa* (jaggery) is called '*Gauḍa*'. If it is prepared of the decoction of *dhātakī* (boiled by adding water) and *śarkarā* (sugar), then this alcoholic preparation is called '*Śārkara*'.

वृद्धशौनकात्

आमेन शीतरसिकसीधुः पक्वरसोद्भवः ।

मध्वासवः[१६५] स विज्ञेयो धातकीक्वाथमाक्षिकात् ।।३१०।।

आसवस्य सुरायाश्च द्वयोरेकत्र भाजने ।

संधानं तद्विजानीयान्मैरेयमुभयात्मकम् ।।३११।।

Varieties of Alcoholic Preparation

According to Vṛddha Śaunaka

If an alcoholic preparation is made out of uncooked material, then it is called '*Śīta-rasika*'. If prepared of boiled material, then it is called '*Sīdhu*'. If prepared of the decoction of *dhātakī* by adding *madhu* (honey) then it is called '*Madhvāsava*'. If *āsava* and *surā* are taken together in a jar and fermented, then the preparation is called '*Maireya*' which has the effects of both these preparations.

चन्द्रिका

मृद्वीकाभिः कृतं मद्यं मार्द्वीकमिति चोच्यते ।

मृद्वीकानां सुपक्वानां यः स्वयं[१६६] गालितः पटात् ।।३१२।।

रसस्तेन हि कृन्मद्यं[१६७] कषायरहितेन यत् ।
मार्द्वीकं कापिशं भीमविक्रान्तं कापिशापनम् ।।३१३।।

According to Candrikā

If an alcoholic prerparation is made out of *mṛdvīkā* (dry grapes), then it is called '*Mārdvīka*'. For this preparation, dry grapes are to be cooked well and the juice should be strained out through a piece of cloth. This juice should be free from astringent taste and this should be used for fermentation. This alcoholic preparation is called *Mārdvīka*, *Kāpiśa*, *Bhīmavikrānta* or *Kāpiśāpana*.

पिंडखर्जूरविकृतिभवं खार्जूरमुच्यते ।।३१४।।

The alcoholic preparation made out of *piṇḍa kharjūra* is called '*Khārjūra*'.

मतान्तरं[१६८]
तालहिन्तालखर्जूरमूर्धन्युच्छिद्य[१६९] गृह्यते ।
तालीति[१७०] सा समाख्याता विज्ञेयं तत्परायणैः ।।३१५।।

Another View

The juice that is collected by making a cut at the top of trees of *tāla*, *hintāla* or *kharjūra* is called *'Tālī'*.

वाचस्पतिः
मैरेयं धातकीपुष्पं गुडधान्याम्लसाधितम् ।
सचातुर्जातकाजाजी[१७१] सकुष्ठोषणनागरम् ।।३१६।।

According to Vācaspati

Maireya is prepared of *dhātakī* flowers, jaggery and *dhānyāmla* (a type of vinegar) along with *cāturjātaka*, *ajājī*, *kuṣṭha*, *ūṣaṇa* and *nāgara*.

यवमाषादिपिष्टोत्था कान्तोली कोहली सुरा ।
कोहलः सक्तुभिर्देशे वाह्लीके क्रियते यवैः ।।३१७।।

The alcoholic preparation made out of the paste of *yava*, *māṣa*, etc., is called *'Kāntolī'*, *'Kohalī'* or *'Surā'*. In the country of *Vāhlīka*, *Kohala* type of alcoholic preparation is made out of barley-flour.

आक्षिकी तु सुरा ज्ञेया अक्षत्वक्शालितण्डुलैः ।
जाम्बवः क्षौद्रसहितो जम्बूरसगुडोद्भवः ॥३१८॥

The alcoholic preparation made out of the bark of *akṣa* and rice grains is called *'Ākṣikī'*. The alcoholic preparation made out of the juice of *jambū*, jaggery and honey is called *'Jāmbava'*.

वृद्धसुश्रुतः
सर्वं मद्यमसंजातं[१७२] मधूलकमुदाहृतम् ।
प्रसन्ना स्यात्सुरामण्डस्तस्मात्कादम्बरी घना ॥३१९॥

According to Vṛddha Suśruta

All types of *madya* (alcoholic preparation), when not properly fermented, is called *Madhūlaka*. The upper layer of the alcoholic preparation (*surā*) is called *'Prasannā'* and the lower thick portion of it is called *'Kādambarī'*.

[प्रसन्नादिः]
मद्यस्याद्यविभागोऽसौ प्रसन्ना प्रोच्यते बुधैः ।
जगलस्तदधः प्रोक्तो मेदको जगलादधः ॥३२०॥
सद्यः पिण्डनकल्कोऽयं वक्कसः स उदाहृतः ।
तस्यावशिष्टं यत् प्रोक्तं सुराबीजं तु किण्वकम् ।
परिपक्वान्नसंधानं समुद्भूता सुरा मता ॥३२१॥

Varieties

The upper layer of the *madya-s* (alcoholic preparations) is called *'Prasannā'*. Its lower part is called *'Jagala'*. The layer still below it is called *'Medaka'*. The lowest layer of it containing the paste of drugs is called *'Vakkasa'*. The remnant of the alcoholic preparation is called *'Surābīja'* or *'Kiṇva'*. The preparation made out by fermenting cooked cereals is called *'Surā'*.

कुम्भं नदनदीतीरे सौम्यजातमृदाऽथवा[७३] ।
सुस्निग्धं बहलं श्लक्ष्णं निश्छिद्रं विशदं लघु ।।३२२।।
आनाहश्च भवेन्मध्ये द्विचत्वारिंशदङ्गुलम् ।
त्रिचत्वारिंशदुत्सेधं घनमेकाङ्गुलं भवेत् ।।३२३।।
आकृत्या च भवेत्कुम्भो बकुलस्य फलं यथा ।
एवंविधो घटश्चैव सलिलादिषु शस्यते ।।३२४।।

Preparation of Jar

A jar should be prepared of the soft mud collected from the silt in the bank of a lake or river. It should be greasy, thick, light and smooth. It should be free from holes (and cracks) and homogenous. Echo should come out from inside this jar. Its circumference in the middle should be 42 *aṅgula-s* and its height should be 43 *aṅgula-s*. Its wall should be one *aṅgula* in thickness and compact. In shape, it should be like the fruit of *bakula*. Such a jar should be used for keeping water, etc.

चुक्र

गुडमाक्षिकधान्याम्लमस्त्वंबुद्विगुणं क्रमात् ।
शंसन्ति चुक्रसिद्ध्यर्थं किञ्चित्त्रिकटुकान्वितम्[७४] ।
यन्मस्त्वादिः[७५] शुचौ भाण्डे सगुडं क्षौद्रकाञ्जिकम् ।
यथर्तुधान्यराशिस्थं शुक्तं चुक्रं तदुच्यते ।।३२५।।

Cukra (A Type of Vinegar)

Cukra is prepared by one part of jaggery, two parts of honey, four parts of *dhānyāmla* (a sour preparation of cereals), eight parts of *mastu* (butter-milk) and sixteen parts of water. To this, a small quantity of the powder of *trikaṭu* should be added.

Mastu, etc., should be kept in a clean jar along with jaggery, honey and *kāñjī* (a type of sour drink). The jar should be kept inside a heap of cereals of the concerned season. This is called *'Śukta'* or *'Cukra'*.

'गुडांबुवसातैलेन[७६] संधानं संस्कृतं च यत् ।
कन्द-शाक-फलैर्युक्तं गुडशुक्तं तदुच्यते' ।।३२६।।

Guḍa Śukta

Jaggery, water, *vasā* (muscle fat) and oil should be fermented and sizzled by adding roots, leaves and fruits. This preparation is called *'Guḍa śukta*.

जम्बीरस्य फलरसं पिप्पलीमूलसंयुतम्[१७७] ।
मधुभाण्डे विनिक्षिप्य धान्यराशौ निधापयेत् ।
त्र्यहेन तज्जातरसं मधुशुक्तं तमादिशेत् ।।३२७।।

Madhu Śukta

Juice of *jambīra* fruit should be added with *pippalī mūla* and kept in a jar containing honey. The jar should then be kept inside a heap of cereals for three days. The fermented liquid, thus obtained, is called *'Madhu śukta'*

[काञ्जिक]
कन्द-मूल-फलोपेतं संधानीकृतमाश्रितम्[१७८] ।
कुल्माषधान्यमण्डादिसाधितं काञ्जिकं मतम् ।।३२८।।

Kāñjika

The preparation made by fermenting rhizomes, roots, fruits, *kulmāṣa*, *dhānya maṇḍa*, etc., is called *kāñjika*.

तुषाम्बुसन्धितं ज्ञेयं आमैर्विदलितैर्यवैः ।।३२९।।

Tuṣāmbu

Tuṣāmbu is prepared by fermenting uncooked and dehusked barley.

सौवीरकं सुवीराम्लं ज्ञेयं गोधूमसम्भवम् ।
निस्तुषैस्तु यवैः केचित्प्राहुः सौवीरकं बुधाः ।।३३०।।

Sauvīraka

Sauvīraka or *suvīrāmla* is prepared by fermenting wheat. According to some physicians, it is prepared by fermenting the dehusked barley.

यवैस्तु निस्तुषैः पक्वैः सौवीरं साधितं क्वचित् ।
यवादष्टगुणं तोयं दापयन्ति चिकित्सकाः ॥३३१॥

For the preparation of *sauvīraka,* dehusked barley should be cooked by adding eight times of water and then fermented.

घनात्यये तथा ग्रीष्मे संधानं षड्दिनं भवेत् ।
हेमन्ते शिशिरे स्थाप्यं भिषकूदशदिनं [च[१७९]] वै ।
प्रावृट् - वसन्ते संधानं भवेदष्टदिनेन वै ॥३३२॥

॥इत्यासवादिपरिभाषा॥

Process of Fermentation

During autumn and summer seasons, fermentation takes place in six days. In early and late winters, the recipe should be kept for 10 days for the completion of the process of fermentation. During rainy season and spring, fermentation takes place in eight days.

Thus, ends the description of *āsava*, etc.

नलः

क्वाथ्यमानं तु निर्वेगं निष्फेनं निर्मलं च यत् ।
अर्धावशिष्टं भवति तदुष्णोदकमुच्यते ॥३३३॥

॥ उष्णोदकं[१८०] लक्षणम् ॥

Uṣṇodaka : According to Nala

Water should be boiled till it becomes free from bubbles (*nirvega*) and foam, clean and reduced to half the quantity. This is called *Uṣṇodaka* (boiled water).

Thus, ends the description of *uṣṇodaka*.

हेमन्ते शिशिरे चैव मध्याह्नेऽञ्जनमिष्यते ।
पूर्वाह्ने वाऽपराह्ने ग्रीष्मे शरदि चेष्यते ।
वर्षास्वनभ्रे वात्युष्णे वसन्ते च सदैव हि ॥३३४॥

Añjana (Collyrium)
Time of Application

During *hemanta* (early winter) and *śiśira* (late winter), collyrium should be applied to the eyes during the mid-day.

During summer and autumn, it should be applied during forenoon or afternoon. During rainy season, it should be applied to the eyes when the sky is free from clouds and when the temperature is high. In the spring, collyrium can be applied over the eyes during any time of the day.

हरेणुमात्रां कुर्वीत वर्तिमुष्णाञ्जने भिषक् ।
प्रमाणं मध्यमे द्वे स्यात्त्रिगुणा तु मृदौ भवेत् ।।३३५।।

Size of the Varti

Collyrium is of three types, viz., (1) *uṣṇa* (hot or sharp), (2) *madhyama* (moderate), and (3) *mṛdu* (mild). The size of the *varti* (elongated pill) of the *uṣṇa* (hot or sharp) type should be like that of one *hareṇu*. Of the moderate type, the *varti* should be of the size of two *hareṇu-s* and of the mild type, the size of the *varti* should be that of three *hareṇu-s*.

रसक्रिया विधातव्या त्रिविडंगसमोत्तमा ।।३३६।।

Rasakriyā

At times, collyrium is prepared in the form of *rasakriyā* (solid extract). The excellent dose of this type of collyrium is like three fruits of *viḍaṅga*.

लेखनं रोपणं चैव तथा स्यात्स्नेहनाञ्जनम् ।।३३७।।

Varieties (On the Basis of Therapeutic Effects)

Collyrium is of three varieties, viz., (1) *lekhana* (which scrapes out dirt, etc., from the eyes), (2) *ropaṇa* (which helps in the healing of ulcers in the eyes), and (3) *snehana* or *prasādana* (which provides nourishment to the eye-tissues).

लेखनं क्षारतीक्ष्णाम्लरसैरञ्जनमुच्यते ।
कषायतिक्तसंयुक्तं[१८१] सस्नेहं रोपणं मतम् ।
मधुरस्नेहसम्पन्नमञ्जनं तु प्रसादनम् ।।३३८।।

Lekhana type of collyrium is prepared out of alkalies and drugs having sharpness and sour taste. *Ropaṇa* type of collyrium is prepared of astringent and bitter drugs mixed with oil, ghee, etc. *Snehana* or *prasādana* type of collyrium is prepared out of drugs having sweet taste mixed with oil, ghee, etc.

गुटिका-रस-चूर्णानि त्रिविधान्यञ्जनानि च ।
वैरेचनिकं चूर्णं तु द्विशलाकं विधीयते ।
मृदौ च द्विशलाकं स्याच्चतस्रः स्नैहिकेऽञ्जने ।।३३९।।

Varieties (On the Basis of Pharmaceutical Processes)

Collyrium can be prepared in three different ways, viz., in tablet form, in the form of *rasakriyā* (solid extract) and in the form of powder. *Vairecanika* (which causes lachrimation) type of collyrium in powder form should be applied through a rod (*śalākā*) for two times. Similarly, mild type of collyrium should be applied twice. The *snaihika* (nourishing) type of a collyrium should be applied with the help of rod for four times.

दशाङ्गुला तनुर्मध्या शलाका मुकुलानना ।
अस्थिजा[१८२] धातुजा वापि कलायपरिमण्डला ।।३४०।।

Preparation of Śalākā (Rod)

The *śalākā* (rod) for applying collyrium should be 10 *aṅgula-s* in length with a thin stem and bud-like heads. It can be made of bone or metals and its head should be of the size and shape of a pea.

वृद्धसुश्रुतः
ताम्रलोहाश्मसंजाता शलाका लेखने मता ।
सुवर्णरजतोद्भूतशलाका[१८३] स्नेहने मता ।
अङ्गुलीत्वक्मृदुत्वेन रोपणे कथिता बुधैः ।।३४१।।

According to Vṛddha Suśruta

For the purpose of *lekhana* (scraping out dirt from the eyes), the collyrium-rod should be prepared of copper, iron or stone. For the purpose of *snehana* (nourishment), the collyrium-rod should be prepared of gold or silver. For the purpose of *ropaṇa* (healing of ulcers, etc.), the collyrium should be applied with the help of finger because the finger-skin is soft.

वामे करतले कृत्वा सजलं निकषोपलम् ।
दक्षिणेनाञ्जनं नीत्वा[१८४] करेण निकषेच्छनैः ।
तेन कल्केन मतिमान् शलाकामभिलिप्य च ।।३४२।।
उच्छाप्य[१८५] चोत्तरं वर्त्म वामेनाङ्गुष्ठपर्वणा[१८६] ।
वर्त्मशुक्लान्तरे चैव शलाकामुपवर्त्तयेत् ।
कृष्णभागादधः कुर्यादपाङ्गं यावदञ्जनम् ।।३४३।।

Mode of Application

The *nikaṣa* (a hard and black stone used for testing purity of gold, etc.) with a little water at its upper surface, should be taken in the left hand and with the help of right hand the recipe of collyrium should be taken and gently rubbed by adding the water over the stone. The paste, thus prepared, should be applied over the [head of the] collyrium-rod. The upper eyelid should then the be pulled out with the help of the phalage of left thumb and rod containing collyrium should be rubbed (applied) between the eyelid and the sclera (*śukla*). Similarly, collyrium should be applied to the lower-lid below the black-circle (cornea with irish at the back) upto the periferal angle of the eyes.

शंखटङ्कणकादीनामदग्धं चाञ्जने क्षिपेत् ।।३४४।।

Śaṅkha (conch shell), *ṭaṅkaṇa* (borax), etc. should be used in a recipe of collyrium in raw powder form without calcination i.e. not in *bhasma* form.

वृद्धभोजः
लेखनमञ्जनं रजतपात्रे[१८७] धार्यम् । रोपणं सुवर्णशंखान्यतमेन प्रसाद्यं[१८८] चंदनान्यतमेन एवं ह्यञ्जनमव्यापन्नगुणं भवति ।।३४५।।

।। अञ्जनम् ।।

According to Vṛddha Bhoja

Lekhana (scraping) type of collyrium should be stored in a vessel of silver. *Ropaṇa* (healing) type of collyrium should be stored in a vessel of gold or in conch-shell. *Prasādya* (nourishing) type of collyrium should be stored in a vessel made out of sandal wood or similar other substance. If stored like this, the collyrium becomes more effective therapeutically.

Thus, ends the description of collyrium.

सेकश्चाश्च्योतनं पिण्डी विडालस्तर्पणं तथा ।
पुटपाकोऽञ्जनं नेत्रे यथावस्थं प्रयोजयेत् ।।३४६।।

Eye-spray, etc.

For the treatment of eye diseases, appropriately *seka* (spray), *āścyotana* (eye-drop), *piṇḍī* (application of paste of drugs over the eyes and tying a bandage over it), *viḍāla* (external application of paste of drugs excluding eye-lashes), *tarpaṇa* (application of nourishing drugs), *puṭapāka* (pouring juice of specially cooked drugs) and *añjana* (collyrium) should be administered.

सेकश्च[१८९] सूक्ष्मधाराभिः सर्वस्मिन्नयने हितः ।
नेत्रं निमीलनं कृत्वा प्रदेयश्चतुरङ्गुलात् ।।३४७।।
षड्वाक्शतैः स्नेहने रोपणे च चतुःशतम् ।
लेखने द्विशतं मात्रा दिवा कार्याऽथवा निशि ।।३४८।।

।। सेक ।।

Seka (Eye-Spray)

Eyes should be sprayed with liquids having fine streams. The spray should be over the entire eyes. The eyes should be closed and spraying should be conducted from a level of four *aṅgula-s* above the eyes. For the purpose of *snehana* (nourishment), spraying should be done till six hundred words are uttered. For the purpose of *ropaṇa* (healing), spraying should be done till four hundred words are uttered. For the purpose of *lekhana* (scraping), spraying should be done till two hundred words are uttered. Spraying therapy should be done either during day or at night.

Thus, ends the description of eye-spraying.

शौनकः

पिष्टं वस्त्रान्तरगतं पीडितं बिन्दुमात्रया ।

नेत्रेषु दीयते तस्य संज्ञा स्यादाश्च्योतनं मता ।।३४९।।
तस्य कालो दिवा ज्ञेयो यामश्च प्रथमो निशि ।
बिन्दवोऽष्टौ लेखने च स्नेहने दशबिन्दवः ।।३५०।।
रोपणे द्वादश ज्ञेया वातपित्तकफे तथा ।
एकवारं द्विवारं च त्रिवारं[१०] वा प्रदापयेत् ।।३५१।।

।। आश्च्योतनम् ।।

Āścyotana : According to Śaunaka

The paste of drugs should be kept in a piece of cloth and squeezed so that the liquid falls over the eyes in drops. This is called *āścyotana*. It should be administered during the day or during the first three hours (*yāma*) of the night. For the purpose of *lekhana* (scraping), eight drops should be poured into the eyes; for the purpose of *snehana* (nourishment), ten drops should be administered, and for the purpose of *ropaṇa* (healing), twelve drops should be poured into the eyes. For *vātika* type of eye-diseases, such drops should be administered once, for *paittika* eye-diseases, it should be done twice; and for *kaphaja* eye-diseases, it should be done three times.

Thus, ends the description of *āścyotana*.

पिण्डिका वलिका प्रोक्ता बध्यते वस्त्रपट्टकैः ।
नेत्राभिष्यन्दरोगेषु व्रणे चैव विशेषतः ।
शुक्तिप्रमाणा सा पिण्डी सार्द्रा योज्या सदैव हि ।।३५२।।

।। पिण्डी ।।

Piṇḍī (Application of Paste)

In *piṇḍī* which is also called *valikā*, the paste of drugs is tied over the eyes with the help of a piece of cloth. It is specially useful in the treatment of *netrābhiṣyanda* (conjunctivitis) and ulcers in the eyes. The *piṇḍī* or paste of drugs should be used in the quantity of one *śukti*. Drugs used for this purpose should always be wet.

Thus, ends the description of *piṇḍī*.

विडालको बहिर्लेपो नेत्रे पक्ष्मादिवर्जिते ।
तस्य मात्रा मता विज्ञैर्मुखलेपस्य या हि सा ।।३५३।।

।। विडालक ।।

Viḍālaka

In *viḍālaka*, paste of drugs is applied over the eye-lids excluding eye-lashes. Its quantity should be like that of *mukhalepa* (ointment used over the face).

Thus, ends the description of *viḍālaka*.

नेत्रसंतर्पणार्थं च नेत्रे बस्तिं प्रकल्पयेत् ।
वातातपरजोहीने[११] देशे चोत्तानशायिनः ॥३५४॥
नेत्रक्षेत्रं परित्यज्य सार्धं च द्वयमङ्गुलम् ।
सर्वतश्चाथ चमसीं जलं दत्वा प्रमर्दयेत्[१२] ॥३५५॥
तेन पिण्डनालवालं दृढं संधिविवर्जितम् ।
कृत्वा नवीनदक्षाण्डं शुक्लभागद्रवेण वै ॥३५६॥
पूरयेच्च यथा पक्ष्मपूरितश्चैव जायते ।
नेत्रे यत्नं प्रकुर्वीत विकाशस्तु यथा[१३] भवेत् ॥३५७॥
क्षीरोत्थितघृते नैव शतधौतेन वा भवेत् ॥३५८॥

Netra Basti (Netra Tarpaṇa)

For the nourishment of eyes, *netra basti* is used. It should be done in a place free from strong wind, hot sun-rays and dust. The patient should lie over his back. Excluding the eye-balls and the area around it of 2 $^1/_2$ *aṅgula-s* radius, water should be poured with the help of a big spoon (*camas*) and rubbed. Around this area, a compact ridge should be raised with the help of flour-paste and into this pit white portion of the egg should be powdered till the eye-lashes get covered up. Effort should be made to open the eyes. This pit alternatively, can be filled with ghee taken out of the cream of milk or with *Śatadhauta ghṛta* (ghee washed with water for one hundred times).

धारयेद्वर्त्मरोगेषु वाङ्मात्रशतमेव च ।
स्वस्थे कफे सन्धिरोगे मात्रा पञ्चशतं विदुः ॥३५९॥
कफे वाते कृष्णे रोगे मात्रा सप्तशतं मतम् ।
दृष्टिरोगेऽष्टशतमधिमन्थे सहस्रकम् ॥३६०॥
शुक्लेऽतिकुटिले[१४] ह्रस्वे स्याद् द्वादशशती मता[१५] ।

पित्तरोगे नवशतं सहस्रं वातरोगिणाम् ।
एकाहं वा त्र्यहं वापि पञ्चाहं चेष्यतेऽथवा ॥३६१॥

In the diseases of eye-lids, the above mentioned recipes should be kept over the eyes, till 100 words are uttered. For a healthy person and in the eye diseases caused by *kapha* and in diseases of eye-joints, these recipes should be kept over the eyes till five hundred words are uttered. In the diseases caused by *kapha* and *vāyu* and in the diseases of the black-circle of the eyes, these recipes should be retained till seven hundred words are uttered. In *dṛṣṭi roga* (diseases of the eye-sight involving pupils), it should be kept till eight hundred words are uttered. In *adhimantha* (a type of eye disease), it should be kept till one thousand words are uttered. If the sclera of eyes has become excessively wrinkled and small, then it should be retained till twelve hundred words are uttered. In *paittika* eye-diseases, it should be retained till nine hundred words are uttered. In *vātika* eye-diseases, it should be retained till one thousand words are retained. The duration of the course is either one day or three days or five days.

द्रवं चापाङ्गतो नीत्वा नीलद्रव्यं विलोक्य च ।
सुखं निरीक्षयेत्पश्चान्नेत्रबस्तिविधिस्त्वयम् ॥३६२॥

When the liquid taken from the periferal angle of the eye looks blue and when the patient is able to see things with comfort, the recipe over the eye should be removed. This is the procedure of using *netra basti*.

निवृत्तिर्व्याधिशान्तिश्च क्रियालाघवमेव च ।
सम्यग्योगे सुखं प्राप्ति वैशद्यं वर्णपाटवम् ॥३६३॥

Appropriate Application

If *netra basti* is appropriately applied, then the eye diseases will be either cured or alleviated, and the patient feels lightness in his eyes, happiness, clarity and good complexion.

शोफाश्रुपातगुरुता स्नैग्ध्यं स्यादतितर्पिते ।
रूक्षाविलं सरक्तं च नेत्रं स्याद्धीनतर्पितम् ॥३६४॥

Excessive & Less Application

If *netra basti* is applied in excess, then there will be oedema, lachrimation, heaviness and unctuousness. If it is less applied, then the eyes will become dry, cloudy and red.

रूक्षः स्निग्धः क्रमश्चात्र प्रयोज्यः संप्रदायतः ।।३६५।।

।। नेत्रबस्तिक्रमः ।।

Alternatively, ununctuous and unctuous recipes should be used for *netra basti.*

Thus, ends the description of the application of *netra basti.*

बृहदात्रेयः

अभ्यंगः परिषेकश्च पिचुर्बस्तिरिति क्रमात् ।

[एवं[१६]]चतुर्विधं मूर्ध्नि तैलं बलवच्चोत्तरोत्तरम् ।।३६६ ।।

Application of Oil Over the Head According to Bṛhadātreya

Oil application over the head is of four types, viz.,

(1) *abhyaṅga* (massage);
(2) *pariṣeka* (sprinkling of oil over head);
(3) *picu* (application of cotton-swab soaked in oil); and
(4) *basti* (keeping oil over the head).

The latter ones are therapeutically more effective than the former ones.

एतेषां हि परा मात्रा यावत् स्रावश्च नेत्रयोः ।

सूचीभिरिव तोदश्च[१७] केशभूमिषु जायते ।।३६७।।

The excellent time limit upto which these therapies are to be administered is indicated by lachrimation from the eyes and feeling of pricking pain in the hair roots.

स्नेहं पिचुप्लुतं कृत्वा प्रदद्यान्मस्तकोपरि ।

ऊर्ध्वजत्रुविकारेषु पिचुतैलं[१८] प्रशस्यते ।।३६८।।

Picu

A cotton-swab should be soaked in oil and applied over the

head. This type of applying oil over the head is very useful for curing diseases of head and neck.

शिरोबस्तिश्चर्मकृतो द्विमुखो द्वादशाङ्गुलः ।
शिरःप्रमाणं तं कृत्वा चर्मबन्धेन यन्त्रयेत् ।।३६९।।
अथवा संधिरोधं च चमसीभिः [?] प्रयोजयेत्[१९९] ।
ततस्तैलं न्यसेत्तत्र यावत्सम्पूर्णता भवेत् ।
तावद्धार्यस्तु यावत्स्यात्कर्णनासामुखस्रुतिः ।।३७०।।
वेदनोपशमो वापि मात्राणां वा सहस्रकम् ।।३७१।।
विना भोजनमेवात्र शिरोबस्तिर्विधीयते ।
विमोच्याथ शिरोबस्तिं युगपत्[२००] विमर्दयेत् ।
ऊर्ध्वकायं ततः कोष्णैर्जलैः स्नानं समाचरेत् ।।३७२।।
मस्तकंमुण्डयित्वा वा शिरोबस्तिं प्रकल्पयेत्[२०१] ।।३७३।।

।।शिरोबस्तिविधिः।।

Śiro Basti

A leather cap of 12 *angula-s* length and having both its ends open should be placed over the head and made tight with the help of a leather strap tied around it. The joint between the head and the leather cap should be sealed with the help of paste of flour. Into this cap oil should be poured till its top. It should be retained till there is flow of secretion from the ears, nose and mouth or till the pain is relieved or till one thousand *mātrā-s* (for details of *mātrā* see below). *Śiro basti* should be administered when the patient is in empty stomach. Thereafter, the oil and the leather cap should be removed and the head should be kneaded from all sides. Thereafter, the patient should take bath and the upper part of the body should be washed with luke-warm water. It is better to administer *śiro basti* after shaving hair from the head.

Thus, ends the description of the procedure for administering *śiro basti*.

दक्षजानुकरावर्त्तं कुर्याच्छोटिकया युतम् ।
निमेषोन्मेषकालो वा एषा मात्रा मता बुधैः ।

बस्त्यवगाहमभ्यङ्गकार्ये योग्यतमा मता[२०२] ।।३७४।।

।।बस्त्यवगाहादिमात्रा[२०३] ।।

Definition of Mātrā

The person should squat with his knees raised and folded. The right hand should be taken around the right leg and snapping should be done with the help of the right thumb and the right middle finger. The time taken for snapping the finger is called *mātrā* [which is a unit of time according to ancient Indian tradition]. This is same as the time taken for closing and opening of the eye-lids (*akṣi nimeṣa* = twinkling). This unit of time should be followed in measuring the duration of *basti*, *avagāha* (bath) and *abhyaṅga* (massage).

Thus, ends the description of *mātrā* (unit of time) for measuring the duration of *basti, avagāha,* etc.

अथावगाहे

'नाभेः[२०४] षडंगुलं यावदूर्ध्वं मग्नमिति स्थितिः' ।।३७५।।

Bath

Keeping the body deeped upto 6 *aṅgula-s* above the umbilicus is called *magna.*

रोमान्तेष्वनुकूमेषु स्थित्वा मात्रा शतत्रयम् ।
ततः प्रविशति स्नेहश्चतुर्भिर्गच्छति त्वचाम्[२०५] ।।३७६।।
पञ्चभिश्च भवेद्रक्तं षड्भिर्मांसं प्रपद्यते ।
मेदःस्थाने सप्तशतैरष्टभिश्चास्थिषु व्रजेत् ।।३७७।।
नवभिर्याति मज्जानं ततो मात्रा न कारयेत् ।
ततस्तु हरते रोगान् वातपित्तकफोद्भवान् ।।३७८।।

।।इति बस्त्यवगाहनमात्रा[२०६] ।।

Time Taken for Absorption of Oil

The oil when applied over the body remains in the roots of hair for three hundred *mātrā-s*. Thereafter, in four hundred *mātrā-s* it enters into the skin. In five hundred *mātrā-s* it enters into the blood.

In six hundred *mātrā-s,* it enters into the muscles. In seven hundred *mātrā-s,* it enters into the fat-tissue. In eight hundred *mātrā-s*, it enters into the bone-tissue. In nine hundred *mātrā-s*, it enters into the bone-marrow. Thereafter, the unit of time does not hold good.

After this period, the oil cures diseases caused by *vāyu*, *pitta* and *kapha*.

Thus, ends the description of the *mātrā* (unit of time) for *basti*, *avagāha* (bath), etc.

[पादाभ्यङ्ग]
स्रोतसां मार्दवकरः कफवातविनाशनः ।
धातूनां पुष्टिजननो[२०७] मृजावर्णबलप्रदः ॥३७९॥
निद्राकरो देहसुखश्चक्षुष्यः पादरोगहा ।
पादत्वक्मृदुकर्त्ता च पादाभ्यङ्गः प्रशस्यते ॥३८०॥

Pādābhyaṅga (Massage Over Soles of Feet)

Oil massage over the soles of feet is very useful inasmuch as it softens the channels of circulation, alleviates *kapha* and *vāyu*, provides nourishment to tissue elements, promotes energy, complexion and strength, induces sleep, gives a feeling of comfort to the body, stimulates eye-sight, cures foot-diseases and produces softens of the skin of the feet.

[कर्णपूरणम्]
कर्णं प्रपूरयेत्सम्यक् स्नेहाद्यैर्मात्रया भिषक् ।
नोच्चैःश्रुतिर्न बाधिर्यं स्यान्नित्यं कर्णपूरणम् ॥३८१॥

Filling the Ears with Oil (Ear-drop)

The physician should suitably fill the ears with oil, etc., in appropriate dose. Regularly filling the ears with oil prevents hard of hearing and deafness.

प्रयोगपारिजाते
तद्विशेषो नखाभ्यङ्गः शिरोनासास्थितापजित् ।
ओष्टस्फुटनपारुष्यं नाभ्यभ्यङ्गेन च शाम्यति ॥३८२॥

According to Prayoga Pārijāta

Massaging the nails with oil, specially cures heat in the head, nose and bones. Massaging the umbilicus with oil cures cracking and roughness of the lips.

[अभ्यङ्ग]
मृदौ समे सुपर्यङ्के गतः स्वस्थः[२०८] सदा नरः ।
उत्तानशायी सम्भूय तैलाभ्यङ्गं समाचरेत् ।
शिरोभ्यक्तेन तैलेन नाङ्गं किञ्चिदुपस्पृशेत् ।।३८३।।
तपो विद्यां धनं चक्षुरायुः कीर्तिं प्रजां हरेत् ।
श्रोत्राक्षिबलदं पित्त-श्रम-तृड्-दाह-मेहनुत् ।।३८४।।

Body Massage

For body massage, the patient (even a healthy person) should lie on his back in a bed which is soft and even and he should be in peace and happy. Thereafter, his body should be massaged. After massaging the head, the residual oil should never be used for body massage because this deplets the power of penance, learning, wealth, eye sight, longevity, fame and progeny. Body massage promotes strength of ears, eyes, etc., and alleviates *pitta* , fatigue, morbid thirst, burning sensation and *meha* (obstinate urinary disorders including diabetes).

वाते पित्ते कफे रक्ते सन्निपाते कृशाङ्गके ।
मदमूर्च्छाप्रलापेषु तृष्णादाहज्वरेषु च ।।३८५।।
संतप्ते संतते जीर्णे ह्यध्वश्रान्ते विशेषतः ।
बालमध्यमजीर्णानां घृताभ्यङ्गः प्रशस्यंते ।।३८६।।

Body Massage with Ghee

In the diseases caused by *vāyu*, *pitta*, *kapha* and vitiated blood, in *sannipāta* (when all the three *doṣa-s* are simultaneously aggravated), in emaciation of the body, in intoxication (*mada*), fainting, delirium, morbid sensation, feeling of hot sensation in the body, remittent fever, chronic fever and specially in fatigue because of long walk, the body massage with [medicated] ghee is very useful. Massage with ghee is indicated for infants, middle aged persons and old persons.

गुल्मं प्लीहाग्निसदनं कमलासातिसारिषु ।
श्वासकासोदरच्छर्दिपाण्डुसर्वाङ्गशोफिषु ।
विद्रधौ पार्श्वशूले च गण्डमालार्बुदादिषु ।
शीतज्वरे[२०९] प्रमेहे च घृताभ्यङ्गं न शस्यते ।।३८७।।

Contra-indications

Massage with ghee is contra-indicated in *gulma* (phantom tumour), splenic disorders, suppression of the power of digestion, jaundice, diarrhoea, asthma, bronchitis, *udara* (obstinate abdominal disorders including ascites), vomiting, anemia, general anasarca, abscess, pain in the sides of the chest, cervical adenitis, tumour, etc., fever with cold (*śītajvara*) and *prameha* (obstinate urinary diseases including diabetes).

'रसाद्यैः[२१०] पूरणं कर्णे भोजनात्प्राक् प्रशस्यते' ।
तैलाद्यैः पूरणं कर्णे भास्करे समुपागते[२११]। ।३८८।।

Time of Karṇa Pūraṇa

Filling the ears with juice, etc., should be performed before taking food. Filling the ears with oil, etc., should be performed after sun-rise.

स्वेदयेत्कर्णदेशं तु परिवर्तनशायिनः ।
मूत्रैः[२१२] स्नेहैः रसैः कोष्णैः पूरयेच्च ततो भिषक् ।।३८९ ।।

Method of Karṇa Pūraṇa

The patient, first of all should lie down in his side and fomentation should be applied to his ears. Thereafter, his ears should be filled with urine, oil, ghee, etc., and juice when these are luke-warm.

स्वस्थस्य पूरितं रक्षेन्मात्रा शतमवेदने ।
शतत्रयं श्रोत्रगदे शिरोरोगे तथैव च ।।३९०।।

।। प्रयोगपारिजाते[२१३] कर्णपूरणमात्रा ।।

According to Prayoga Pārijāta, Time of Karṇa Pūraṇa

In a healthy person, the liquid, after filling up in the ear, should be retained in it for one hundred *mātrā-s* or till the person does not feel any pain in the ear. In a patient suffering from ear diseases and head-diseases, the liquid after filling up into the ear should be retained in it for three hundred *mātrā-s*.

Thus, ends the description of the time of *karṇa pūraṇa* according to *Prayoga pārijāta*.

रंगमातां कंसमितां पलाश-बदरीभवाम् ।
कुट्टयित्वा जलद्रोणे दत्वा[214] लोध्रसुचूर्णितम् ।।३९१।।
कुडवं शुक्तिमात्रां च स्वर्जिकां तत्र निक्षिपेत् ।
किञ्चिच्च बदरीपत्रं दत्वा क्वाथं प्रकल्पयेत् ।
पादावशेषं च जलं ग्राहयेदुक्तकर्मणि ।।३९२।।

।। लाक्षारसग्रहणम् ।।

Preparation of Lākṣā Rasa (Lac-Water)

Lac growing in the trees of *palāśa* and *badarī* trees should be collected. One *kaṃsa* of this lac should be pounded, added with one *droṇa* of water, one *kuḍava* of the fine powder of *lodhra* and one *śukti* of *svarji kṣāra*. Thereafter, some leaves of *badarī* should be added to it and a decoction of the whole thing should be prepared [by boiling] till one fourth of the liquid remains. This decoction (called *Lākṣā rasa*) should be used in therapeutics.

Thus, ends the description of *Lākṣā rasa*.

घृततैलावलेहादीनेकाह्नी नैव साधयेत् ।
उषितास्तु प्रकुर्वन्ति विशेषेण गुणान्बहून ।।३९३।।

Duration of Cooking Medicated Ghee, etc.

Medicated ghee, medicated oil and medicines in linctus form should not be cooked just in one day. If these preparations are slowly cooked for several days, then they become therapeutically more effective.

आत्रेयः
पक्षे सिद्ध्यति तैलं च सप्ताहात्सिद्ध्यति घृतम् ।
कषायं प्रहरेणापि यत्नेनैवं[215] प्रसाधयेत् ।।३९४।।

According to Ātreya

Medicated oil becomes more effective if the cooking is completed in 15 days. Similarly, cooking of medicated ghee should be completed in seven days to obtain the prescribed effects. A decoction should be prepared by cooking for one *prahara* (four hours).

शौनकः

प्रसारण्यादि[२१६]निर्दिष्टं शतमेकं पृथक् पृथक् ।
जलद्रोणेन चैकैकं साधयेच्छुष्ककुट्टितम् ।।३९५।।
सम्यग्वीर्यं न मुञ्चति वारिस्वल्पेन निश्चितम् ।
व्रीहिप्राण्यंगयोः क्वाथं व्युषितं[२१७] दोषलं मतम् ।।३९६।।

According to Śaunaka

For the preparation of *Prasāraṇyādi taila*, each of the hundreds of ingredients of this recipe should be dried and pounded, and cooked by adding one *droṇa* of water separately for the preparation of decoction. If less of water is used, then the essence of these drugs does not come into the decoctions. In the case of cereals and animal products, preparation of the decoction should be finished on the same day. If this process continues for the next day, then it becomes stale and harmful.

वृद्धसुश्रुतात्[२१८], आत्रेयात्

व्रीहिश्यामाकनीवारादयो न तु माषादयः ।।३९७।।

उक्तं च

माषयूषं पर्युषितं तैलपाके प्रयोजयेत् ।
अम्लत्वात्स्वप्रभावाच्च वातपीडां जयेद् ध्रुवम् ।।३९८।।

According to Vṛddha Suśruta and Ātreya

In the above text, the term *vrīhi* (cereal) refers to *śyāmāka, nīvāra*, etc., and not to *māṣa*. It is said "The decoction of *māṣa* should be kept over night and when stale, it is to be used in the cooking of medicated oil. By doing so, the decoction becomes sour and the potency of the drug increases. This helps in alleviating pain caused by aggravated *vāyu*."

तैलाच्चतुर्गुणक्वाथ्यं धान्यं क्वाथ्यार्धमेव च[२१९] ।
धान्यार्धमामिषं प्रोक्तं पारंपर्योपदेशतः ।।३९९।।

Ratio

For preparing a medicated oil, according to tradition, oil should be one part, ingredients for the preparation of decoction should be four parts, cereals should be two parts and animal products should be one part.

'भद्रशौनकः[२२०]

स्नेहः सिद्धयति शुद्धाम्बुनिःक्वाथस्वरसैः क्रमात्'।
कल्कस्य योजयेदंशं चतुर्थषष्ठमाष्टमम् ॥४००॥

According to Bhadra Śaunaka

If a medicated oil is to be prepared by adding either water or decoction or juice, the quantities of the paste (of drugs) should be one fourth, one sixth and one eighth respectively.

अग्निवेशः

स्नेहपादः स्मृतः कल्कः कल्कवन्मधुशर्करा ॥४०१॥

॥प्रसिद्धः[२२१]॥

According to Agniveśa

The quantity of paste (of drugs) [in a recipe of medicated oil] should be one fourth of the quantity of oil. The quantities of honey and sugar should be similar to that of the paste. This rule is popularly followed.

शणस्य कोविदारस्य वृषस्य ककुभस्य च ।
पुष्पाढ्यत्वात्प्रशंसन्ति पुष्पकल्के चतुर्गुणम् ॥४०२॥

If a recipe of medicated oil is described to be prepared by adding, *śaṇa, kovidāra, vāsaka* or *arjuna*, then while preparing this recipe four times of water should be added because the above mentioned plants have more of flowers.

शिवमेखला

पुष्पकल्कस्य यः स्नेहः तत्र तोयं[२२२] चतुर्गुणम् ।
कल्कः स्नेहाष्टमांशः स्यादिति सर्वत्र निश्चितम् ॥४०३॥

According to Śivamekhalā

If a medicated oil or ghee is to be prepared with the paste of flowers, then in such a recipe four times of water should be added and the paste (of flowers) should invariably be added in one eighth of the fat.

यतः क्वाथस्ततः कल्कः केवलं क्वाथभाषिते ।
क्वाथ्याच्चतुर्गुणं[२२३] वारि स्नेहात्क्वाथ्यं चतुर्गुणम् ।
क्षीरं स्नेहसमं दद्यात् कल्कश्च[२२४] स्नेहपादिकः ॥४०४॥

If in a recipe of medicated ghee, ingredients for the decoction only are described [and those of paste are not described], then the paste should be prepared of the very ingredients described for decoction.

Ingredients for decoction (*kvāthya*) should be boiled by adding four times of water, [reduced to one fourth and strained to obtain the decoction]. For a medicated oil, these ingredients should be four parts, oil should be one part, milk should be one part and paste should be one fourth of the oil in quantity.

द्रवेण केवलेनैव स्नेहपाके भवेद् यदि ।
तत्राम्बुपिष्टः कल्कः स्याज्जलं चापि चतुर्गुणम् ॥४०५॥

If a medicated oil is described to be prepared only with liquids (water), then four times of water should be added to the recipe and the paste should be prepared by triturating ingredients with water.

कषायात्कल्पयेत्कल्कं कल्कात्क्वाथं न कल्पयेत्[२२५] ॥४०६॥

For a medicated oil, ingredients described for decoction should be used for the preparation of the paste (if such ingredients are not specified). But the ingredients specifically described for the preparation of paste cannot be used for preparing the decoction.

तदाह कृष्णात्रेयः
'अनिर्दिष्टकल्पनं[२२६] भैषज्यं कल्कं कुर्यादिति यदि विशेषनिर्देशो भवति तदोभयं कल्प्यते' ॥४०७॥

According to Kṛṣṇātreya

If in a recipe of medicated oil, ingredients described are not specified with reference to their use as decoction or paste but use of paste (*kalka*) is mentioned, then such ingredients may be used both for decoction and paste.

तदाह
सर्पिर्गुडूचीवृषकण्टकारीक्वाथेन कल्केन च सिद्धमेतत् ।
पेयं पुराणज्वरकासशूलश्वासाग्निमान्द्यग्रहणीगदेषु ।।४०८।।
न तु सर्वत्र ।।४०९।।

For Example

The medicated ghee prepared of the decoction and the paste of *guḍūcī*, *vāsaka* and *kaṇṭakārī* should be administered internally which cures chronic fever, bronchitis, colic pain, asthma, *agnimāndya* (suppression of the power of digestion) and *grahaṇī* (sprue syndrome). In this recipe, the ingredients described for decoction can be used for the preparation of paste. But this rule does not hold good always.

यत्राधिकरणेनोक्तिर्गणे स्यात्स्नेहसंविधौ ।
तत्रैव कल्कनिर्यूहाविष्येते स्नेहवादिभिः ।।४१०।।

When a medicated oil is described to be prepared with a group (*gaṇa*) of drugs, then the drugs of this group are to be used both for decoction and paste while preparing the oil.

गुग्गुलुप्रचुरे गर्भे चार्धसिद्धेऽवतारिते ।
कल्कं त्यक्त्वा पुनः पाच्यं सारः स्नेहे प्रतिष्ठति ।
अन्यथा च[227] भवेद्धानिः स्नेहे वीर्य[228] ध्रुवं वचः ।।४११।।

Use of Guggulu

In a recipe of medicated oil, if large quantity of *guggulu* is prescribed to be added then by adding this *guggulu*, the oil should be boiled till it becomes half-cooked. Thereafter, the paste should be strained out and the oil should be cooked again. In this way, the essence of *guggulu* is retained in the medicated oil. Otherwise [if the oil is cooked by keeping the whole amount of *guggulu* till the end], the potency (therapeutic utility) of the medicated oil is lost.

क्षीराढके स्नेहसमं पचेन्मन्देन वह्निना ।
फेनोद्गमोऽस्य निष्पत्तिर्नष्टदुग्धसमाकृतिः ।
स एव तस्य पाकस्य पाको नेतरलक्षणः ।।४१२।।

।। क्षीरपाक।।

Kṣīrapāka

One *āḍhaka* of milk should be cooked with equal quantity of oil over mild fire so that foam does not arise. If there is foam, then the recipe is to be treated as spoiled milk. This is the only way of cooking oil with milk.

Thus, ends the description of cooking oil with milk.

दध्नि क्षीरे च रुधिरे ह्यारनालेऽथ पुष्पजे ।
रसे तथेक्षुधात्रीणां मधुमस्त्वासवादिकान् ।।४१३।।
एतानि सर्ववस्तूनि स्नेहयोगे विशेषतः ।
सम्यग्वीर्यं न मुञ्चन्ति जलं देयं चतुर्गुणम् ।।४१४।।

Curd, milk, blood, *āranāla* (vinegar), juice of flower, sugarcane and *āmalakī*, honey, *mastu* (butter-milk), *āsava* (fermented liquid), etc. — all these ingredients do not appropriately release their potencies specially when mixed with oil, ghee, etc. Therefore, when such ingredients are included in a recipe of medicated oil, it should be cooked by adding four times of water [which will help in making the product therapeutically effective].

घृततैलवसामज्जामांसास्रलशुनादिकैः ।
द्वात्रिंशत्पलिकैः प्रस्थं भवेद्वाग्भटसंमतम् ।।४१५।।

Prastha

According to Vāgbhaṭa, in respect of ghee, oil, muscle fat (*vasā*), bone-marrow, meat, blood, *laśuna*, etc., thirty two *pala-s* constitute one *prastha*.

व्रीहिधान्यं तथोत्सेधं यथा विकसितं भवेत् ।।४१६।।

Vrihi dhānya-s (cereals), while getting boiled, become swollen and their volume increases. Thus, a large size vessel should be used for their cooking.

चरकः

जलस्नेहौषधानां च प्रमाणं यत्र नोदितम् ।
तत्र स्यादौषधात्स्नेहः स्नेहात्तोयं चतुर्गुणम् ।।४१७।।
[चरकः कल्पस्थान १२:१०१]

According to Caraka

If in a recipe of medicated oil, the proportion of water, oil and drugs are not specified, then one part of the drugs, four parts of oil and sixteen parts of water should be used for making the preparation.

स्नेहाच्चतुर्गुणं द्रव्यमादाय स्नेहसंविधौ ।
चतुर्गुणं जलं दत्वा क्वाथः क्वाथ्यः समो मतः ।।४१८।।

Preparation of Decoction

For the preparation of a medicated oil, ingredients for decoction should be taken four times of the quantity of oil. To these ingredients, four times of water should be added, boiled and reduced to one fourth. Thus, the quantity of decoction should be the same as that of the drugs.

स्नेहाच्चतुर्गुणं क्वाथ्यं क्वाथ्यात्तोयं चतुर्गुणम् ।
क्वाथः क्वाथ्यसमः कार्यः कल्कश्च स्नेहपादिकः ।
इत्येषा स्नेहपाकार्थं प्रोक्ता क्वाथस्य कल्पना ।।४१९।।

In brief, drugs for decoction should be four times of oil; water should be four times of these drugs; the decoction, thus obtained, should be equal to the drugs [because after boiling, the water is reduced to one fourth] and the paste should be one fourth of the oil. This is how a decoction should be prepared for cooking a medicated oil.

अग्निवेशः

शकृन्मांसरसं चैव मूत्रं सौवीरकादिकम् ।
स्नेहतुल्यं दधिक्षीरं जलं चापि चतुर्गुणम् ।।४२०।।

According to Agniveśa

Juice of stool, meat soup, urine, *sauvīra* (vinegar), etc., should be taken in the same quantity as that of oil. Curd, milk and water should be four times of the quantity of oil in preparing medicated oil.

वज्रोदकेन यत्रैव स्नेहपाकः प्रजायते ।
स्नेहादष्टगुणं देयं जलं च द्विगुणं क्षिपेत् ।।४२१।।

If a medicated oil is to be prepared with *vajrodaka*, then the latter should be eight times of oil and water should be double in quantity of the oil.

पञ्चप्रभृति यत्र स्युर्द्रवाणि स्नेहसंविधौ ।
तत्र स्नेहसमान्याहुरर्वाक् तस्माच्चतुर्गुणम् ।।४२२।।
अस्यामर्थः, यत्रैको द्रवस्तत्रैकेन चातुर्गुण्यम् ।
द्वाभ्यामपि चातुर्गुण्यं त्रिभिरपि चातुर्गुण्यमिति ।।४२३।।

If in the recipe of medicated oil or ghee, five or more liquids are included, then each one of these liquids should be equal to the oil or ghee. If these liquids are four or less than four in number, then each one of these liquids should be four times of the oil or ghee. By implication, if there is only one liquid it should be four times; if there are two liquids each one of these should be four times; and if there are three liquids then each one of these should also be four times of the oil in quantity.

तत्र जैज्जटः[२२९]
'यत्र द्वित्रिद्रवैर्द्रव्यैः कुर्यात्स्नेहाच्चतुर्गुणम् ।
क्षीरं स्नेहसमं दद्याच्चतुर्भिश्च चतुर्गुणम् ।।४२४।।
यत्र द्रवान्तरेषूक्तं क्षीरमेव'[२३०] चतुर्गुणम् ।
द्रवान्तरेण योगो हि चतुर्गुणमितो भवेत् ।।४२५।।

According to Jaijjaṭa

In a recipe of medicated oil, if two or three liquids are described then each one of these liquids should be four times of the oil. If milk is one of these liquids, then it should be equal to oil in quantity. If, however, four liquids are described then each one of these should be four times of the oil. If along with other liquids milk is described to be added in the quantity of four times, then this should be interpreted that milk and the other liquids taken together should be four times of the oil.

गन्धाम्बुचन्दनाम्बुभ्यां पृथक् पाको विधीयते ।
अर्धावशेषः[२३१] कर्त्तव्यः पाको गन्धाम्बुकर्मणि ।
सौगन्धार्थे प्रदातव्यमर्द्धसिद्धे भिषक्तमः ॥४२६॥

Aromatic Liquids

If in a recipe of medicated oil, aromatic liquids or sandal wood water is mentioned to be added, then such liquids or decoctions should be prepared differently by adding water to these drugs, boiling and reducing to half [not one fourth] only. For the purpose of aroma, these liquids should be added to the recipe while, it is half-cooked.

मुहुर्मुहुर्वस्त्रपूतं कृत्वा पाकं प्रकल्पयेत् ।
पुष्पाणि गन्धनिर्यासः सिद्धे शीतेऽवतारिते ॥४२७॥
प्रयोज्यं गंधवृद्ध्यर्थं यत्र कल्कं प्रयुज्यते ।
'चन्द्रकस्तूरिकादीनां[२३२] सहस्रांशं प्रयोजयेत् ॥४२८॥
शालूकपत्नी काश्मीरं कपितैलादिकं[२३३] तथा' ।
शतांशं योजयेत्तत्र तैलेन परिभाषितम् ॥४२९॥

If the aromatic flowers or aromatic exudates are to be added to a preparation of medicated oil, then these, in liquid (decoction or infusion) form should be strained through a cloth repeatedly and added to the medicated oil after it is cooked, taken out of the oven and cooled.

Addition of Camphor and Musk

Camphor and musk should be added in paste form to the medicated oil in 1/1000th part (of the prepared oil). The paste of *śālūka patnī*, saffron, *kapi taila (śilā rasa)*, etc., should be added to the medicated oil $^{1}/_{100}$th in quantity of the prepared oil.

[पाककर्म]
घृतस्य फेनोपशमस्तैलस्य च तदुद्भवः ॥४३०॥

Signs of Proper Cooking of Medicated Oil, etc.

When a medicated ghee is properly cooked, at the end, foam (bubbles) will arise. On the other hand, when a medicated oil is properly cooked, at the end, the foam will disappear.

स्नेहपाकस्तथा मन्दचिक्कणः खरचिक्कणः ।
मंदः किट्टसमः कल्के मर्दिते महनोपमः ।
वरं पाके मृदुः कार्यो द्रव्यस्य न खरो मतः ।
किञ्चित्सवीर्यमादत्ते तज्जहाति खरः सदा ।।४३१।।

Varieties of Cooking

Cooking of medicated oil or ghee is of [two types, viz.,] *manda-cikkaṇa* and *khara-cikkaṇa*. In the former type, when the paste is rubbed between two fingers it feels like a waste product or wax [i.e. soft and sticky]. Between these two types, *manda* or *mṛdu pāka* is better than the *khara pāka* because in the former, therapeutic potency is retained into some extent whereas the latter is therapeutically useless.

ईषत्सरसकल्कस्तु स्नेहपाके मृदुर्भवेत् ।
मध्यपाकस्तु सिक्थाभः कल्के नीरसकोमले ।
किञ्चित्सिध्यति कृष्णश्च निर्गन्धश्च खरो मतः ।।४३२।।

The other types of cooking are three viz., *mṛdu*, *madhya* and *khara*. In *mṛdu pāka* or mild cooking, the paste contains certain amount of water. In *madhyama pāka* or moderate cooking, the paste feels like wax and it is free from water and soft. When the paste becomes black and free from any smell, it is called *khara pāka* (over cooking). Such type of medicated oil is therapeutically useless.

मृदुर्नस्ये[२३४] खरोऽभ्यंगे पाने बस्तौ च मध्यमः ।।४३३।।

Medicated oil of *mṛdu pāka* (mild cooking) is useful for *nasya* (inhalation therapy); the one of *khara pāka* (over cooking) is useful for massage; and the one *of madhyama pāka* (moderate cooking) is useful for *pāna* (taking internally) and *basti* (medicated enema).

सर्वेषामेव पाकानां मध्यपाकः प्रशस्यते ।।४३४।।

Among all the different types of *pāka*, *madhyama pāka* (moderate cooking) is therapeutically more useful.

स्नेहकल्को यदाङ्गुल्या वर्त्तितो वर्त्तिवद्भवेत् ।
शब्दहीनोऽग्निनिःक्षिप्तस्तदा पाकोत्तमोत्तमः ।।४३५।।

Test

When the paste from the recipe is rolled between two fingers and it becomes like a *vartti* (elongated pill), and if this paste is placed over fire and no cracking sound is produced, then it should be treated as properly cooked.

"तन्त्रान्तरे[१३५]

सद्गन्धिसद्वर्णा विभक्तमाद्यं, यत्कल्कमग्नौ न करोति शब्दम् ।
निष्फेननिःशब्दवदेवं भूतं वर्त्तित्वमायाति च पक्वलिङ्गम् ।।४३६ ।।

।। इति रूपायनात् ।।

According to Another Text Called Rūpāyana

The signs of proper cooking are as follows :

(1) Appearance of proper smell;
(2) Appearance of proper colour;
(3) Separation of the paste from the oil;
(4) There is no cracking sound when the paste is placed over fire.
(5) Absence of foam and bubbling sound; and
(6) The paste when rolled between two fingers becomes like a *vartti* (elongated pill).

विघ्नेशं क्षेत्रपालौ वटुकमपि शुभे वासरे पूजयित्वा ।
तैलस्याज्यस्य किंवा रचयतु निपुणः संस्कृतिसंप्रदायात् ।।४३७।।

Rituals

After offering prayer to Gaṇeśa, two *Kṣetrapāla-s* and *vaṭuka*, in an auspicious day, the expert physician should start cooking a medicated oil or medicated ghee according to traditional method.

आदौ वह्निं प्रदद्याद्यदवधि शनैः फेनशब्दव्ययः स्यात् ।
पश्चान्मृत्पिण्डकैस्तद्दशभिरलघुभिः नातिपानं विशोध्यम् ।।४३८।।

एकं संस्थाप्य यन्त्रं विधिवदथ पचेद्वासरादग्निभाच्च ।
क्वाथैः कल्कैः पयोभिस्तदनुसुरभिशोधनीयैश्च शोध्यम् ।।४३९ ।।
कस्तूरीचण्डनलो जलजलदशटीरपुष्पत्वङ्मंजिष्ठा ।
तुरुष्कागुरुनखजलदकंकोलमुख्यैः सारसंग्रहः ।।४४० ।।

In the beginning, fire should be given below the oil-containing-pan slowly till the foam and bubbling noise subsides. Thereafter, 10 hot and heavy bolus made of mud should be immersed into the oil for purification. Then the oil pan should be appropriately placed over the oven and cooked by adding decoctions, pastes, milk or water. Thereafter, aromatic and purifying drugs should be added to the oil. These aromatic drugs are *kastūrī*, *caṇda*, *nala*, *jala* (*hrībera*), *jalada* (*mustā*), *śaṭhīra*, flower, *tvak*, *mañjiṣṭhā*, *turuṣka*, *aguru*, *nakha*, *jalada* (?) and *kaṅkola* in brief.

तैलं कृत्वा कटाहे दृढतरविले मन्द-मन्दानलैस्तत् ।
पक्वं निष्फेनभावं गतमिह हि यदा शैत्यभावं ततस्तु ।।४४१ ।।
मंजिष्ठारात्रिलोध्रैर्जलधरनलकैः सामलैः साक्षपथ्यैः ।
सूचीपुष्पांघ्रिनीरैरुपहितमथितैस्तैलगंधं जहाति ।।४४२ ।।

Oil should be kept in a strong and clean pan and cooked with mild fire. When the foam disappears and the oil becomes cool, then the paste or decoction of *mañjiṣṭhā*, *haridrā*, *lodhra*, *mustā*, *nalaka*, *āmalakī*, *bibhītaka*, *harītaka* and the root of *sūcīpuṣpa* should be added and stirred which imparts aroma to the oil.

तैलस्य तु कलां एकैकविकसां भागस्तु तस्यांशकः ।
ये चान्येन्दीवरी पयोदरजनीह्रीबेररोध्रान्विता" ।।४४३ ।।

Similarly, other aromatic drugs like *indīvara, payoda, haridrā, hrībera* and *rodhra* should be added in the quantity of 1/16th part of the oil.

[Note: There are many mistakes in the paragraph nos. 438-443.]

येनैव विधिना तैलं घृतं तेनैव साधयेत् ।।४४४ ।।

।। इति स्नेहपाकविधिः[२३६] ।।

The method prescribed for cooking a medicated oil should be followed for preparing a medicated ghee.

Thus, ends the description of cooking medicated oil or medicated ghee.

अथ रसकरणम् (MERCURY)

रसार्णवात्

उत्तरायणगते सूर्ये रसकर्मारभेद्बुधः ।
शुभेऽह्नि शुभनक्षत्रे ताराचन्द्रवले तथा ।।४४५।।

Processing of Mercury
According to Rasārṇava

A wise physician should start processing mercury during *uttarāyaṇa* (northern solstice) on an auspicious day having an auspicious constellation where the stars and moon are powerful.

पञ्चाशत् पञ्चविंश वा दशपञ्चैकमेव वा[२३७] ।
पलादूनं न कर्त्तव्यं रससंस्कारमुत्तमम् ।।४४६।।

Quantity of Mercury

For processing, the physician should take 50 or 25 or 10 or 5 or 1 *pala-s* of mercury. The quantity of mercury should never be less than one *pala* for the purpose of proper processing.

अथ रसावतारे

सूतार्कतालाम्बुभवत्रपुरंगशिलावलीनामिह शोधने तु ।
या षट्पली वा द्विपली चतुष्पली मात्रोत्तमा
स्यादधमापिमध्यमा ।।४४७।।
तस्यार्द्धभागः[२३८] सितरुक्मपोरतोवैक्रांतमुक्ताफलशोधनेषु ।
लोहादिकानां द्विगुणाः क्रमात्तु हीनाधिकश्चेद्गुणदात्र न भवेत् ।
व्योमस्य मात्रा रसवत्प्रदिष्टा किंचित्तथा वज्ररसोनिकादिषु ।।४४८।।

According to Rasāvatāra

Mercury, copper, realgar, mica, lead, tin, orpiment and sulphur, for the purpose of *śodhana* (processing), should be either six *pala-s*, two *pala-s* or four *pala-s* which constitute *uttama* (excellent), *adhama* (inferior) and *madhyama* (moderate) in quantity respectively.

Silver, gold, *pora*, *vaikrānta* and *muktā* (pearl) should be taken half of the above mentioned quantity for the purpose of purification. Iron, etc., should, however, be taken double the above mentioned quantity for purification. More or less of this prescribed quantity does not produce the prescribed therapeutic effects. Mica should be taken in the quantity prescribed for mercury. Diamond, *rasonikā* etc., may, however, be taken in small quantity for purification.

अथ नागार्जुनात्

नाधः पञ्चपलात् त्रयोदशपलादूर्ध्वं न लोहं पचेत् ।
तत्राद्यः[२३९] पलपञ्चकस्य पचने निर्वापनादिक्रमे ।।४४९ ।।
उद्दिश्य त्रिफलापलानि शनकै [?] र्निःक्वाथयेत्षोडश ।
प्रक्षिप्याष्टगुणं जलं परिमितं पादेन तच्चोद्धरेत् ।।४५० ।।

According to Nāgārjuna

For processing, iron, etc., should not be taken in less than five *pala-s* or more than thirteen *pala-s*. For boiling and *nirvāpana* (hot-immersion) of five *pala-s* of iron, sixteen *pala-s* of *triphalā* should be boiled by adding eight times of water and reduced to one fourth.

एवं कुर्याद्रसकर्म मारणे शोधने भिषक्[४०] ।
न कर्माणि[२४१] भिषक्कुर्याद्विधिज्ञो[२४२]ऽप्यलसो भिषक् ।।४५१ ।।

Māraṇa (calcination) and *śodhana* (purification) of *rasa* (mercury and other metals) should be done by the physician in the above mentioned manner. A lazy physician, even though he knows the process, should not attempt processing mercury, etc.

अभ्रादिसर्वधातूनां भवेदौषधयोगतः ।
ध्मातश्च निर्गतः सारः सत्त्व इत्यभिधीयते ।।४५२ ।।

Sattva

All the minerals like *abhraka* (mica), when added with drugs and blown in a crucible over fire exude their essence which is called *sattva*.

धातुभिर्गन्धकाद्यैश्च निर्द्रवो मर्दितो रसः ।
सुश्लक्ष्णः कज्जलाभोऽसौ कज्जलीत्यभिधीयते ।।४५३ ।।

Kajjalī

Trituration of mercury and other minerals like sulphur, without adding any liquid, produces a collyrium-like fine powder which is called *kajjalī.*

गन्धकेन समं सूतं ऊर्ध्वमायसपात्रके ।
सजले पतितः सूतः उमायोनिरिति स्मृतः ।।४५४ ।।

Umāyoni

Sulphur and mercury taken in equal quantities should be kept in an iron plate, [covered with another iron plate, joint of these two plates should be sealed and heat should be applied from the above]. The liquefied mercury and sulphur will come down through a hole in the lower plate and collected in another vessel containing water. This is called *Umā yoni*.

कालिकारहितं शुल्वलक्षणम्
शुकचंचुहिंगुलाभं कोमलं भिद्यते[२४३] लघु ।
खानिदोषविनिर्मुक्तं शुल्वं कालिकावर्जितम्[२४४] ।।४५५ ।।

Signs of Copper Without Blackness

When copper is cleaned of the other mineral impurities which got mixed up in the mine, then it looks like *śuka cañcu hiṅgula* (cinnabar having the colour of parrot's beak). This type of copper is soft, breakable, light and free from blackness (*kālikā*).

मृतस्य पुनरुद्भूतिस्तप्तोत्थोत्थापनक्रिया ।
द्रुतद्रव्यस्य निक्षेपो द्रवे तत्क्षालनं मतम् ।।४५६ ।।

Utthāpana & Kṣālana

When a calcined powder is [added with drugs and] heated, it comes back to its original metallic form. This process is called *utthāpana* (retrieval). When a melted material is poured into another liquid, the process is called *kṣālana* (washing).

रसांकुशात्
वह्नितापितलोहानामौषधीभिः सुसाधिते ।
सलिले तु परिक्षेपः सोऽभिषेक इति स्मृतः ।।४५७।।

Abhiṣeka : According to Rasāṅkuśa

When heated metals are immersed into the decoction of drugs, the process is called *abhiṣeka* (immersion).

विष्टां भूनागसंभूतां प्रक्षाल्य बहुभिर्जलैः ।
समाहृत्य रजः कृत्स्नं धौतमित्यभिधीयते ।।४५८।।

Dhauta

When the faeces of earth-worm is washed with a lot of water and the sand particles of this stool are collected, this is called *dhauta* (cleaning).

रत्नाकरात्
मूलिकामारितः सूतो जारणः क्रमवर्जितः ।
न क्रमेद्देहलोहाभ्यां रोगहर्त्ता प्रजायते ।।४५९।।

According to Ratnākara

If the *bhasma* (calcined powder) of mercury is prepared with the help of herbal roots, etc., then this does not help in the transmutation of metals and the body. It, however, helps in curing diseases.

स्वच्छन्दात्
गुञ्जैकमात्रं तु नरस्य भुज्यते गद्याणकं प्रोत्तमं वाजिपुङ्गवे ।
गद्याणसार्धं करिपुङ्गवेषु देयं सदा व्याध्यनुपानयोगात् ।।४६०।।

According to Svacchanda

The dose of mercury *bhasma* is one *guñjā* for human beings, one *gadyāṇaka* for horses, and one and half *gadyāṇaka* for elephants. Mercury *bhasma* should always be administered along with *anupāna* (vehicle) appropriate for the disease.

रसार्णवात्
"गुञ्जमात्रं रसं देवि! हेमजीर्णं तु भक्षयेत् ।

द्विगुञ्जं तारजीर्णं[245] स्याद्रविजीर्णस्य च त्रयम् ।।४६१।।
तीक्ष्णाभ्रकान्तमाक्षिकं[246] गुञ्जैकैकं च भक्षयेत्[247] ।
वज्रवैक्रान्तजीर्णं तु भक्षयेत्सर्षपोपमम्[248] ।।४६२।।

According to Rasārṇava

Mercury *bhasma* prepared by the *jāraṇa* (impregnation) of gold should be administered in the dose of one *guñjā*; the dose of mercury *bhasma* prepared by the *jāraṇa* of silver is two *guñjā-s*; the dose of mercury *bhasma* prepared by the *jāraṇa* of copper is three *guñjā-s*; the dose of mercury *bhasma* prepared by *jāraṇa* with *tīkṣṇa lauha*, mica, *kānta lauha* or *mākṣika* should be administered in the dose of one *guñjā*, and the dose of mercury *bhasma* prepared by *jāraṇa* of diamond and *vaikrānta* is one *sarṣapa* (weight of mustard seed).

नागवंगवसाविड्विषोपविषसंयुतम्[249] ।
मूत्रयुक्तं[250] हठाद्बद्धं त्यजेल्कल्कं रसायने[251] ।।४६३।।
[रसार्णव : अष्टादशपटल : ३३-३५]

If the *bhasma* of mercury is prepared by *jāraṇa*of lead, tin, fat, stool, poisons, semi-poisonous drugs or urine or from *haṭhabaddha* (solidified immediately by adding drugs) type of mercury, then such a product should not be used ~~for~~ the purpose of rejuvenation.

"हेमजीर्णे भस्मसूते त्रिपले भक्षिते क्रमात्" ।
[रसार्णव : अष्टादश पटल : ४४]
क्षयकुष्टप्रमेहार्शो ग्रहणीं च जयेत्तथा ।
ज्वरं च बहुवर्षोत्थं जयेद् दीर्घायुषं नयेत् ।।४६४।।

If the *bhasma* of mercury is prepared by the gradual *jāraṇa* of three *pala-s* of gold, then it cures tuberculosis, *kuṣṭha* (obstinate skin diseases including leprosy), *prameha* (obstinate urinary diseases including diabetes), piles and sprue syndrome. It also cures chronic fever of many years. It promotes longevity.

एवं च द्वादशपलं तीक्ष्णजीर्णं च[252] भक्षयेत् ।
"चतुष्पलं[253] शुल्वजीर्णं तारजीर्णं तथैव च" ।

वज्रवैक्रान्तजीर्णं च शुक्तिमात्रं च भक्षयेत् ।।४६५।।

Bhasma of mercury prepared by *jāraṇa* with *tīkṣṇa lauha* should be given in the quantity of twelve *pala-s* [in total]. *Bhasma* of mercury prepared by *jāraṇa* with copper or silver should be given in the quantity of four *pala-s* [in total]. *Bhasma* of mercury prepared by *jāraṇa* with diamond or *vaikrānta* should be given in the quantity of one *śukti* [in total].

गुञ्जैकमात्रं देवेशि! ज्ञात्वा चाग्निबलं निजम् ।
घृतेन मधुना सार्धं ताम्बूलं कामिनीं त्यजेत् ।।४६६।।

Bhasma of mercury should be administered in the dose of one *guñjā* on the basis of the power of digestion of the patient. This should be given mixed with honey and the patient while taking this should avoid *tāmbūla* (betel-leaf) and sexual intercourse with woman.

दिनमेकान्तरं कृत्वा निर्विषं योजयेद्रसम् ।
दिनद्वयमतिक्रम्य सविषं योजयेद्रसम् ।।४६७।।

Bhasma of mercury prepared without adding poisonous drugs should be administered on alternate day. If prepared by adding poisonous drugs, then the *bhasma* of mercury should be administered leaving a gap of two days.

विष [POISONS]

रसदर्पणात्
अङ्गवङ्गकलिङ्गे च कार्नाटे[५४] चोरमण्डले ।
सेवने चांध्रदेशे च मात्रार्धं निक्षिपेद्विषम् ।।४६८।।
म्लेच्छदेशे च गौडे च हैमाले नारिमण्डले[५५] ।
यावत्मात्रा रसं प्रोक्ता संपूर्णं निक्षिपेद्विषम् ।।४६९।।

According to Rasadarpaṇa

For the patients of Aṅga, Vaṅga, Kaliṅga, Karnāṭa, Cora and Āndhra, poisonous drugs in the *bhasma* of mercury should be added in half of the prescribed quantity. For the patients of Mleccha country, Gauḍa, Himalaya and N(K)āri, poisonous drugs in the *bhasma* of mercury should be added in full quanity as prescribed.

नैपाले चित्रकूटे च सौराष्ट्रे सिन्धुमण्डले ।
मरुमायापुरे चैव चतुर्थांशं क्षिपेद्विषम् ।।४७० ।।
यथादेशं यथाकालं तथामात्रं क्षिपेद्विषम्[२५६] ।
'एकमात्रां[२५७] न कुर्वीत देशकालविभागतः' ।
देहस्तु विविधो भूमिभेदत्वात्तद् विचार्य च ।।४७१ ।।

For the patients of Nepāla, Citrakūṭa, Saurāṣṭra, Sindhu and Māyāpura (which is a desert), the poisonous drugs should be added in the *bhasma* of mercury in one fourth of the prescribed quantity. Depending upon the nature of the country and the time (season), poisonous drugs should be added in different proportions. Same quantity of poisonous drugs should not be added in different countries and seasons because the body of the patient is different in different countreis and it should be kept in view.

प्रथमं भक्षयेद्रोगी विषं सर्षपमात्रकम् ।
नीलकंठेन. मंत्रेण अमर्षायाभिमंत्रितम् ।।४७२ ।।
द्विसर्षपं द्वितीयेऽह्नि तृतीये सर्षपत्रयम् ।
चतुर्थे पञ्चमे षष्ठे सप्तमे च तथाक्रमः ।
सप्तसर्षपमात्रेण प्रथमे सप्तके[२५८] भवेत् ।।४७३ ।।
एवं क्रमेण विज्ञेयं द्वितीये सप्तके[२५९] विषम् ।
यवमात्रं विषं ज्ञेयं तृतीये सप्तके क्रमात् ।।४७४ ।।

Gradual Increase of Dose

To start with, on the first day the patient should take the poisonous drug in the dose of one *sarṣapa* (weight of a mustard seed) which is impregnated with the *Amarṣa mantra* of Lord Śiva. On the second day, the dose should be two *sarṣapa-s*; on the third day the dose should be three *sarṣapa-s* and on the fourth, fifth and sixth days the dose should be four, five and six *sarṣapa-s* respectively. Thus on the seventh day, the dose should be seven *sarṣapa-s*. During the second week, the drug should be continued in the dose of seven *sarṣapa-s*. During the third week, the dose of poison should be one *yava* (weight of a barley grain) each day.

यवमात्रं ग्रसेत्स्वस्थो गुञ्जमात्रं तु कुष्ठिनः ।
तथोदरी माषमात्रं वीक्ष्य देहबलाबलम् ।।४७५।।

Dosage for Different Diseases

A healthy person, [for the promotion of positive health and prevention of diseases], should take the drug (having poisonous ingredients) in the dose of one *yava* (weight of a barley grain). A patient suffering from *kuṣṭha* (obstinate skin diseases including leprosy) should take such a drug in the dose of one *guñjā*. Similarly, the patient suffering from *udara* (obstinate abdominal diseases including ascites) should take it in the dose of one *māṣa* keeping in view his strength ot' 'rwise.

उदरादिषु विप्रं च क्षत्रियं रसशोधने ।
सन्निपाते प्रदेयं च सर्पदष्टे च शूद्रकम् ।।४७६।।
तैलपाकेऽपि शूद्रं स्याद्वैश्यं[२६०] सर्वगदेषु च ।
ग्रन्थिलेपे प्रदेयं च काकचण्डेश्वरोदितम् ।।४७७।।

According to Kākacaṇḍeśvara
Varieties of Poison

In *udara roga* (obstinate abdominal diseases including ascites, etc.,) *brāhmaṇa* type of poison is useful; for the purification of mercury, *kṣatriya* type of poison is useful; in *sannipāta* and snake bite *śūdra* type of poison is useful; in *taila pāka*, *śūdra* type of poison is also useful and in all the diseases specially for application over the glands, *vaiśya* type of poison is useful. This is described in *Kākacaṇḍeśvara tantra*.

ब्राह्मणः पाण्डुरो ज्ञेयः क्षत्रियो रक्तवर्णकः ।
वैश्यः पीतप्रभः शूद्रः कृष्णाभो बिन्दुभेदतः ।।४७८।।

Colour of Different Types of Poison

Brāhmaṇa type of poison is pale yellow in colour; *kṣatriya* type is red in colour; *vaiśya* type is yellow in colour; and *śūdra* type is black in colour and spotted with drops.

न दातव्यं न भोक्तव्यं विषं वादे कदाचन ।
आत्मना चैव भोक्तव्यं शिष्यप्रत्ययकारणात्[२६] ।।४७९।।

For the purpose of competition, poison should neither be given to others nor taken by oneself. Only to convince and demonstrate to the students, the physician may take the poison himself.

दातव्यं सर्वरोगेषु हिताशिनी घृताशिनी ।
क्षीराशिने प्रयोक्तव्यं रसायनरतेषु च ।।४८०।।

Poison may be administered for all types of diseases; but the patient should take wholesome food added with ghee and milk. It can also be given to persons interested in *rasāyana* (rejuvenation therapy).

न क्रोधिते पिपासार्ते न क्लीबे राजयक्ष्मसु ।
क्षुत्तृष्णाश्रमघर्माध्वसेविने क्षीणरोगिणे ।
गर्भिणीबालवृद्धेषु न विषं राजमन्दिरे ।।४८१।।

।। रसरत्नाकरात् ।।

।।इति विषपरिभाषा ।।

According to Rasaratnākara
Contra-indications

Poison should not be administered to a wrathful patient and to one sufffering from morbid thirst, impotency and tuberculosis. Similarly poison should not be given to persons with hunger, thirst, fatigue, exposure to sun, exposure to long walk and emaciation. It should not be given to a pregnant woman, to infants, to old people and to inmates of royal palace.

Thus, ends the description of *viṣa* (poisons).

अभावे द्रव्यग्रहणम् [SUBSTITUTES]

अग्निवेशात्

न हि सर्वमनुष्याणां सन्ति सर्वपरिच्छदाः ।
न हि रोगाः न सेवन्ते दरिद्रमतिदारुणाः ।।४८२।।

यद्यच्छक्यं मनुष्येण कर्तुमौषधमापदि ।
तत्तत्सेव्यं यथाशक्तिर्भेषजान्यशनानि च ।।४८३।।

According to Agniveśa

All the persons are not endowed with all the requirements of life and poor people are not spared of the suffering from serious diseases. Therefore, in the event of misfortunate, whatever medicament and diet are procurable by the person should be appropriately used.

शैवालभक्षमतात्[२६२]
वज्राभावे तु वैक्रान्तं स्वर्णाभावे तु माक्षिकम्[२६३] ।।४८४।।

According to Śaivālabhakṣa

If diamond is not available, then *vaikrānta* may be used as a substitute. Similarly, in the place of gold, *mākṣika* (copper pyrite) may be used.

गोरक्षमतात्
हेममाक्षिकजं सत्त्वं मृतहेमसमं ध्रुवम् ।
विमलामाक्षिकं ज्ञेयं ध्रुवं रजतवद्गुणैः ।।४८५।।
मुक्ताभावे क्षिपेन्नित्यं मुक्ताशुक्तिं न संशयः ।
अभावेऽभ्रकसत्त्वस्य कान्तलोहं प्रयोजयेत् ।
कान्ताभावे तीक्ष्णलोहमित्युक्तं रसदर्पणे ।।४८६।।
मधु यत्र न लभ्येत[२६४] तत्र जीर्णगुडो मतः ।
सिताभावे भवेत्खण्डं शाल्यभावे च षष्टिकः ।।४८७।।
असंभवे तु द्राक्षायाः प्रदेयं काश्मरीफलम् ।
वृक्षाम्लो न भवेद्यत्र दाडिमाम्लं प्रयोजयेत् ।।४८८।।
वेतसाम्लस्य चाभावे हरिमन्थाम्लमादिशेत् ।
मुस्ता चातिविषाभावे शिवाभावे शिवं मतम् ।।४८९।।
कुष्ठं च तगराभावे मेलयेत्संप्रदायवित् ।
अभावे चन्दनस्यापि निक्षिपेद्रक्तचन्दनम् ।।४९०।।

अभावे सति पित्तानां रसादौ भावनाविधौ ।
विषमुष्टीकषायेण षड्गुणा भावना भवेत् ।।४९१।।

Substitutes
According to Gorakṣa

The *sattva* (metallic essence) of *svarṇa mākṣika* is certainly useful like the *bhasma* of gold. *Raupya mākṣika* is similar in properties to silver. If pearl is not available, then *muktā śukti* (mother of pearl) can undoubtedly be used in its place. If the *sattva* (metallic essence) of mica is not available, the physician should use *kānta lauha*. According to *Rasadarpaṇa* if *kānta lauha* is not available, then *tīkṣṇa lauha* should be used in its place. If honey is not available then old jaggery should be used in its place. If *sitā* (purified sugar) is not available, then *khaṇḍa* (brown sugar) should be used in its place. If *śāli* type of rice is not available then *ṣaṣṭika* type of rice should be used in its place. If grape is not available, in its place, fruit of *kāśmarī* should be used. If *vṛkṣāmla* is not available, then *dāḍimāmla* may be used in its place. If *vetasāmla* is not available, then physician may use *harimanthāmla* in its place. *Mustā* may be used in the place of *ativiṣā*. In the place of *śivā*, *śiva* can be used. *Kuṣṭha* may be used in the place of *tagara* according to tradition. If white variety of sandal wood is not available, then red variety of sandal wood may be used in its place. For impregnation (*bhāvanā*), if *pitta* (bile) is not available, then six times of the decoction of *viṣamuṣṭī* can be used in its place.

वैद्यालंकारात्
मेदा-जीवक-काकोली-द्वन्द्वाभावे प्रयोजयेत् ।
यष्टी-विदार्यश्वगन्धा-बला-वाराहिकाः नवाः ।।४९२।।

According to Vaidyālaṅkāra

In the place of *medā*, *mahāmedā*, *jīvaka*, *ṛṣabhaka*, *kākolī* and *kṣira kākolī* one should use *yaṣṭī*, *vidārī*, *aśvagandhā*, *balā* and *vārāhī*. [There seems to be an error in the second line of the verse inasmuch as the name of the substitute is missing and in its place '*navāḥ*' meaning 'fresh' is used].

रसाञ्जनाभावे योज्यं द्रुमपतिकद्विगुणम् ।
भिषक् करिकणाभावे योजयेत् कुक्कुटमस्तकम् ।

भिषक् मलीमसाभावे चूलिकालवणं क्षिपेत् ।।४९३।।

In the place of *rasāñjana*, double the quantity of *drumapatika* may be used. In the place of *gaja pippalī*, the physician may use *kukkuṭa mastaka*. If *malīmasa* is not available, the physician may use *cūlikā lavaṇa* in its place.

फलमात्रमपुष्टं च त्यजेद्विल्वादृते सदा ।
द्राक्षाबिल्वशिवादीनां फलं शुष्कं गुणोत्तरम् ।।४९४।।
आदिशब्देन परूषकबिभीतकादीनाम् ।।४९५।।

Matured and Immature Fruits

Immature fruits except those of *bilva* should always be avoided. *Drākṣā*, *bilva* and *harītakī*, etc., are more useful when these fruits are dried. Similarly, the dry fruits of *parūṣaka* and *bibhītaka* are more useful.

धन्वन्तरीभागः [PHYSICIAN'S SHARE]

अर्द्धं सिद्धरसस्य तैलघृतयोर्लेहस्य भागोऽष्टमः ।
संसिद्धाखिललोहचूर्णवटकादीनां तथा सप्तमः ।।४९६।।
यो दद्याच्च भिषग्वराय सरुजा निर्दिश्य धन्वन्तरिम् ।
देहारोग्यसुखाप्तये निगदितो भागः स धन्वन्तरेः ।।४९७।।
स एवाश्विनीकुमारभागः ।।४९८।।

Dhanvantarī Bhāga

When the physician prepares a medicine for a patient, then a part of these medicines should be given by the patient to the physician free of cost. This is called *dhanvantarī bhāga*. If a medicine containing mercury and metals is prepared then half of this goes to the physician. One eighth of medicated oil, medicated ghee and *leha* (linctus) should be given to the physician. One seventh of all the preparations of *lauha* (containing iron), powders, pills, etc., should also be given to the physician. This share to the physician is determined by the sage Dhanvantari. This gift endows the patient with freedom from disease and health. This is called *Dhanvantarī bhāga* or *Aśvinīkumāra bhāga*.

रौद्रांशः[२६५]

भैषज्यक्रीतद्रव्यस्य भागश्चैकादशो हि यः ।
वणिग्भ्यो गृह्यते वैद्यैः रुद्रभागः स कथ्यते ।।४९९।।

Rudrabhāga

When a physician is deputed to purchase drugs from a business man, the latter gives 1/11th of these drugs to the physician gratis. This is called *Rudra-bhāga*.

गृहीत्वाऽधिकं रुद्रांशाद् यो समीचीतमौषधम् ।
दापयेल्लुब्धहृत्' वैद्यः स स्याद्विश्वासघातकः ।।५००।।
विश्वासघातिनां पुंसां न शुद्धिर्मरणं विना ।
शास्त्रेषु विहिता शुद्धिर्ब्रह्महत्याकृतामपि ।।५०१।।

If a physician accepts more than *Rudrāṃśa* (or *Rudra-bhāga*) while purchasing drugs for the patient, then physician commits a breach of faith. Those who commit this breach of faith never get rid of the sin without death. In scriptures, measures are prescribed to anihilate the sins of killer of brahmins but for those who commit breach of faith, there is no remedy.

बालपरिभाषा [DOSE FOR INFANTS]

बालस्य प्रथमे मासि देया भेषजरक्तिका ।
अवलेही कृता सम्यक् क्षीरक्षौद्रघृतेन वा ।।५०२।।
वर्धयेत्तावदेकैकां यावत्संवत्सरो भवेत् ।
माषवृद्धिस्तदूर्द्ध्वं स्याद्यावत्षोडशवत्सराः ।।५०३।।
एवं च स्थापयेत्तावद्यावद्वर्षाणि सप्ततिः ।
ततो बालकवन्मात्रां ह्रासनीया शनैः शनैः ।
मात्रेयं कल्कचूर्णानां कषायाणां यथाविधिः ।।५०४।।

।। इति वृद्धहारीतात् बालपरिभाषा ।।

Dosage for Infants
According to Vṛddha Hārita

During the 1st month of age, the infant should be given medicine in the dose of one *ratti*. The medicine should be mixed with either milk or honey or ghee and made to a linctus (*avaleha*) form appropriately and then administered. The dose should then be increased by one *māṣa* [every year] till the child becomes 16 year old. This dose should be maintained till the person becomes 70 year old. Thereafter, the dose of medicine should be gradually reduced like the dose of children. This dose is in respect of drugs in paste, powder and decoction forms.

पादेन वा त्रिभागेन दशांशेनाथवा रसात् ।
ताम्रचूर्णं समादाय पिष्टीं कृत्वाऽथ पातयेत् ।।५०५।।
सूताधिक्याद्यदा नैव पिष्टी साधु प्रजायते ।
तदा विनिक्षिपेत्तुत्थं संप्रदायपरायणः ।।५०६।।

।।इत्यूर्ध्वाधःपातने ताम्रमात्रा ।।

Quantity of Copper for Ūrdhva and Adhaḥ Pātana

The *bhasma* of copper should be added to mercury in 1/4th, 1/3rd or 1/10th in quantity of the latter, made to a paste form and then the recipe should be used for (*ūrdhva* or *adhaḥ*) *pātana*. If because of the excess quantity of mercury, the paste is not formed properly, then according to tradition, some quantity of copper sulphate (*tuttha*) should be added to it till the paste is formed.

रसजारण [JĀRAṆA OF MERCURY]

अथ रससाराद्रसजारणमात्रा

आदौ संजारयेद्बीजं पश्चाद्गन्धं च जारयेत् ।
रसे रसायने चापि यावद्बीजं न जारयेत् ।
तावत् वृथा द्रव्यहानिं करोति ब्रह्महा भिषक् ।।५०७।।
तप्तखल्वे रसं दत्वा खदिराङ्गारतापिते[266] ।
चतुःषष्ट्यंशकं सूताद्बीजं सूते नियोजयेत् ।।५०८।।
संधानकाम्ललवणं चूलिकालवणेन च ।
दीपनीदीपिते सूतं मर्दयेन्मर्दकेन वै ।।५०९।।

तप्तेन तु श्रमात्रं [?] च मर्दितं योजयेद्रसम् ।
उध्र्वाधश्च पिंडं दत्त्वा यन्त्रे भैरवसंज्ञके ।
विडं सूतादष्टमांशमितं पश्चाद्दिनत्रयम् ।।५१०।।
'मन्दं[२६७] सञ्चालयेदग्निं संप्रदायपरायणः' ।
चतुर्थेऽह्नि रसं प्रोष्णं कांजिके क्षालितं[२६८] पुनः ।।५११।।
पूर्ववद् दापयेद्बीजमेवं वारचतुष्टयम्[२६९] ।।५१२।।
पलांशं[२७०] जीर्येत बीजं दोलायामथ जारयेत् ।
अथवा कच्छपे यन्त्रे जारयेद्बीजमुत्तमम् ।।५१३।।
ततः[२७१] परं गन्धकंच[२७२] जारयेत्तु पूर्वतः[२७३] ।
सबीजं सूतकं कृत्वा जारयेत्षड्गुणं बलिम् ।।५१४।।
एवं युक्त्या गंधकंच जारयेत् षड्गुणं[२७४] बुधः ।
गन्धकं जारयेद्धीमान् रक्तचित्रकभावितम् ।।५१५।।
अङ्कोलतैलतो वापि रक्तवर्गेण वा तथा ।
किंशुकतैलतो वापि हेमभृङ्गरसेन वा ।।५१६।।
काकमाचीरसेनापि अथवा वेणिकारसैः ।
चूलिकालवणोपेतं यन्त्रे भूधरसंज्ञके ।।५१७।।

Jāraṇa of Mercury
According to Rasasāra

In mercury, in the beginning *bīja* should be used for *jāraṇa,* and thereafter, *jāraṇa* should be done by *gandhaka* (sulphur). In the preparation of *rasa-s* (medicines containing mercury, etc.), and *rasāyana-s* (rejuvenating drugs), *jāraṇa* with *bīja* is essential. Otherwise, the whole preparation goes waste and becomes useless and the physician incurs the sin of killing a brahmin.

In a pestle and mortar, made hot (*tapta khalva*) with the charcoal of *khadira*, mercury and *bīja* in the quantity of $^1/_{64}$th of mercury should be added together. To this, *sandhānakāmla* (vinegar), *lavaṇa* (ordinary salt) and *cūlikā lavaṇa* (a special type of salt) should be added. This drug promotes the digestive power (power to assimilate other metals) of the mercury. After adding these drugs, the mercury should be triturated with the help of a pestle and mortar. After making the pestle & mortar hot, mercury should be added to other durgs for trituration.

Thereafte, in *Bhairava yantra*, mercury should be kept with the paste of drugs below and above it. To the mercury, *viḍa* 1/8th in quantity [of mercury] should be added and cooked for three days. Accroding to tradition, only mild fire should be employed for cooking. On the foruth day, the mercury should be removed from the *Bhairava yantra* and when still warm, it should be washed with *kāñjī* (a type of vinegar). To this, *bīja* should be added again and cooked as before. This process of cooking should be repeated for four times. In this way, one *pala* of the *bīja* gets digested. This process of *jāraṇa* can be done in *Dolā yantra* or *Kacchapa yantra*.

Thereafter, *jāraṇa* should be done with the help of sulphur. As before, *bīja* should be added to mercury and *jāraṇa* should be done with the help of six times of sulphur. Sulphur should first of all be impregnated with the decoction of the red variety of *citraka* or the oil of *aṅkola* or decoction of plants belonging to *rakta varga* (group having red colour) or oil of *kiṃśuka* or the juice of *hema* (*nāga kesara*) or juice of *bhṛṅgarāja* or juice of *kākamācī* or the juice of *veṇikā*. For *jāraṇa*, mercury should be added with *cūlikā lavaṇa* and cooking should be done in *Bhūdhara yantra*.

तद्यथा

निर्माय गोस्तनाकारां वज्रमूषां दशाङ्गुलाम् ।
अर्धपक्वां पटुक्षारस्नुहीदुग्धार्कदुग्धतः ॥५१८॥
विषाम्लक्लृप्तां[२७५] संशुष्कां तत्र सूतं निवेशयेत् ।
धरण्यामवटं कृत्वा वितस्तिद्वयमानतः ॥५१९॥
तत्र मूषां प्रतिष्ठाप्य रसयुक्तां ततः क्षिपेत् ।
गन्धकं राजिकामात्रं प्रागुक्तौषधभावितम् ॥५२०॥
अभिधाय पिधायाथ पुटं दद्यादरण्यजैः ।
छानैः कुक्कुटसंज्ञं च स्वांगशीतैस्ततः क्षिपेत् ॥५२१॥
राजिकाद्वयमानेन गन्धकं पूर्ववन्मतम्[२७६] ।
इच्छन्द्वित्रिचतुःपञ्चक्रमेण[२७७] परिवर्धयेत् ॥५२२॥
यथा गन्धो न निर्याति धूमो वापि कथंचन ।

एवं प्रवर्धयेत्तावद्यावत्स्यात्षोडशांशकम् ।।५२३।।
न वर्धयेत्ततः पश्चाद्वर्धितं न गुणावहम् ।
रसस्य मारकत्वाच्च वर्धनं परिवर्जयेत् ।
एवं युक्त्या गन्धकं हि जारयेत्षड्गुणं प्रिये ।।५२४।।

।। इति जारणमात्रा ।।

Process of Jāraṇa

Vajramūṣā (a type of crucible) of 10 *aṅgula-s* in length and having shape of a nipple of the cow should be prepared of salt, alkalies, latex of *snuhī* and the latex of *arka*. It should be used when half-baked. This crucible should then be smeared with poisonous drugs and sour liquids, and dried. Mercury should be poured into this crucible. In the earth, a hole of the diameter of two *vitasti-s* should be dug and the crucible containing mercury should be placed in it. To this, one *rājikā* of sulphur impregnated with drugs described earlier [in verse nos. 515-516], should be added and the mouth of the crucible should be closed with the lid. This should then be cooked in *Kukkuṭa puṭa* with the help of cowdung cakes collected from the forest. After the cooking is over and the crucible is slightly warm, two *rājikā-s* of sulphur should be added to the mercury and cooked again. In subsequent cookings, the dose of sulphur does not come out. Thus, in subsequent cookings, the dose of should be gradually increased from two to three, four and five *rājikā-s*. The cooking should be done in such a way that the fume of sulphur should be gradually increased till it becomes 1/16th of mercury. The quantity of sulphur should not be increased thereafter, because it does not enhance or maintain the therapeutic effect of mercury.

Since excess of sulphur used in the *jāraṇa* of mercury destroys the effect of mercury, increase in the quantity of sulphur should be avoided. Therefore, *jāraṇa* of mercury should be done with six times of sulphur.

Thus, ends the description of the quantity of sulphur to be used for *jāraṇa* of mercury.

स्वछन्दात्

स्वीकृत्य सर्वाः सरितो यथा गंगाम्बु संविशेत् ।
धातुलोहगुणांल्लब्ध्वा सर्वान् हेमरसे विशेत् ।।५२५।।

दह्यन्ते धातवो वह्नौ मणिरत्नाभ्रकादयः ।
न क्षीयते न दिह्येत सुवर्णमजरामरम् ।
तस्मान्मृतोत्थितं चापि भक्षयेन्न विचारयेत् ।।५२६।।
हेम्नः प्रमाणं प्रथमं हि गुंजा दिनान्तरात्तत्प्रतिमैव वृद्धिः ।
द्व्यहादतः काञ्चनकंतु वृद्धैर्योज्यं प्रयत्नात्प्रतिपञ्च-गुञ्जाम् ।।५२७।।
अर्धत्रिंशत्तमा प्राप्ता गुंजानां विंशतेः परम् ।
नैव वृद्धिर्विधेया स्यादिति वृद्धपरंपरा ।।५२८।।
तथा कान्तायसादीनां मात्रा चैव हि मता ।
रसायनस्य मात्रेयं रोगिणां माषमात्रकम् ।
लोहादीनां प्रयोक्तव्यं देशकालविभागवित् ।।५२९।।

।। हेमादीनां मात्रा ।।

The Dosage of Gold etc., According to Svacchanda

As all the rivulets ultimately enter into the water of the river Ganges of their own, similarly all the metals with their attributes enter into the gold. Gems, costly stones and minerlas like mica get burnt in fire. But gold does not get diminished or burnt in fire and it is free from ageing & death. Therefore, the *bhasma* of gold should be used without any reservation.

The dose of gold on the first day is one *guñjā* and every consecutive days, the dose should be increased by one *guñjā*. Therefore, from the second day onwards, gold should be given in increased dose till five *guñjā-s* with care. According to the tradition of senior (old) physicians, the dose of gold should be given upto 15 *guñjā-s* and it should not exceed twenty *guñjā-s*.

Similar is the dose *of kānta lauha*, ordinary iron, etc.

This dose should be followed for the purpose of rejuvenation therapy. For patients, iron,etc., should be administered in the dose of one *māṣa* depending upon the nature of the country and season.

Thus, ends the description of the dose of gold, etc.

नागार्जुनात्
भिषगाद्ये द्वितीये च दिने गुंजाद्वयं हितम् ।
तृतीयेषु चतुर्गुंजा चतुर्थेषु तथैव च ।।५३०।।

एवं द्व्यहाद् द्व्ययहादूर्ध्वं द्विगुञ्जं विधिवर्धनम् ।
विवृद्ध्या विंशतिर्यावत्पुनरूर्द्ध्वं न वर्धयेत् ।।५३१।।
बद्धकोष्ठाग्निदीप्तस्तु पिबेत्छ्यामाशृतं पयः ।
कुर्वीत चानुलोमार्थं बहुताम्बूलभक्षणम् ।।५३२।।
अप्रवृत्तौ च लोहस्य शर्करावृद्धदारकम् ।
चूर्णयित्वा तु पानार्थं दापयेत्कर्मविद्भिषक् ।।५३३।।
क्वाथं गुडूच्या त्रिफलोद्भवं च क्षौद्रेण[२७८] गोमूत्रपयोष्णधारम् ।
अजापयस्तोकमथांबुसिद्धं पिबेत्तथायुष्यमथाल्पवह्निः ।।५३४।।
क्षुत्वा तु पत्रं पुष्पं वा विज्जलस्यांभसि क्षिपेत् ।
अनुपेयं ततश्चाम्लो ह्यनुरक्तातिसारनुत् ।।५३५।।
पिबेल्लोहभवे शूले वान्ते वाम्भोधिवृक्षजैः ।
सप्तभिः क्वथितं पत्रैः सलिलं पूर्वदोषनुत् ।।५३६।।
प्रभाते सह भक्तेन कुर्यान्मात्रां विभज्य वा ।
लोहं लिह्यात्प्रभातेऽर्धमर्धं समशनेन च ।
द्वौ वा लिह्यात्प्रातरसाविति नागार्जुनोऽब्रवीत् ।।५३७।।
ततो लोहाच्चतुःषष्टिगुणं गव्यं पयः पिबेत् ।
धारोष्णं तदलाभे तु क्वाथ्यं क्षीरं समोदकम् ।।५३८।।
येषां क्षीरमसात्म्यं स्याद्ये च मन्दाग्नयो भृशम् ।
तेषां क्षीरानुपानस्य मात्रेयं कथिता सदा ।
लोहात्तत्पेयमन्ये तु पयः पञ्चाशतं गुणैः ।।५३९।।
ततो मुस्तां घर्षयित्वा त्यजेत्किट्टं पिबेद्रसम् ।
तथा चास्य प्रसन्नात्मा वामपार्श्वेन संविशेत् ।।५४०।।
अप्रवृतौ तु लोहस्य त्यजेत्क्षीराम्बुतापितम् ।।५४१।।
वर्जयेत्सततं चिन्तामध्वानं मारुतातपौ ।
हर्षशोकौ वेगरोधं स्नानमभ्यङ्गमर्दनम् ।
दिवास्वप्नं विदाह्यम्लकन्दांश्च लशुनानि च ।।५४२।।

नवसप्तकमध्ये तु विधिरेष प्रशस्यते ।
तृतीयसप्तकादूर्ध्वं गुणं दापयति ध्रुवम् ।।५४३।।
एकविंशतिसंख्येभ्यः सप्तकेभ्योऽप्यनन्तरम्[२७९] ।
हन्ति वातं कफं पित्तं प्रमेहमवबाहुकम् ।।५४४।।
रक्ताढ्यवातं शोषं च कुष्टानि विषमज्वरान् ।
गुल्मांश्च पाण्डुरोगं च वह्निमान्द्यमरोचकम् ।।५४५।।
शूलं च परिणामं च निद्रां दुर्नामकानि च ।।५४६।।
स्वरभेदोदरं मेदं जीर्णज्वरहरं परम् ।
ग्रहणीरक्तपित्तघ्नं नेत्रामयगरापहम् ।।५४७।।
नैवाद्याद् द्विदलं तक्रं न तैलं लवणं न हि ।
एभिः सिद्धं न वाश्नीयान्नाश्नीयाद्बीजपूरकम् ।
न नारङ्गं सूरणं न नालाबु न च तुम्बकम् ।।५४८।।
'न[२८०] विना भावनात्प्रोक्तं विनाप्यभ्रकयोजनात्' ।
विना भैषज्यचूर्णैश्च विनापि त्रिफलाम्भसात् ।।५४९।।
विपक्वं विधिवल्लिह्यात् द्वितीयोऽयं विधिः स्मृतः ।।५५०।।
पुटैर्विना भावनाभिः केवलाभिस्तु संस्कृतम् ।
आयसं अथवा लिह्यात् तृतीयोऽयं विधिः स्मृतः ।।५५१।।
निरच्छं न दिनं लोहं विनाऽपि क्वथितात्पुटात् ।
विपक्वंविधिवल्लिह्याच्चतुर्थोऽयं विधिः स्मृतः ।।५५२।।
पुटैर्वा केवलैरेव संस्कृतं[२८१] शुद्धमभ्रकम् ।
विपक्वं विधिवल्लिह्यात्पञ्चमोऽयं विधिः स्मृतः ।।५५३।।
लोहं विनौषधैरेव पूर्वोक्तैरभ्रमिश्रितैः ।
विपक्वमभ्रकं दद्यात्षष्ठोऽयं विधिरीरितः ।।५५४।।
नाभ्रकेन विना लोहं न लोहेन विनाभ्रकम् ।
लोहाभ्रकप्रयोगो[२८२] हि जरामरणघातकः ।
लोहाभ्रकप्रकारं हि वक्ष्ये क्षयचिकित्सिते ।।५५५।।

यथारोगौषधेनैव पुटं दद्याद्विचक्षणः[२८३] ।
भावना सापि दातव्या[२८४] तत्रादौ गन्धकेन वै ।।५५६।।

।।इति लोहमात्राक्रमः[२८५]।।

The Dose and Mode of Administration of Loha According to Nāgārjuna

Loha-s (iron and other metallic preparations) should be given in the dose of two *guñjā-s* on each of the first and second days. On the third and fourth days, the dose should be four *guñjā-s*. In this way, on every two subsequent days the dose should be increased by two *guñjā-s* till the dose becomes twenty *guñjā-s* per day. Thereafter, the dose should not be increased.

Management of Complications

If there is constipation and if the power of digestion is strong, then the patient should be given milk boiled *with śyāmā*. For the downward movement (*anulomana*) of *vāyu*, the patient should be given large quantity of betel-leaf to chew. If the *loha-s* (iron and other metallic preparations) do not get eliminiated, then the patient should be given the powder of sugar and *vṛddhadāraka* [mixed with water] to drink.

If the power of digestion is low, the patient should take the decoction of *guḍūcī* or *triphalā* along with honey, cow's urine or hot cow's milk or goat's milk boiled by adding the small quantity of water. These recipes help in the promotion of longevity.

The leaf and flower of *vijjala* should be cut into small pieces and soaked in water. Intake of this water followed by a sour drink cures blood-diarrhoea.

Seven leaves of *ambhodhi* tree should be boiled with water. Intake of this decoction cures colic pain and vomiting caused by the intake of *loha-s* (iron and other metallic preparations).

Division of Dose

Loha-s (iron and other metallic preparations) may be administered in the morning with food or it can be given in divided doses during the whole day. Half of the recipe can be given in the morning and the other half along with food. According to Nāgārjuna, two divided doses of the recipe can be given in the morning itself.

Post-Prandial Drink

After the intake of *loha* (iron or other metallic preparation), the patient should drink sixty four times of cow's milk when it is warm immediately after milking (*dhāroṣṇa*). If this type of *dhāroṣṇa* milk is not available, milk should be boiled by adding equal quantity of water and given to the patient.

The quantity of milk and its mode of intake described above is applicable to patients who have very low power of digestion and for whom milk is not otherwise wholesome. Others should take milk which should be fifty times of the quantity of *loha* (iron and other metallic preparations).

Vehicle

Mustā should be made to a paste by trituration, and the fibrous part of the paste should be strained out. The juice of it should be given to the patient after he has taken milk. Therafter, he should be made to sleep in left side with happiness of the spirit (mind). If inspite of these measures, the *loha* (iron and other metallic preparations) does not get assimilated, then the patient should take milk boiled by adding water.

Prohibitions

A person taking *loha* should always avoid worry, long walk, exposure to wind and sun, excitement, grief, suppression of natural urges, bath, masssage, kneading, sleep during day time, *vidāhī* food (ingredients causing burning sensation), sour things, rhizomes, garlic, etc.

Course of Treatment & Therapeutic Effects

The above mentioned regimens should be followed for nine weeks. The recipe will certainly exhibit its therapeutic effects after the third week of treatment. After 21 weeks of use, the recipe cures diseases of *vāyu*, *kapha* and *pitta*, *prameha* (obstinate urinary diseases including diabetes), *avabāhuka* (brachial-nuralgia), blood-diseases, *āḍhya vāta* (gout), consumption, *kuṣṭha* (obstinate skin diseases including leprosy), *viṣama jvara* (irregular fever), *gulma* (phantom tumour), *pāṇḍu* (anemia), *agnimāndya* (suppression of the power of digestion), *arocaka* (anorexia), *śūla* (colic pain), *pariṇāma śūla* (colic pain caused by duodenal ulcer), excessive sleep, piles, hoarseness of voice, *udara* (obstinate abdominal diseases including ascites), adiposity, chronic fever, *grahaṇī* (sprue syndrome), *rakta pitta* (a disease characterised by bleeding from different parts of the body), eye-diseases and ailments caused by poisons.

Diet

A person using *loha-s* (preparations of iron and other metals) should not eat *dvidala* (dicotyledons or pulses), butter-milk, oil, salt, food prepared by boiling with these ingredients, *bījapūraka*, *nāraṅga*, *sūraṇa*, *alābu* and *tumbī*.

Second Process

Loha-s (iron and other metallic preparations) can be cooked in *puṭa* after *bhāvanā* (impregnation) and without adding *abhraka* (mica), powder of drugs and decoction of *triphalā*. This can be given to the patient in the form of a *lehya* (linctus). This is the second method of processing.

Third Process

Loha-s (iron and other metallic preparations) can be prepared just by *bhāvanā* (impregnation) [and trituration] without cooking in *puṭa*. This recipe can then be used in the form of a linctus. This is the third process.

Fourth Process

[There seems to be errors in this text; hence left untranslated.]

Fifth Process

Loha (iron and other metallic preparations) mixed with purified *abhraka* (mica) can be cooked only by *puṭa* appropriately, and thereafter, used in the form of a lincus. This is the fifth process.

Sixth Process

Loha (iron and other metallic preparations) added with purified mica (stated before) should be cooked (not by *puṭa*) without adding any other drug and given to the patient. This is the sixth process.

Loha-s (iron and other metals) are not effective without mica and the latter is not effective unless it is added with the former. The recipe containing both *loha* (iron and other metals) and mica prevents ageing process and death.

Different recipes containing *loha* and mica will be described (in detail) in the chapter dealing with the treatment of *kṣaya* (tuberculosis) [of the Nāgārjuna's work].

For the treatment of different diseases, *bhāvanā* (impregnation) of the recipe of *loha* should be done with different appropriate drugs and then cooked by *puṭa pāka*. But in the beginning, the recipe should always be mixed with sulphur.

Thus, ends the description of the processing and dosage of *loha-s* (iron and other metallic preparations).

बीजम् [SEED FOR TRANSMUTATION]

यल्लक्षणं रसमात्रा [?]

ताम्रसुमारितं कृत्वा सुवर्णं च सुमारितम् ।
मूषायां मित्रवर्गेण पुनरुज्जीवयेत्ततः ।।५५७।।
एकीकृत्वा चाधरोर्द्ध्वं ताप्यं दत्वा समं भवेत् ।
अंछयित्वा हेमशेषमेष एवंविधैः शतम् ।।५५८।।
वारान्तादुत्तमं बीजं पञ्चाशन्मध्यमं मतम् ।
अधमस्तत्त्रयस्त्रिंशद् दश चैवाधमाधमम् ।
महारसेषु सर्वेषु सत्वं शतगुणं भवेत् ।।५५९।।
लोहभस्म तथा सत्वं रसानपि महारसान् ।
संप्रदायविदा साक्षात्छतमेवावपेद्बुधः ।।५६०।।
सर्वथैवाप्यशक्तश्चेत्सप्तवारं[१८६] मृतोत्थितम् ।
अन्यथा सर्वथा सिद्धिर्न भवत्येव निश्चितम् ।।५६१।।

Preparation of Bīja

Properly prepared *bhasma* of copper and *bhasma* of gold should be added with the drugs belonging to *Mitra varga* and kept inside a *mūṣā* (crucible). By the application of strong-heat, the copper and gold in their original metallic form should be obtained. These, taken together, should be cooked again by adding *tāpya* (copper pyrite) over and below. Thereafter, the residual gold should be taken out which is called *bīja*. Repeating this process for one hundred times gives the best type of *bīja*. If it is repeated for 33 times then the *bīja* is of medium quality and if the process is repeated only for ten times then it gives rise to *bīja* of inferior quality.

The *sattva* (essence) of all the *mahārasa-s* is one hundred times more effective than the original metals. A person aquainted with the medical tradition should do *āvāpa* (hot immersion) for one hundred times of *lauha bhasma*, *sattva*, *rasa* and *mahārasa*.

If it is not possible to follow all these elaborate procedures, then the *bhasma* of the metal, etc. should be revived to the original metallic form for at least seven times. Otherwise, the recipe will certainly be ineffective.

रससिद्धान्तात्

आरोटसंज्ञां लभते एकवारं मृतस्तु यः ।
न तेन बीजकर्मस्यान्न तथा व्याधिनाशनः ।।५६२।।

According to Rasasiddhānta

If a metal is reduced to *bhasma* form (lit. killed) for once only, it is called *āroṭa*. This is useful neither as *bīja* nor for curing diseases.

रसदर्पणे

सुशोधितो रसः सम्यक् युक्तो योगेन केनचित् ।
आरोटसंज्ञाख्यो यो[२८७] हि स क्षेत्रीकरणे मतः ।।५६३।।

According to Rasadarpaṇa

If the purified mercury is added to any recipe appropriately, it is called *āroṭa* and it is useful for *kṣetrīkaraṇa* (preparation of the base).

वल्मीकमृत्तिका धूमं गैरिकं चेष्टिका[२८८] पटुम् ।
इत्येताः मृत्तिकाः पञ्च प्रोक्तस्थाने प्रयोगिकाः ।।५६४।।

।। इति पञ्चमृत्तिकाः ।।

Five Types of Mud (Earth)

The earth of the ant-hill, house-soot, *gairika* (red ochre), brick and *paṭu* (salt)-these five types of earth taken together are called *pañca-mṛttikā*. These are to be used in the place of *pañca-mṛttikā* prescribed in a recipe.

खल्व [PESTLE & MORTAR]

खल्वयन्त्रं त्रिधा प्रोक्तं मर्दनादिषु कर्मणि ।
पाषाणदारुसंभूतं तृतीयं लोहसंभवम् ।।५६५।।

उत्सेधं[२८९] च नवाङ्गुलं शशिकलातुल्यांगुलायाम् ।
विस्तारेण नवांगुलं रसमितैर्निम्नं तथैवाङ्गुलैः ।।५६६ ।।
कण्ठे द्व्यंगुलं विस्तरं च मसृणं द्रोण्यर्धचन्द्रोदयम् ।
पेष्यं[२९०] चैव दशाङ्गुलं चलदिदं खल्वाख्ययन्त्रं मतम् ।।५६७ ।।

Khalva Yantra (Pestle & Mortar)

Khalva yantra is of three types and these are used for trituration. These are prepared of either stone or wood or metal (iron). In height, it is nine *aṅgula-s;* in length, it is fifteen *aṅgula-s;* in width it is nine *aṅgula-s*; in depth it is six *aṅgula-s* and in thickness, it is two *aṅgula-s*. It is smooth and the shape of its cavity is like half-moon (cresent shaped.) The pestle should be of ten *aṅgula-s* and mobile. This type of instrument is called *Khalva yantra*.

अस्मिन्पञ्च पलः सूतो मर्दनीयो विशुद्धये ।
तत्तदौचित्ययोगेन खल्वेष्वन्येषु शोधयेत् ।।५६८ ।।

In such a mortar (*khalva*), five *pala-s* of mercury should be triturated for the purpose of purification. Such purification can also be appropriately carried out in other types of *khalva yantra*.

द्वादशाङ्गुलविस्तारः खल्वो भवति वर्तुलः ।
चतुरङ्गुलनिम्नश्च मर्दकोऽष्टांगुलायतः ।।५६९ ।।

Round type of *khalva yantra* is twelve *aṅgula-s* in radius. Its depth is four *aṅgula-s* and the pestle is eight *aṅgula-s* in length.

लोहेन च भवेद्यस्तु तप्तखल्वः स उच्यते ।
कृते कान्तायसे खल्वे भवेत्कोटिगुणो रसः ।।५७० ।।

।। इति खल्वलक्षणम्[२९१] ।।

The pestle and mortar prepared of iron is called *tapta khalva*. If mercury is processed in a mortar prepared of *kānta lauha* then it becomes one crore times more effective.

न देया यस्य कस्येयं परिभाषा मयोदिता ।
सुशिष्याय सुपुत्राय प्रदेया ब्राह्मणाय वै ।।५७१ ।।

।। इति परिभाषा ।।

This *paribhāṣā* (explanation of technical terms) described by me should not be given (taught) to any body except to a worthy disciple or to one's own son or to a brahmin.

Thus, ends the descrption of *paribhāṣā* (explanation of technical terms).

इति[२१२] श्रीमहाराजाधिराजटोडरमल्लविरचिते टोडरानन्दे आयुर्वेदसौख्ये परिभाषा-कथनं नाम सप्तमो हर्षः'।।

Thus, ends the seventh chapter dealing with *paribhāṣā* of the *Āyurveda saukhya* in *Ṭodarānanda* composed by the great king Ṭodaramalla.

NOTES AND REFERENCES

1. This is the beginning of seventh chapter of *Āyurveda saukhya* in Toḍarānanda and the invocation reads as follows :

'वत्साभिर्लीलास्वनुरक्तपित्तो ब्रह्मांडसर्गादिकटाक्षमोक्षान्।
यस्यास्ति भूतिं च तनोतु भूपे श्रीटोडरेन्द्रे सुखदोस्तु लोके'।।

२. "कलिङ्गमानः" पाठोऽयं प्रथमपुस्तके अधिकमुपलभ्यते।

३. पाठोऽयं प्रथमपंचमपुस्तकयोः अधिकमुपलभ्यते।

४. 'त्रसरेणुर्बुधैः ----- परमाणुभिः' पाठोऽयं षष्ठपुस्तके नोपलभ्यते।

५. कर्षः इति षष्ठपुस्तके पाठः।

६. क्षुद्रको इति आकरे पाठः।

७. अक्षः इति आकरे पाठः।

८. करमध्यो इति द्वितीयपुस्तके आकरे च पाठः।

९. प्रकुञ्चं इति प्रथममपुस्तके पाठः।

१०. कीर्तिते इति पंचमपुस्तके पाठः।

११. प्रसृतिश्च इति पंचमपुस्तके पाठः।

१२. 'प्रमानकः इति षष्ठपुस्तके पाठः।

१३. अर्द्धमानं इति आदर्शपुस्तकेषु पाठः।

१४. संज्ञेया इति आदर्शपुस्तकेषु पाठः।

१५. पलश्च सः इति आदर्शपुस्तकेषु पाठः।

१६. संज्ञितः इति आदर्शपुस्तकेषु पाठः।

१७. मता इति द्वितीयपुस्तके पाठः।

१८. सर्वत्रैष विनिश्चयः इति प्रथमपुस्तके पाठः।

१९. बलं वयम् इति प्रथमपुस्तके पाठः।

२०. देशदोषौ इति द्वितीयपुस्तके पाठः।

२१. यद् द्रव्यं इति आकरे पाठः।

२२. तु इति द्वितीयपुस्तके पाठः।

२३. ज्ञेयं इति द्वितीयपुस्तके पाठः।

२४. श्चैव सं पूज्याद्रक्तचन्दनम् इति षष्ठपुस्तके पाठः।

२५. हीनवीर्यत्वमाप्नुते इति प्रथमपुस्तके पाठः।

२६. 'हीना------वत्सरात्परम्' पाठोऽयं प्रथमपुस्तकेनोपलभ्यते

२७. °साधिकस्तथा इति आकरे पाठः।

२८. 'वज्राभावे तु गुणोत्तरम्' पाठोऽयं षष्ठपुस्तके अधिकमुपलभ्यते।

२९. द्रष्टव्यम् : भावप्रकाश : पू. ख. ५:१६८।

३०. रसदर्पणात् इति षष्ठपुस्तके पाठः।

३१. षोडशभिः क्षुधा इति द्वितीयपुस्तके पाठः।

३२. द्वयेन सर्षपो रक्तस्ते इति द्वितीयपुस्तके पाठः।

३३. स्यात् तद् त्रयं इति प्रथमपुस्तके पाठः।

३४. 'रक्तिका........ विशारदैः' पाठोऽयं द्वितीयपुस्तके नोपलभ्यते।

३५. क्वचिन्माषद्वयेन हि इति प्रथमपुस्तके पाठः।

३६. 'त्रिभिर्माषैर्वा-शाण इत्युच्यते' पाठोऽयं प्रथमपुस्तके अधिकमुपलभ्यते।

३७. गद्यनो इति षष्ठपुस्तके पाठः।

३८. घटकश्चैव इति द्वितीयपुस्तके पाठः।

३९. 'रसार्णव.----- विदुः।' पाठोऽयं रसार्णवतन्त्रे नोपलभ्यते'।

४०. तथा इति प्रथमपंचमपुस्तकयोः पाठः।

४१. षोडशिका तथा व मणि मानिका इति प्रथमपंचमपुस्तकयोः पाठः।

४२. मूर्धबस्तौ इति द्वितीयपुस्तके पाठः।

४३. मात्रेयमिति मे निश्चिता मतिः इति प्रथमपंचमपुस्तकयोः पाठः।

४४. इति प्रथमपंचमपुस्तकयोः पाठः।

४५. इति प्रसंगाद् विन्दुमात्रा इति प्रथमपंचमपुस्तकयोः पाठः।

४६. शुक्तिद्वयनामा इति प्रथमपुस्तके पाठः।

४७. स्यान्माणिकाष्टफलं इति प्रथमपंचमपुस्तकयोः पाठः।

४८. प्रस्थैर्भवेत्कंसः इति प्रथमपंचमपुस्तकयोः पाठः।

४९. पात्रं सूर्याष्टकं इति प्रथमपंचमपुस्तकयोः पाठः।

५०. सूर्पाच्चतुर्गुणा गोणी खारीबाहस्ततस्ततः इति प्रथमपुस्तकेपाठः।

५१. द्रोणी वाहः परिकेति यथासंख्यं चतुर्गुणाः पाठोऽयं प्रथमपंचमपुस्तकयोः अधिकमुपलभ्यते।

५२. राशि. ------ चतुर्गुणम् पाठोऽयं प्रथमपुस्तकेनोपलभ्यते।

५३. यवः प्रोक्तो कथितं तव इति आदर्शपुस्तकेषु पाठः।

५४. साक्षा यवः षड्सर्षपैर्भवेत् इति प्रथमपुस्तके पाठः।

५५. षड्यवैरेक इति प्रथमपुस्तके पाठः।

५६. "शेषं पूर्ववत्" पाठोऽयं प्रथमपुस्तके अधिकमुपलभ्यते।

५७. .मध्यपुरुषादि. इति प्रथमपंचमपुस्तकयोः पाठः।

५८. '.कषायादि... परिकीर्त्तितः' पाठोऽयं प्रथमपंचमपुस्तकयोः नोपलभ्यते।

५९. 'लोहरत्नादि... माषक' पाठोऽयं षष्ठपुस्तके नोपलभ्यते।

६०. द्विगुणा मता इति द्वितीयपुस्तके पाठः।

६१. प्रकीर्त्तितं इति प्रथमपंचमपुस्तकयोः पाठः।

६२. श्रतनामतः इति द्वितीयपुस्तके पाठः।

६३. पाठोऽयं प्रथमपंचमपुस्तकयोः नोपलभ्यते।

६४. भोजः इति पाठः षष्ठपुस्तके अधिकमुपलभ्यते।

६५. ग्राह्यास्तत्क्षुणमेव इति प्रथमपंचमपुस्तकयोः पाठः।

६६. भेडः इति प्रथमपंचमपुस्तकयोः पाठः।

६७. क क्षारहिङ्गुवजमोदाम्लवेतसैस्तान्न केवलाम् इति प्रथमपुस्तकेपाठः।

ख. क्षारहिङ्ग्वम्ललवणवेतसाम्लं न केवलम् इति पंचमपुस्तकेपाठः।

६८. क्लिनावस्थादिभागवित् इति पंचमपुस्तके पाठः।

६९. कार्यमेव इति प्रथमपंचमपुस्तकयोः पाठः।

७०. कारयेत्तद्विपर्ययम् इति प्रथमपुस्तके पाठः।

७१. द्रष्टव्यम् : शार्ङ्गधर : पूर्वखण्ड १ : ६०।

७२. 'स्थाने...... मोदा' पाठोऽयं प्रथमपुस्तके अधिकमुपलभ्यते।

७३. 'अंतः...... कुशलो भिषक्' पाठोऽयं षष्ठपुस्तके अधिकमुपलभ्यते।

७४. भद्रशौनक इति पंचमपुस्तके पाठः।

७५. पाठोऽयं षष्ठपुस्तके अधिकमुपलभ्यते।

७६. 'यथायोगं...... द्रव्यं' पाठोऽयं प्रथमपुस्तके अधिकमुपलभ्यते।

७७. यौगिकम् इति आदर्शपुस्तकेषु पाठः।

७८. 'सर्पिः.........विजानता' पाठोऽयं प्रथमपुस्तके अधिकमुपलभ्यते।

७९. जानता इति प्रथमपुस्तके अधिक पाठ :।

८०. द्रष्टव्यम् : शार्ङ्गधर : पूर्वखण्ड १ : ३७-३८।

८१. सिद्धं इति षष्ठपुस्तके पाठः।

८२. पाठोऽयं षष्टपुस्तके नोपलभ्यते।

८३. स्वरस विधिः इति प्रथमपुस्तके पाठः।

८४. पेयश्चतुर्गुणः इति द्वितीयपुस्तके पाठः।

८५. वह्नि सन्निभम् इति द्वितीयपुस्तके पाठः।

८६. 'मृतपात्रे----पिबेत्' पाठोऽयं प्रथमपंचमपुस्तकयोः नोपलभ्यते।

८७. गुडादीनां इति प्रथमपुस्तके पाठः।

८८. 'तोये----पलद्वयम्' पाठोऽयं पंचमपुस्तकेनोपलभ्यते।

८९. पाठोऽयं प्रथमपुस्तके अधिकमुपलभ्यते।

९०. स्नेहक्वाथौषधेषु वा इति प्रथमपुस्तके पाठः।

९१. चतुर्भागावशिष्टं इति प्रथमपुस्तके पाठः।

९२. प्रसृतं तु चिकित्सक इति द्वितीयपुस्तके पाठः।

९३. भेडः इति प्रथमपुस्तके पाठः।
९४. द्रष्टव्यम् : शार्ङ्गधर : मध्यमखण्डः १:१।
९५. क्लेदी इति प्रथमपुस्तके पाठः।
९६. सायं इति द्वितीयपुस्तके पाठः।
९७. रोगमुक्तौ इति टिप्पणी द्वितीयपुस्तके उपलभ्यते।
९८. वा पयो गुडा इति द्वितीयपुस्तके पाठः।
९९. भवेद्यदि इति पंचमपुस्तके पाठः।
१००. क्वथते पात्रभाजनम् इति षष्ठपुस्तके पाठः।
१०१. माषकम् इति पंचमपुस्तके पाठः।
१०२. माक्षिकम् इति द्वितीयपुस्तके पाठः।
१०३. 'आर्येन---कर्त्तव्यमाह' पाठोऽयं द्वितीयषष्ठपुस्तकयोः नोपलभ्यते।
१०४. स्नपनं इति प्रथमपुस्तके पाठः।
१०५. शीतलेन इति प्रथमपुस्तके पाठः।
१०६. माहभेडः इति प्रथमपुस्तके पाठः।
१०७. यदा इति षष्ठपुस्तके पाठः।
१०८. प्रयोजयेत् इति द्वितीयपुस्तके पाठः।
१०९. पलार्द्धमुपभुञ्जीत कनीयस्तु इति प्रथमपुस्तके पाठः।
११०. विरेचनपरिभाषा इति प्रथमपुस्तके पाठः।
१११. मदनानि प्रयोजयेत् इति प्रथमपुस्तके पाठः।
११२. वातादिके इति द्वितीयपुस्तके पाठः।
११३. मूलं इति द्वितीयपुस्तके पाठः।
११४. यस्मिन्दोषादिकं इति प्रथमपुस्तके पाठः।
११५. पृथग्बस्तिश्चतुर्विंशकैः इति प्रथमपुस्तके पाठः।
११६. समीधान्य इति प्रथमपुस्तके पाठः।
११७. आद्यं इति द्वितीयपुस्तके पाठः।
११८. 'अत्र-----गुणत्वात्कर्मः' पाठोऽयं प्रथमपंचमपुस्तकयोः अधिकमुपलभ्यते।

११९. पाठोऽयं षष्ठपुस्तके नोपलभ्यते।
१२०. कृतो कृतः इति षष्ठपुस्तके पाठः।
१२१. न सा दोषबलं प्रति इति षष्ठपुस्तके पाठः।
१२२. गुडलेहः उपागतः इति षष्ठपुस्तके पाठः।
१२३. भेडः इति द्वितीयपुस्तके पाठः।
१२४. द्रष्टव्यम्— शार्ङ्गधर : मध्यमखण्ड : ८:१-३।
१२५. पाठोऽयं द्वितीयपुस्तके नोपलभ्यते।
१२६. रसावर्त्तिवदेति इति षष्ठपुस्तके पाठः।
१२७. पुराणं न च भावितम् इति आकरे पाठः।
१२८. व्यापद्येतौषधं द्रुतम् इति आकरे पाठः।
१२९. द्रष्टव्यम् — चरकः चिकित्सा :१:३:५५-६१।
१३०. 'वृदाः धूपादिकल्पना ग्रंथांतरादवगन्तव्या' पाठोऽयं प्रथमपंचमपुस्तकयोः अधिकमुपलभयते।
१३१. उक्ते तु इति द्वितीयपुस्तके पाठः।
१३२. पात्रादपरन्तु भूयः इति पंचमपुस्तके पाठः।
१३३. प्रसन्नभावान्मलयेत्यधस्तात् इति द्वितीयपुस्तकेपाठः।
१३४. परं इति षष्ठपुस्तके पाठः।
१३५. चतुर्थभागो इति प्रथमपुस्तके पाठः।
१३६. निःशर्करममृत्स्नं इति द्वितीयपुस्तके पाठः।
१३७. प्रक्षिपेद्रसे भूयः इति आकरे पाठः।
१३८. पाठोऽयं प्रथमपंचमपुस्तकयोः अधिकमुपलभ्यते।
१३९. एकत्रिसप्तसप्ताहं कर्षमर्धपलं इति आकरे पाठः।
१४०. क्रमान्मतः इति आकरे पाठः।
१४१. विशोधनं इति द्वितीयपुस्तके पाठः।
१४२. छेदनं इति प्रथमपुस्तके पाठः।
१४३. सुसंहिता इति प्रथमपंचमपुस्तकयोः पाठः।
१४४. ०साधितम् इति प्रथमपुस्तके पाठः।

१४५. त्रिधा इति प्रथमपुस्तके पाठः।
१४६. स्यात् प्रदेहोष्णस्तथैव च इति प्रथमपुस्तके पाठः।
१४७. चर्म तस्योत्सेधनलेपनम् इति द्वितीयपुस्तके पाठः।
१४८. दद्याद् दन्तं न्निपतितं तथा इति प्रथमपुस्तके पाठः।
१४९. शुष्कमानं इति आदर्शपुस्तकेषु पाठः तत्तु शुष्यमानं इति सम्यक् प्रतिभाति।
१५०. सुश्रुतात् इति प्रथमपुस्तके पाठः।
१५१. त्यपार्थके इति षष्ठपुस्तके पाठः।
१५२. अथ शिरोलेपनविधिः इति द्वितीयपुस्तके पाठः।
१५३. प्रशस्यते इति प्रथमपुस्तके पाठः।
१५४. 'कल्केन' पाठोऽयं द्वितीयपुस्तके अधिकमुपलभ्यते।
१५५. पाठोऽयं षष्ठपुस्तके अधिकमुपलभ्यते।
१५६. अस्य श्लोकार्धं षष्ठपुस्तके नोपलभ्यते।
१५७. संमिता इति षष्ठपुस्तके पाठः।
१५८. न इति षष्ठपुस्तके पाठः।
१५९. क्वाथ्यौषधसमं इति प्रथमपुस्तके पाठः।
१६०. माद्य. इति द्वितीयचतुर्थपंचमपुस्तकेषु पाठः।
१६१. यदा इति द्वितीयषष्ठपुस्तकयोः पाठः।
१६२. श्रावणार्थेषु इति द्वितीयपुस्तके पाठः।
१६३. संधानं श्रावणार्थेषु इति पंचमपुस्तके पाठः।
१६४. दाहं इति षष्ठपुस्तके पाठः।
१६५. पाठोऽयं द्वितीयपुस्तके नोपलभ्यते।
१६६. रसं इति षष्ठपुस्तके पाठः।
१६७. रसस्तेन कृतं मद्यं इति प्रथमपुस्तके पाठः।
१६८. पाठोऽयं द्वितीयपुस्तके नोपलभ्यते।
१६९. तालसिन्दोलखर्जूर. इति द्वितीयपुस्तके पाठः।
१७०. यद्रसं तत्तदाख्यं च विज्ञेयं तत्परायणैः इति प्रथमपंचमषष्ठपुस्तकेषु पाठः।

१७१. चातुर्जातकजाती इति षष्ठपुस्तके पाठः।
१७२. मद्यसमं जातं इति द्वितीयपुस्तके पाठः।
१७३. सौम्यजातं मृदाऽथवा इति प्रथमपुस्तके पाठः।
१७४. किञ्चित्त्रिमधुरान्वितम् इति प्रथमपुस्तके पाठः।
१७५. यनमध्वादि इति द्वितीयपुस्तके पाठः।
१७६. 'गुडांबु------तदुच्यते' पाठोऽयं द्वितीयपुस्तकेनोपलभ्यते।
१७७. पिप्पलीमधुसंयुतम् इति षष्ठपुस्तके पाठः।
१७८. संधानीमाश्रुतम् इति पंचमपुस्तके पाठः।
१७९. न इति आदर्शपुस्तकेषु पाठः।
१८०. पाठोऽयं प्रथमपुस्तके अधिकमुपलभ्यते।
१८१. कषायस्नेहसंयुक्तं इति प्रथमपुस्तके पाठः।
१८२. अस्मजा इति प्रथमपुस्तके पाठः।
१८३. 'सुवर्ण......मता' पाठोऽयं द्वितीयपुस्तके नोपलभ्यते।
१८४. कृत्वा इति षष्ठपुस्तके पाठः।
१८५. दुत्थाय इति प्रथमपुस्तके पाठः।
१८६. वामेनाङ्गुष्ठवर्म्मणा इति षष्ठपुस्तके पाठः।
१८७. रजतसुवर्णपात्रे इति द्वितीयपुस्तके पाठः।
१८८. पाठोऽयं प्रथमपुस्तके अधिकमुपलभ्यते।
१८९ सेकस्तु इति प्रथमपंचमपुस्तकयोः पाठः।
१९०. वारं वारं इति द्वितीयपुस्तके पाठः।
१९१. वातायनरजोहीनदेशे इति प्रथमपुस्तके पाठः।
१९२. प्रमर्द्य च इति प्रथमपंचमपुस्तकयोः पाठः।
१९३. तथैव च इति द्वितीयपुस्तके पाठः।
१९४. शुष्के इति पंचमपुस्तके पाठः।
१९५. मिता इति प्रथमपुस्तके पाठः।
१९६. पाठोऽयं प्रथमपंचमपुस्तकयोः अधिकमुपलभ्यते।
१९७. निस्तोदोश्च इति पंचमपुस्तके पाठः।

१९८. पिचुयुतं कृत्वा इति षष्ठपुस्तके पाठः।

१९९. प्रकल्पयेत् इति प्रथमपुस्तके पाठः।

२००. .मूर्द्धजत्रुं इति प्रथमपुस्तके पाठः।

२०१. 'कटहे मृन्मये पात्रे किंवा पक्वकुसुम्भके।
ताम्रादिजेऽथवा पात्रे किंवा पाषाणसंभवे'।।
पाठोऽयं षष्ठपुस्तके अधिकमुपलभ्यते।

२०२. आकंधमगोनिक्सेत् प्रचुरं प्रातरेव वैः। पाठोऽयं षष्ठपुस्तके अधिकमुपलभ्यते।

२०३. पाठोऽयं प्रथमपुस्तके अधिकमुपलभ्ययते।

२०४. 'नाभेः..... स्थितिः' पाठोऽयं पंचमषष्ठपुस्तकयोः नोपलभ्यते।

२०५. क स्वयम् इति द्वितीयपुस्तके पाठः।
ख. त्वयम् इति पंचमपुस्तके पाठः।

२०६. अवगाहमात्रा इति प्रथमपुस्तके पाठः।

२०७. °जनको मृदुवर्णबलप्रदः इति षष्ठपुस्तके पाठः।

२०८. सुस्थः इति द्वितीयपुस्तके पाठः।

२०९. क जीर्णे नवज्वरे शीते च इति प्रथमपुस्तके पाठः।
ख. नवज्वरे शीत च इति पंचमपुस्तके पाठः।

२१०. 'रसाद्यैः----प्रशस्यते' पाठोऽयं द्वितीयपुस्तकेनोपलभ्यते।

२११. स्तमुपागते इति प्रथमपुस्तके पाठः।

२१२. सस्नेहैः इति द्वितीयपुस्तके पाठः।

२१३. पाठोऽयं षष्ठपुस्तके अधिकमुपलभ्यते।

२१४. कृत्वा इति षष्ठपुस्तके पाठ।

२१५. जलेनैवं इति षष्ठपुस्तके पाठः।

२१६. प्रसारिण्यादि इति षष्ठपुस्तके पाठः।

२१७. ध्युषितं इति द्वितीयपुस्तके पाठः।

२१८. वृद्धसुश्रुतः इति द्वितीयपुस्तके पाठः।

२१९. वा इति द्वितीयपुस्तके पाठः।
२२०. 'भद्रशौनक------क्रमात्' पाठोऽयं द्वितीयषष्ठपुस्तकयोः नोपलभ्यते।
२२१. पाठोऽयं प्रथमपुस्तके अधिकमुपलभ्यते।
२२२. कल्कचतुर्गुणं इति द्वितीयपुस्तके पाठः।
२२३. क्वाथाच्चतुर्गुणं इति द्वितीयपुस्तके पाठः।
२२४. दह्याक्षीरश्च इति षष्ठपुस्तके पाठः।
२२५. कल्पते इति प्रथमपुस्तके पाठः।
२२६. 'अनिर्दिष्ट------कल्प्यते' पाठोऽयं प्रथमपंचमपुस्तकयोः नोपलभ्यते।
२२७. न इति प्रथमपुस्तके पाठः।
२२८. वीर्ये इति द्वितीयपुस्तके पाठः।
२२९. जैयटः इति द्वितीयपुस्तके पाठः।
२३०. 'यत्र-------क्षीरमेव' पाठोऽयं षष्ठपुस्तकेनोपलभ्यते।
२३१. अर्धावशिष्टः इति प्रथमपंचमपुस्तकयोः पाठः।
२३२. 'चन्द्र......... तथा' पाठोऽयं प्रथमपुस्तके नोपलभ्यते।
२३३. कपितैलं शिलारस इत्यर्थः इति द्वितीयपुस्तके टिप्पणी।
२३४. द्रष्टव्यम् - चरकः कल्पस्थान १२:१०८।
२३५. "तन्त्रान्तरे रोधान्विता" पाठोऽयं षष्ठपुस्तके अधिकमुपलभ्यते।
२३६. इति तैलघृतपाकविधि इति प्रथमपुस्तके पाठः।
२३७. च इति प्रथमपुस्तके पाठः।
२३८. सितार्कभागः शितरुक् इति प्रथमपुस्तके पाठः।
२३९. तत्रायः इति द्वितीयपुस्तके पाठः।
२४०. तथा इति द्वितीयपुस्तके पाठः।
२४१. विधि इति द्वितीयपुस्तके पाठः।
२४२. कुर्यात् नालसः कर्मकौ विधिज्ञः इति प्रथमपुस्तके पाठः।
२४३. छिद्यते इति प्रथमपुस्तके पाठः।

२४४. कालिकावर्जितम् इति प्रथमपुस्तके पाठः।
२४५. तारजीर्णस्य रविजीर्णस्य तत् त्रयम् इति आकरे पाठः।
२४६. तीक्ष्णाभ्रकान्तमाषैकं इति आकरे प्रथमपुस्तके च पाठः।
२४७. गुञ्जैका द्राविका भवेत् इति आकरे पाठः।
२४८. ०सर्पिषान्वितम् इति आकरे पाठः।
२४९. नागं वङ्गं रसं भस्म इति आकरे पाठः।
२५०. मात्रायुक्तं ततश्चैव भक्षयेच्च रसायने इति आकरे पाठः।
२५१. रसायनं इति प्रथमपुस्तके पाठः।
२५२. तथैव च इति द्वितीयपुस्तके पाठः।
२५३. "चतुः.. तथैव च" पाठोऽयं प्रथमपंचमपुस्तकयोः अधिकमुपलभ्यते।
२५४. कर्णाटि इति द्वितीयपुस्तके पाठः।
२५५. क कारि. इति प्रथमपुस्तके पाठः।
ख. भ्कारि. इति पंचमपुस्तके पाठः।
२५६. विभागतः इति द्वितीयपुस्तके पाठः।
२५७. 'एकमात्रां....... विभागतः' पाठोऽयं प्रथमद्वितीयपुस्तकयोः अधिकमुपलभ्यते।
२५८. सप्तमे इति प्रथमपुस्तके पाठः।
२५९. सप्तकं इति द्वितीयपुस्तके पाठः।
२६०. स्याद्वैस्य इति प्रथमपुस्तके पाठः।
२६१. कारयेत् इति प्रथमपुस्तके पाठः।
२६२. सैवालभक्षमतात् इति प्रथमपुस्तके पाठः।
२६३. सुमाक्षिकम् इति पंचमपुस्तके पाठः।
२६४. विद्यते इति प्रथमपुस्तके पाठः।
२६५. वैद्यांशः इति प्रथमपुस्तके पाठः।
२६६. खदिराङ्गारपूरिते इति प्रथमपुस्तके पाठः।
२६७. 'मंदं....... परायणः' पाठोऽयं प्रथमपंचमपुस्तकयोः उपलभ्यते। द्वितीयपुस्तके अस्मिन् स्थाने 'प्रक्षिप्य मर्दयेत् सम्यक्

सम्प्रदायपरायणः' इति पाठः उपलभ्यते।

२६८. क्षालयेत्पुनः इति द्वितीयपुस्तके पाठः।

२६९. वारचतुष्टयात् इति द्वितीयपुस्तके पाठः।

२७०. दत्वा पलांशं जीर्येत दोलायमथ जारयेत् इति द्विततीयपुस्तकेपाठः।

२७१. अतः इति प्रथमपुस्तके पाठः।

२७२. हि इति प्रथमपुस्तके पाठः।

२७३. पूर्वसः इति पंचमपुस्तके पाठः।

२७४. जारयेत् गन्धकं बुधः इति द्वितीयपुस्तके पाठः।

२७५. विषाम्ललिप्तां इति प्रथमपुस्तके पाठः।

२७६. पूर्ववत्पुटं इति प्रथमपुस्तके पाठः।

२७७. इत्थं द्वि त्रि चतु इति पंचमपुस्तके पाठः।

२७८. क्षौद्रेण गोमूत्रमथोषणधारणम् इति द्वितीयपुस्तके पाठः।

२७९. सप्तकेभ्योऽथानन्तरम् इति प्रथमपुस्तके पाठः।

२८०. 'न----योजनात्' पाठोऽयं द्वितीयषष्ठपुस्तकयोः नोपलभ्यते।

२८१. संस्थितं इति प्रथमपुस्तके पाठः।

२८२. खादेद्युक्तं प्रयोगो हि इति द्वितीयपुस्तके पाठः।

२८३. पुटपाकपरायणः इति द्वितीयपुस्तके पाठः।

२८४. ज्ञातव्या इति द्वितीयपुस्तके पाठः।

२८५. इति लोहमात्राक्रमः जल्लक्षणं रसरत्नाकरतन्त्रात्।।

२८६. सर्वथैवाथ शक्तश्चेत्सप्तवारं मृतोच्छ्रितम् इति द्वितीयपुस्तकेपाठः।

२८७. ०संज्ञाख्यातो इति द्वितीयपुस्तकेपाठः।

२८८. षटी इति द्वितीयपुस्तके पाठः।

उत्सेधेन इति द्वितीयपुस्तके पाठः।

२८९. उत्सेधेन इति द्वितीयपुस्तके पाठः।

२९०. व्रेषां इति प्रथमपुस्तके पाठः।

२९१. द्वादशांगुलः इति प्रथमपुस्तके पाठः।

२९२. 'इति ----हर्षः' पाठोऽयं प्रथमपुस्तकेएव उपलभ्यते।

CHAPTER-II

अथ रसादीनां शोधनं मारणं च

(PROCESSING OF MERCURY, ETC.)

रसविद्या[1] दृढगोप्या मातृगुह्यमिव ध्रुवम् ।
भवेद्वीर्यवती गुप्ता निर्वीर्याऽऽतिप्रकाशनात् ।।१।।

Need for Secrecy

Rasa vidyā (science of mercury or Alchemy) should always be kept as a closely guarded secret like the genital organs of the mother. When kept secret, the knowledge becomes more powerful (effective) and its disclosure leads to loss of potency.

यः श्लेष्मानिलपित्तदोषशमनो रोगापहो मूर्च्छितः ।
पञ्चत्वं च गतो ददाति विपुलं राज्यं चिरं जीवितम् ।।२।।
बद्धः खे गमनं करोत्यमरतां विद्याधरत्वं नृणाम् ।
सोऽयं पातु सुरासुरेन्द्रनमितः श्रीसूतराजः प्रभुः ।।३।।

Prayer of Mercury

Let mercury, the Lord Sūtarāja, which in its state of *mūrcchanā* (lit. fainting = a type of purification process) alleviates *kapha*, *vāyu* and *pitta* and cures diseases, which in its state of *mārana* (lit. killed = *bhasma* or calcination) endows a person with great wealth (lit.

kingdom) and longevity (lit. deathlessness) which in its state of *baddha* (lit. binding = solidification) helps a person to move in the sky and to become *vidyādhara* (abode of all knowledge) and which is revered by the gods and the king of gods, protect [all living creatures].

आत्मा वै पुत्रनामासि न्यायादीश्वरनामभिः ।
कीर्त्यते पार्वतीकान्त इत्यादिभिरयं बुधैः ।।४।।

Synonyms

Mercury is procreated by Lord Śiva. The progeny (lit. son) represents the procreator himself . According to this rule, mercury is known by all the synonyms of Lord Śiva, viz., Īśvara, Pārvatī-kānta, etc.

मृन्मयः कंचुकश्चैको परः पाषाणकंचुकः ।
तृतीयो जलजो ज्ञेयौ द्वौ द्वौ स्तो नागवंगयोः ।
रसेऽहि[१]कंचुकाः सप्त विज्ञेयाः रससागरे ।।५।।

Seven Kañcuka-s (Layers of Adulterants)

According to *Rasasāgara,* there are seven layers of adulterants in the mercury which are called *Kañcuka doṣa*. The first one is of mud, the second one is of stone, the third one is of water, the fourth and fifth ones are *nāga* (lead) and the sixth and seventh ones are of *vaṅga* (tin).

तद्यथा[३]
कपाली[४] कालिका वंगे नागे श्यामा कपालिका ।
दुग्धोपरितरायां तु तद्रूपा[५] स्यात्कपालिका ।
पंकवर्णा भवेच्छ्यामा कपाली कृष्णवर्णिका ।।६।।

Because of *vaṅga doṣa*, the mercury becomes ***kapālī*** and ***kālikā*** and because of ***nāga doṣa***, the mercury becomes *śyāma* and ***kapālikā***. Because of *kapālī* the mercury appears as if smeared with the layer of milk. *Śyāmā* makes the colour of mercury like that of mud and *kapālikā* imparts black colour to mercury.

मलदोषो भवेदेको द्वितीयो वह्निसंज्ञकः ।
भूदोषस्तु तृतीयश्च उन्मत्तश्च चतुर्थकः ।
पञ्चमः शैलदोषश्च पञ्चदोषाः प्रकीर्तिताः ।।७।।

Five Doṣa-s of Mercury

Five defects (*doṣa-s*) of mercury are-(1) *mala doṣa*, (2) *vahni doṣa*, (3) *bhū doṣa*, (4) *unmatta doṣa*, and (5) *śaila doṣa*.

पृथिव्याः कंचुकात्कुष्ठं जाड्यं पाषाणदोषतः ।
वलीपलितखालित्यं वारिदोषात्प्रजायते ।।८।।
दद्रुणि गजचर्माणि करोत्येव कपालिका ।।९।।
कामलां पाण्डुरोगं च महाकुष्ठं तथोदरम् ।
प्रमेहं श्वेतकुष्ठं च श्यामा कंचुकसम्भवम् ।।१०।।
मर्मच्छेदं बस्तिशूलं काली कुर्यादसंशयम्[६] ।
कापाली वीर्यहानिं च कुरुते तान् निवारयेत्[७] ।।११।।

Adverse Effects of Kañcuka-s

(1) Because of *bhū doṣa* (*pṛthivī kañcuka*), the mercury causes *kuṣṭha* (obstinate skin diseases including leprosy).
(2) Because of *pāṣāṇa kañcuka*, mercury causes *jāḍya* (dumbness).
(3) Because of *jala kañcuka*, mercury causes premature wrinkling, premature graying of hair and baldness.
(4) *Kapālikā kañcuka* causes *dadru-s* (ring-worm) and *gaja carma* (a type of skin disease in which the skin of the person becomes like that of the elephant).
(5) Because of *śyāmā kañcuka*, mercury causes jaundice, anemia, *mahā kuṣṭha* (major types of obstinate skin diseases), *udara* (obstinate abdominal diseases including ascites), *prameha* (obstinate urinary diseases including diabetes) and leucoderma.
(6) Because of *kālī kañcuka*, mercury causes *marma cheda* (damage to the vital organs) and pain in urinary bladder.
(7) Because of *kāpālī kañcuka*, mercury destroys semen (*vīrya hāni*). The physician should, therefore, remove all these *kañcuka doṣa-s* of mercury.

मूर्च्छयेन्मलसंयुक्तो वह्नियुक्तश्च तापयेत् ।
धूम्मा[८] च विषदोषेण भूदोषात्तेजनाशनम्[९] ।
दर्पादङ्गं स्फुटत्येवोन्मत्तादुन्मत्तता भवेत् ।।१२ ।।

Adverse Effects of Doṣa-s

(1) Because of *mala doṣa,* mercury causes fainting.
(2) Because of *vahni doṣa*, mercury causes burning sensation.
(3) Because of *viṣa doṣa*, mercury causes *dhūmmā* (?). This is not enumerated in verse no.7.]
(4) Because of *bhū doṣa*, mercury causes loss of complexion.
(5) Because of *darpa doṣa*, mercury causes cracking of limbs. [This is in the place of *śaila doṣa* - vide verse no.7]
(6) Because of *unmatta doṣa*, mercury causes madness.

युक्तं द्वादशभिर्दोषैर्यश्च हन्याद्रसेश्वरम्[१०] ।
ब्रह्महत्यादिकः दोषाः भवेत्तस्य पदे पदे ।।१३ ।

Needs for Correcting Kañcuka-s and Doṣa-s

If a physician attempts to make *bhasma* (*hanyāt*= to kill) of mercury without removing these *kañcuka-s* and *doṣa-s*, he in his every step, incurs the sin of *brahma hatyā* (killing a brahmin).

रत्नाकरात्
आकृष्णश्चपलो रूक्षः कपिलः कालिकावृत्तः ।
वंगसंश्लेषदोषेण रसेन्द्रो वातलः स्मृतः ।।१४ ।।
आपीतः कपिलश्चैव कृष्णराजिकया[११]वृत्तः ।
आरजीर्णं विजानीयात्सूतकं पित्तकोपनम् ।।१५ ।।
श्वेतं च विधि[?] सुस्निग्धं गुरु भाजनभेदिनम् ।
श्लेष्मलं नागजीर्णं च पारदं प्राणहारिणम् ।।१६ ।।
सर्वरूपधरं सान्द्रं अतिशीतमकंपितम् ।
जीर्णेऽपि रसकंमस्य रसेन्द्रः[१२] सान्निपातिकम् ।।१७ ।।
रसेन्द्रं वर्जयेद्यत्नादीदृशं च घनं गुरुम् ।

म्रियन्ते[13] जन्तवः सर्वे भक्षणादपरीक्षणात् ।।१८।।
मुक्तं द्वादशभिर्दोषैर्यस्तु हन्याच्छिवात्मजम् ।
ऐहिके तत्तु पूज्यः स्यात्परत्रे स्वर्गतां भवेत् ।
गुणप्रच्छादकाः 'सप्तकंचुकाः'[14] पारदे मताः ।।१९।।

According to Rasaratnākara

Because of the contact (mixture) of *vaṅga*, mercury becomes blackish, *capala* (more fickle), ununctuous, brownish black, covered with a black layer and aggravator of *vāyu.*

Because of the mixture of *āra*, mercury becomes yellowish, brownish black, covered with black lines and aggravator of *pitta*.

Because of the mixture of the *nāga*, mercury becomes white, excessively unctuous, heavy, *bhājanabhedin* (it penitrates into and causes cracks in the container) and aggravator of *kapha*. If taken in, it causes death of the patient.

Because of the mixture of *rasakampa,* mercury becomes variegated in colour , dense, excessively cold to touch, less of quivering and aggravator of all the three *doṣa-s*.

Mercury of the above mentioned characteristic features and mercury which is thick as well as heavy should be carefully rejected . If not examined properly and taken in, it causes death of all living creatures.

If a physician prepares *bhasma* of mercury which is free from twelve types of defect (seven *kañcuka-s* and five *doṣa-s*), he becomes respected during his lifetime and gets liberation after death.

Seven types of *kañcuka-s* work like sheaths of all the attributes of mercury.

अथ रसराजलक्ष्मीतः[15]

नत्वा गुरुं भैरवं कन्यकां वटुं द्विपाननं सिद्धमनुष्यलक्षितम् ।
अन्तःसुनीलं बहिरुज्ज्वलरसं निवेशयेत् खल्वतले शुभेदिने ।।२०।।
जलमृण्मयपाषाणनाशने सप्तकैस्त्रिभिः ।
वज्रकादिकमालाशकषायेण[16] प्रमर्दयेत् ।।२१।।
चित्रकक्वाथे संघृष्टा कपाली घाति वंगजा ।
वज्रकन्दरसेनैव याति वंगजकालिका ।।२२।।
कटुतुम्बीरसेनैव श्यामा नश्यति नागजा ।

बीजकक्वाथसंपिष्टा क्मालीनागसंभवा ।।२३।।
एकेन लशुनेनापि शुद्धो भवति पारदः[१७] ।
सप्तसप्तदिनं पिष्टः शुद्धो भवति सूतकः ।।२४।।
फलत्रयं चित्रककृष्णसर्षपाः कुमारिका च बृहतीकषाये ।
विमर्द्य सूतं त्रिदिनानि यावद्विमुच्यते पञ्चमलादिदोषैः ।।२५।।
एवं संसाधितः[१८] सूतः स्वेदनार्थं[१९] प्रयोजयेत् ।।२६।।

According to Rasarājalakṣmī

After offering prayer to the teacher, Bhairava, virgin girls, *vaṭu* (young brahmin sons), Gaṇeśa and *siddha-s* (those who have attained perfection), in an auspicious day, the physician should place mercury which is blue in the centre and dazzling outside in a clean mortar (*khalva*). Thereafter, for the removal of defects caused by the mixture of water, earth and stones, it should be triturated by adding the decoction of *vajraka, palāśa,* etc., for twenty one times in each.

Trituration with the decoction of *citraka* removes the *kāpālī doṣa* caused by *vaṅga*.

Trituration with the juice of the rhizome of *vajra* removes the *kālikā doṣa* caused by *vaṅga*.

Trituration with the juice of *kaṭu tumbī* removes the *śyāmā doṣa* caused by *nāga*.

Trituration with the decoction of *bījaka* removes *kapālī doṣa* caused by *nāga*.

Trituration with the juice of *laśuna* alone even removes all these defects and makes the mercury pure.

In each of these ingredients, mercury should be triturated, at least, for seven days to make it pure.

Mercury triturated with the decoction of *triphalā, citraka,* black mustard, *kumārī* and *bṛhatī* for three days becomes free from the five types of *doṣa-s,* viz., *mala,* etc.

Mercury purified in the above mentioned manner should be taken for *svedana* (fomentation).

शैवालभक्षः

भिषग्विमर्दयेच्चूर्णैर्मिलित्वा षोडशांशतः ।
प्रमर्द्योष्णारनालेन[२०] क्षालयेत्काचभाजने ।।२७।।

उष्ण एव रसः कार्यः शीतं सर्वात्मना त्यजेत् ।
शीते च बहवो दोषाः षंढाद्याः[21] संभवन्ति हि ।।२८।।
दृढं प्रमर्दयेत् सूतं रक्षितं द्वित्रिसेवकैः ।।२९।।
सहस्रनिंबूफलतोयघृष्टो रसो भवेद्वह्निसमप्रभावः ।।३०।।
राजिकाचित्रकहिंगुलवणं व्योषसंयुतम् ।।३१।।
सूतपादमितं सर्वं स्वर्जिकाक्षारसंयुतम् ।।३२।।
शिग्रुपत्ररसेनैव पिष्ट्वा कुण्डलिकाकृतिम् ।
कुर्याद्भूर्जदले सम्यगथवा कदलीदले ।।३३।।
सुपक्वे सुदृढे वापि वस्त्रखण्डे चतुर्गुणे[22] ।।३४।।
रसं मध्ये विनिक्षिप्य बध्नीयात्तु सुपोटलिम् ।।३५।।
क्षीराम्लमूत्रवर्गेण स्वेदयेच्च दिनत्रयम् ।
तथा स्वेदः प्रकर्तव्यो मज्जिता पोटली यथा ।।३६।।
भवेन्न च तलस्पर्शो भाण्डस्यापि कदाचन ।।३७।।

Svedana of Mercury
According to Śaivālabhakṣa

The physician should add all the powders of drugs in the quantity of 1/16th of mercury and triturate. Thereafter, keeping the mercury in a glass pan, it should be washed with hot *āranāla* (a type of vinegar). For processing mercury, washing should always be done with hot liquids . Washing with cold liquids give rise to several defects like *ṣaṇḍha* (impotency of mercury), etc.

Trituration should be done with the strong hands and for this purpose, the pyhsician should engage two or three attendants.

Trituration with the juice of one thousand lemons, makes the mercury very powerful like fire.

Rājikā, *citraka*, *hiṅgu*, *lavaṇa*, *vyoṣa (trikaṭu)* and *svarjikṣāra* should be taken in the total quantity of one fourth of mercury, and by adding the juice of *śigru*-leaf it should be triturated. The paste should be made to a round bolus form and kept appropriately over the bark of *bhūrja* or leaf of *kadalī*. This should then be wrapped with the four layers of thick and strong cloth. In the centre of the paste, mercury shuold be kept and the wrapped cloth should thereafter be tied with a string. This should then be given fomentation (*svedana*) for three days with milk, vinegar and cow's urine (ingredients belonging to the groups of milk, vinegar and urine). During fomentation, it should be ensured that the *poṭṭalī* (round mass) is fully submerged in the liquid and it does not touch the bottom of the vessel.

रसार्णवात्
'अथ द्रवेण भाण्डस्य पूरितार्धस्य तस्य च।
मुखे तिर्यक् कृते दण्डे रसं सूत्रेण लम्बितम्।
तं स्वेदयेत्तलगतं दोलायन्त्रमिति स्मृतम्' ।।३८।।
[रसार्णव : चतुर्थपटल : ७]

Svedana of Mercury and Dolā Yantra According to Rasārṇava

Half of the jar [of *dolā yantra*] should be filled with the [prescribed] liquid, and over the jar, a rod should be placed in transverse position. On this rod, the *poṭṭalī* (round bolus) should be hanged with the help of a string till it is submerged in the liquid at the bottom of the jar. Thereafter, fomentation (*svedana*) should be given [through fuel below the jar]. This is called *dolā yantra*.

भवेदेकैकसंस्कारप्रान्ते सुदृढमर्दनम्।
मर्दितः स्थापयेद्धर्मे यावच्छुष्कतरो भवेत् ।।३९।।
ततो रसं समानीय क्षालयेदिति सर्वतः।
तथा यत्नं प्रकुर्वीत यथा न क्षीयते रसः ।।४०।।

Method of Processing After Saṃskāra

After each *saṃskāra* (special methods of processing), mercury should be strongly triturated. After that, it should be kept exposed to sun till it gets well dried up. Then the mercury should be well washed taking due care to avoid any wastage of it.

रसार्णवात्
कार्पासपत्रनिर्यासैः स्विन्नस्त्रिकटुकान्वितः।
सप्तकंचुकनिर्मुक्तो सप्ताहाज्जायते रसः।

अत्यम्लकाञ्जिकेनापि सोष्णेन[२३] क्षालनं तथा ।।४१ ।।

।। इति स्वेदनम् ।।

Svedana Saṃskāra

According to Rasārṇava

Mercury mixed with *trikaṭu* should be boiled [in a *dolā yantra*] with the juice of *kārpāsa*-leaf for one week. This makes the mercury free from the seven *kañcuka-s*. Thereafter, it should be washed with exceedingly sour and hot vinegar (*kāñjī*).

Thus, ends the description of *svedana* (fomentation) *saṃskāra*.

आश्रयांसरसं वा सुरदाली स्मारणी गजबला च शृगाली' ।
धावनी रजनी वह्निं कुमारी मर्दनाद्भवति दोषविदारी ।।४२ ।।

Mardana Saṃskāra

Trituration with the juice of *āśrayāṃsa, suradālī, smāraṇī, gajabalā, śṛgālī, dhāvanī, rajanī, vahni* and *kumārī* makes mercury free from its defects.

अथ रसदर्पणात्

क्षाराम्लैर्लवणैर्मूत्रैर्विषैरुपविषैस्तथा ।
दिव्यौषधिसमूहेन मर्दयेत्[२४] दिवसत्रयम् ।
पारदस्य कलांशेन भेषजेन प्रमर्दयेत् ।।४३ ।।

।। इति मर्दनम् ।।

[रसकामधेनु : पृष्ठ ३३८ : ५३-५४]

According to Rasadarpaṇa

Mercury, added with 1/16th in quantity of *kṣāra-s* (alkalies), *amla-s* (sour drugs), *lavaṇa-s* (salts), *viṣa-s* (poisonous drugs), *upaviṣa-s* (subsidiary poisonous drugs) and *divyauṣadhi-s* (celestial drugs) for three days should be triturated.

Thus, ends the description of *mardana saṃskāra*.

मलं विषं तथा वह्निदोषा नैसर्गिकास्त्रयः ।
मरणं दाहमोहौ च यथासंख्यं प्रजायते ।।४४ ।।

कुमारीत्रिफलावह्निजटामर्दितमूर्च्छितः ।
प्रकाशते स्वरूपं च रसः परमदुर्लभः ।।४५।।

Mūrchana Saṃskāra

The three *naisargika doṣa-s* (natural defects) of mercury are *mala*, *viṣa* and *vahni* which cause death, burning sensation and unconsciousness respectively. Trituration with *kumārī*, *triphalā* and root of *citraka* causes *mūrcchana* (unconsciousness) of mercury giving rise to its original complexion of excellence.

रसदर्पणात्

सूतः क्षाराम्लमूत्रैर्वसनपरिवृत्तः[२५] स्वेदितोऽष्टौ च यामा ।
कन्यावह्न्यर्कदुग्धैस्त्रिफलजलयुतैः[२६] मूर्च्छितः सप्तवारान् ।।४६।।
पादांशार्केण युक्तः समगगनयुतः तुत्थताप्येन च स्या-
दूर्ध्वं पात्यस्त्रिवारं भवति किल ततः सर्वदोषैर्विमुक्तः ।।४७।।

According to Rasadarpaṇa

Mercury should be wrapped in a cloth and given *svedana* (fomentation) with the help of *kṣāra-s* (alkalies), *amla-s* (sour drugs) and *mūtra-s* (urines) for eight *yāma-s*.

Thereafter, it should be given *mūrcchana saṃskāra* by triturating with the juice or decoction of *kanyā*, *vahni*, milky latex of *arka* and decoction of *triphalā* for seven times. Then by adding copper 1/4th in quantity, equal quantity of mica, *tuttha* and *tāpya*, it should be triturated. Thereafter, three times of *ūrdhva pātana* (sublimation) *saṃskāra* should be performed which makes mercury free from all the defects.

अथ रसचिन्तामणिः

रुद्ध्वा डमरुके यन्त्रे याममेकं तु वह्निना ।
अमूर्च्छितः प्रदातव्यः कलांशे मूर्च्छिते रसे ।।४८।।
दोलास्वेदं प्रकुर्वीत मधुक्षाराम्लमूत्रकैः ।
उत्थाप्य मूर्च्छयेत्पश्चात् त्रिवारं च पुनः पुनः ।।४९।।

।। इति मूर्च्छनविधिः ।।

According to Rasacintāmaṇi

Mercury, which has not undergone *mūrcchana saṃskāra*, should be kept sealed inside a *ḍamaru yantra* and cooked with fire for one *yāma*. After *mūrcchanā*, mercury should be cooked in *dolā yantra* with honey, alkalies, sour drugs and urines. Thereafter, it should be revived (*utthāpana*). The process of *mūrcchana* and *utthāpana* should be repeated for three times.

Thus, ends the description of *mūrcchana saṃskāra*.

ततः खल्वेन तप्तेन अम्लेनोत्थापयेद्रसम् ।
क्षाराः मुखकराः सर्वे सर्वे अम्लाः प्रबोधकाः ॥५०॥

Utthāpana Saṃskāra

After *mūrcchana saṃskāra*, mercury should be kept in a *tapta khalva* (hot mortar made of iron) and triturated with sour liquids. All the alkalies promote the desire (*mukhakara*) and all the sour liquids stimulate (*prabodhaka*) the power of digestion of mercury.

रसदर्पणात्[१७]

"फलत्रयाग्न्यासुरिशिग्रुसिन्धुजैः कुर्वन्ति सूतं भृशं नष्टपिष्टकम् ।
तेनैव भाण्डस्य पिधानपात्रकंलिपेदधस्तात्तदधः स्थितेऽपि ॥५१॥
जलं क्षिपेत्तत्र पिधानभाण्डकादुपर्यथाग्निं ज्वलयेद्यथाऽप्यधः ।
सूतः पतेन्नूनमोर्द्धपातस्तत्तद्वैपरीत्येन भवेद्रसस्य च ॥५२॥
[रसकामधेनु : पृष्ट ३४० : ८०-८१]

Pātana Saṃskāra

According to Rasadarpaṇa

Mercury triturated by adding *triphalā*, *citraka*, *āsuri*, *śigru* and *saindhava* loses its paste form (*naṣṭa piṣṭa*) and becomes divided into small globules. This mercury should be smeared at the back of the lid. It should be kept over a jar containing water [and the joint of the lid and the jar should be sealed]. Over this lid, fire should be ignited as a result of which the mercury smeared at the back of the upper lid will fall down into the water of the lower jar. This is called *adhaḥ pātana*. If done in the reverse order, the process is called *ūrdhva pātana*.

वह्निं खदिरसारेण मध्यं यामद्वयं कुरु ॥५३॥

[For both the *adhaḥ* and *ūrdhva pātana*], heat should be applied with the fuel of the heart wood of *khadira*. The heat should be of morderate nature and should be applied for two *yāma-s*.

नष्टपिष्टलक्षणम्

स्वरूपस्य विनाशेन पिष्ट्वाऽऽपादनं रसः[28] ।
विषाग्निवर्जितश्चापि नष्टपिष्टः स उच्यते ।।५४।।

Naṣṭa-piṣṭa

Destruction of the original paste form of mercury by trituration [with drugs] is called *naṣṭa piṣṭa*. Such processed mercury is free from *viṣa* and *agni doṣa-s*.

अथ रसरत्नाकरात्

अजाशकृत्तुषाग्निं तु[29] दीपयित्वा विचक्षणः ।
तस्योपरि स्थितं खल्वं तप्तखल्वं[30] विनिर्दिशेत् ।।५५।।

।। इति तप्तखल्वलक्षणम् ।।

[रसरत्नाकर : रसखण्ड : द्वितीयोपदेश : १०]

Tapta Khalva : According to Rasaratnākara

Fire should be made of the stool of goat or the husk of paddy Over this fuel, the mortar (*khalva*) should be placed. This is called *tapta khalva*.

रससिन्धुः

मिश्रितौ तद्रसे नागवंगौ विक्रयहेतुना ।
ताभ्यां स्यात्कृत्रिमो दोषस्तन्मुक्तिः पातनत्रयात् ।
नागवंगविनाशार्थमथ सूतं निपातयेत् ।।५६।।

Pātana Saṃskāra
According to Rasasindhu

For commercial purpose (to get more profit), *nāga* (lead) and *vaṅga* (tin) are added to mercury. Thus, an artificial *doṣa* (impurity) is introduced into the mercury by these two which can be separated by three types of *pātana* (upward sublimation, downward sublimation and distillation). Therefore, to remove *nāga* (lead) and *vaṅga* (tin), mercury should be treated by the process of *pātana*.

रसचिन्तामणिः

भागत्रयं[३१] रसस्यार्कचूर्णं पादांशसंयुतम् ।
दत्त्वाम्लं मर्दयेत्तावद्यावत्पिष्टी प्रजायते ।
"यदा न जायते पिष्टी किञ्चित्तुत्थं तदा क्षिपेत् ।।५७।।

।। इति सर्वत्र[३२] ।।

Preparation of Piṣṭi or Paste According to Rasacintāmaṇi

Three parts of mercury and one part of the *bhasma* of copper should be triturated by adding the juice of lemon or vinegar till a paste is formed. If the paste is not formed then a small quantity of *tuttha* (copper sulphate) should be added and triturated which will help in the formation of the paste. This rule should always be applied.

कटाहं नूतनं कृत्वा तस्याधो लेपयेद्रसम् ।
द्विगुणेन तु वस्त्रेण जटयेद्बुध्नकादधः ।
वस्त्रात्तानि मृदा लिप्त्वा जलस्थाल्युपरि न्यसेत् ।
स्थालीकटाहयोः सन्धिः[३३] लेपयेत्सुदृढं मृदा ।।५८।।
कटाहोपरि कर्त्तव्यमुपलाग्निप्रदीपनम् ।
जलमध्ये रसो याति शुल्वं[३४] तिष्ठति बुध्नके ।।५९।।
'शुल्वाद्रसो[३५] रसात्ताम्रं पातनेयं पृथक्कृतम् ।
ससूतभाण्डवदने मन्याद्गिलति भाण्डकम् ।।६०।।
तथा सन्धिर्द्वयोः कार्यः पातनत्रययन्त्रके[३६]' ।
जलस्थाने कांजिकं च दापयेन्नात्र संशयः ।।६१।।

।। इत्यधःपातनम् ।।

Adhaḥ Pātana (Downward Sublimation)

At the back of a new pan, the paste of mercury and copper should be smeared. Over the paste, two layers of cloth should be wrapped and this cloth should then be smeared with mud. This pan should be placed [with bottom downwards] over a jar containing water. The joint between the jar (below) and the pan (placed over it) should be tightly sealed by smearing mud. Over the pan, fire should be given with the cow-dung cakes. Thus, the mercury will fall down (by the effect of heat) into the water of the jar placed below and the copper will remain in the back of the pan. In this way, mercury gets separated from copper and the copper gets separated from mercury. The shape of the upper pan should be of same size and shape so that it just fits into the brim of the jar below containing water. The joint of these two jars should be tightly sealed in all the three types of *pātana*. In the place of water, *kāñjī* (a type of vinegar) should be kept in the jar below.

Thus, ends the description of *adhaḥ pātana* (downward sublimation).

पुनः पिष्टी प्रकर्त्तव्या दत्वाम्लं ताम्रसंयुतम्[३७]" ।
[रसकामधेनु : पृष्ठ ३४१-३४२ : ९२-९७]
तं पिण्डं तलभाण्डस्थमूर्द्धभाण्डे हि[३८] रोधयेत् ।।६२।।
सन्धिर्मृत्कर्पटैर्लिप्त्वा चुल्यामारोपयेत्ततः ।
शनैर्वह्निं दहेद् दत्वा ऊर्द्धभाण्डे जलं क्षिपेत् ।
कृत्वालवालं केनापि त्रियामात्सूतमुद्धरेत् ।।६३।।

Ūrdhva Pātana (Upward Sublimation)

Mercury, after *adhaḥ pātana* (downward sublimation) should again be made to a paste form by triturating with copper and sour juice. The bolus mercury should be kept in the lower jar and the latter should be covered with another jar. The joint between these two jars should be sealed with mud-smeared cloth and both the jars should be kept over an oven. The fuel should be slowly ignited and water should be poured over the upper jar. The cooking should be done for three *yāma-s* and then the mercury at the bottom should be washed and collected.

तथा च रसप्रदीपे
रसं च भाण्डद्वयगर्भमध्ये पिष्टीं ततः सम्पुटमव्रणान्तम् ।
निवेश्य चुल्यासु शनैः प्रदाय प्रमाणमस्याथ तले विदध्यात् ।।६४।।

अग्निं शिरस्वस्थं जलार्द्रमेकं वस्त्रं क्षिपेदल्पमनुष्यमेवम् ।
वास्त्रयेनो रसवंगसंज्ञौ[39] नष्टः प्रदिष्टो ह्ययमूर्द्धपातः ।।६५।।

।। इत्यूर्द्धपातनम् ।।

According to Rasapradīpa

[The text appears to be corrupt; hence left untranslated.]

'रसार्णवात्[40]

घटे रसं विनिक्षिप्य सजलं घटमन्यकम् ।
तिर्यक् भांडद्वयं कृत्वा सुमुखं रोधयेत् सुधीः ।।६६।।
रसाधो ज्वालयेदग्निं यावत्सूतो[41] जलं विशेत् ।
तिर्यक्पातनमित्युक्तं सिद्धैर्नागार्जुनादिभिः' ।।६७।।

[रसेन्द्रसारसंग्रह : रसशास्त्र : पृष्ठ १२-१३]

रसं रसपिष्टिः ।।६८।।

Tiryak Pātana Saṃskāra (Distillation)

Two jars should be taken. In one of them mercury should be kept and the other should be filled with water. These two jars should be kept in oblique position so that the brims of the both come together and the joint of these brims should be sealed. Below the jar containing mercury, heat should be applied till the mercury kept in it gets vapourised and goes to the second jar containing water. This process is called *tiryak pātana* by Siddha Nāgārjuna, etc.

In the present context, the paste of mercury (*rasa piṣṭī*) should be used for *tiryak pātana* (distillation).

"खर्परं पृथुकं सम्यक् विस्तारस्तस्य[42] मध्यमे ।
आलवालं पुटैः कृत्वा तन्मध्ये[43] पारदं क्षिपेत्" ।।६९।।

[रसकामधेनु : पृष्ठ ९ : ६१]

ऊर्द्धाधस्तु विडं दत्वा मल्लेनारुध्य यत्नतः ।
ऊर्द्ध्वं देयं पुटं तस्य यन्त्रं कच्छपसंज्ञकम् ।
"जारणार्थं रसस्योक्तं गन्धादीनां विशेषतः ।।७०।।
कच्छपयन्त्रम् ।।७१।।

Kacchapa (Tortoise) Yantra

In the middle of a jar [containing water], a piece of *kharpara* (piece of broken jar) should be kept and in the centre of this, mercury wrapped with paste, leaves and cloth should be placed. *Viḍa* should be placed over and under this mercury and the whole thing should be surrounded by *malla* (arsenic). [The jar should then be covered with a lid and the joint should be sealed.] Above this lid, *puṭa* (fire) should be applied. This is called *kacchapa yantra*. This is used for *jāraṇa* of mercury specially by adding sulphur, etc.

तथा च

जलपूर्णं दृढं पात्रं सुविशालं समाहरेत ।
तदन्तः खर्परं दद्यात्सविस्तीर्णं दृढं[44] नवम् ।।७२।।
[रसकामधेनु : पृष्ठ ९ : ६२]
विडं दत्त्वा तदुपरि क्षिपेद्बीजभुजं[45] रसम् ।
उपरिष्टाद्विडं दद्यात्ततो लोहकटोरिकाम् ।।७३ ।।
अयस्कान्तमयीं वापि पत्तलीभूतविग्रहाम् ।
उपरिष्टादधो वक्त्रां दत्वा सम्यग्विलेपयेत् ।।७४ ।।
खटीपुटं शिवां भक्तं सम्यग्निः पिष्यमुद्रयेत् ।
उपरिष्टाद्वनोत्थानैरंगारैः खर्परं धमेत् ।।७५ ।।
[रसकामधेनु : पृष्ठ १० : ६३-६५]

कच्छपयन्त्रः ।। ७६ ।।

Kacchapa (Tortoise) Yantra (Second Description)

A spacious and strong jar should be filled with water. Inside it a wide piece of new *kharpara* should be placed. Over it, *viḍa* should be kept and on it mercury which is to be processed for digesting *bīja* should be placed. It should be covered above with another layer of *viḍa*. The whole thing should be covered with an iron pan or thin pan prepared of *ayaskānta maṇi* with its mouth facing downwards. The joint of the jar and the pan should be appropriately sealed with the paste of chalk, *śivā*, rice, *sami* and *agni*. Cowdung cakes collected from the forest should be ignited over it and blown with the help of a blower. This is called *kacchapa* (tortoise) *yantra*.

वृंताककरमूषे द्वे तयोः कुर्यादधः खलु ।
प्रादेशमात्रनलिकामृदालिप्तसुसन्धिका ।।७७।।
तत्रैकस्यां क्षिपेत्सूतमन्यस्यां गन्धचूर्णकम् ।
निरुध्य मूषयोर्वक्त्रं शलुकायन्त्रके क्षिपेत् ।।७८।।
गन्धाधो[४६] ज्वालयेद्वह्निं तुलायन्त्रमुदाहृतम् ।
तालगन्धाश्मताराणां जारणार्थमुदाहृतम् ।।७९।।

Tulā(Balance) Yantra

Two crucibles of the shape of *vṛntāka* (fruit of egg-plant or brinjel) should be taken and at their lower ends a connecting tube should be inserted. The joints of the crucibles and the tube should be properly sealed with mud. In one of these crucibles mercury should be kept and in the other the powder of sulphur. Then the opening (upper parts) of these two crucibles should be sealed and kept inside a *śalukā-yantra*. Fire should be given at the crucible containing sulphur. This is called *tulā* (balance) *yantra*. It is used for the *jāraṇa* (digestion) of *haritāla*, *gandhaka* and *tāra* in the mercury.

अथवा वेतसं [?] सूतं काकिनीरेतसा दिनम्[४७] ।
मर्दयेच्चेतसा [?] गाढं ऊर्ध्वपातनतो ग्रहेत् ।।८०।।

Bodhana (Rodhana) Saṃskāra

Mercury should be mixed with the *retas* (secretion of the bartholin gland or the menstrual blood) of a ***kākinī*** type of woman and strongly triturated for one day. Thereafter, mercury should be retrieved with the help of *ūrdhva pātana* (upward sublimation).

शिवागमात्
यस्याः स्युः कुटिलाः केशाः श्यामांगी रक्तलोचना ।
अश्वत्थपत्रसदृशो गुह्यदेशो विराजितः[४८] ।
कृष्णपक्षे पुष्पवती सा नारी काकिनी मता ।।८१।।
तस्या देयं त्रिसप्ताहं गन्धकं घृतसंयुतम् ।
तद्रसे च रसं सम्यक् मर्दयेदुक्तकर्मसु ।
बन्धनार्थं विशेषेण [सूतं कस्य?] प्रयोजयेत् ।।८२।।

Identification of Kākinī Woman According to Śivāgama

A woman whose hair are curled, whose complexion is bluish, whose eyes are red, the shape of whose genital organ is like that of the leaf of *aśvattha*, and who menstruates during the dark fortnight (*kṛṣṇa pakṣa*) is called *kākinī*. This type of woman should be given sulphur with ghee to eat for three weeks and along with her menstrual blood, mercury should be triturated for the purpose of further processing. This type of treatment of mercury is specially required for the *bandhana* (prevention of vapourisation) of mercury.

मर्दनमूर्च्छनपातैः कदार्थितो[४९] मन्दवीर्यत्वम् ।
सृष्ट्यंबुजैर्निरोधं लब्ध्वा प्रायो न षंढः स्यात् ।।८३ ।।

Removing Impotency

Because of the *saṃskāra-s* (processes) of *mardana*, *mūrcchana* and *pātana*, the mercury becomes tortured which reduces its potency. Because of this *rodhana saṃskāra* with the help of menstrual blood (*sṛṣṭyambu*) the mercury generally do not become impotent.

अथ सूतं समुद्धृत्य काचकूप्यां विनिःक्षिपेत् ।
शुक्ताम्लेनाथ संपूर्य द्वारे मुद्रां प्रदापयेत् ।।८४ ।।
स्थापयेद्भूधरे यन्त्रे स्वेदयेद्दिनसप्तकम् ।
स्वांगशीतं समुद्धृत्य क्वाथैः स्वेदयेत्पुनः ।।८५ ।।
कर्कोटीकञ्चुकीवह्निसर्पाक्ष्यम्बुजमार्कवैः ।
दिनत्रयं[५०] चारनालैः स्वेद्यश्चापल्यशान्तये ।।८६ ।।

।। इति नियमनसंस्कारः ।।

Niyamana Saṃskāra

After the *rodhana saṃskāra*, mercury should be retrieved and kept in a glass bottle. The remaining empty space of the bottle should be filled with *śukta* (vinegar) and *amla* (sour juice). The mouth of the bottle should then be corcked. It should be kept in a *Bhūdhara yantra* and cooked (fomented) for seven days. After it has cooled down, the mercury should be taken out of the bottle and fomented again with the decoctions of *karkoṭī*, *kañcukī*, *vahni*, *sarpākṣī*, *ambuja* and *mārkava*, and *āranāla* (a type of vinegar) for three days. This reduces the fickleness (*cāpalya*) of mercury.

"लवणराजिकाहिंगुकन्याक्षारचतुष्टयम् ।
त्र्यूषणं लशुनं चैव मातुलुङ्गरसाप्लुतम् ।।८७।।
पिण्डिमध्ये रसं कृत्वा स्वेदयेत्सप्तधा पुनः ।
अनुद्‌गरी भवेत्तेन ग्रासो जीर्णोऽपि जीर्यति" ।।८८।।
[रसकामधेनु : पृष्ठ ३४८ : १५०-१५२]
अनेनैव भवेच्छुद्धः सर्वदोषविवर्जितः ।
निश्चलः स्वच्छरूपश्च कांजिकादिविशोधितः ।।८९।।
क्षारः सर्वं मलं हन्ति लवणं ग्रन्थिभेदनम् ।
स्वेदोप्यजीर्णतां हन्ति षंढत्वं पटुकाम्लकम्" ।।९०।।
।। इति दीपनसंस्कारश्चाष्टमः ।।

Dīpana Saṃskāra

A paste should be prepared of *lavaṇa*, *rājikā*, *hiṅgu*, *kumārī*, four types of *kṣāra*, *trikaṭu* and *laśuna* by adding the juice of *mātuluṅga*. This paste should be made to a bolus form and in the centre of this bolus, mercury should be kept. [In a *dolā yantra*], this bolus including mercury should be cooked for seven times. By doing so, the metals digested by the mercury do not come out and become fully digested.

Being processed in the above manner and being washed with *kāñjika* (a type of vinegar) etc., mercury becomes pure and free from all defects. It remains stable and clean. *Kṣāra-s* (alkalies) remove the *mala doṣa*. *Lavaṇa* removes the knots (*granthi*), *svedana* (fomentation) corrects indigestion, and pungent as well as sour ingredients used for processing mercury remove its impotency.

Thus, ends the eighth *dīpana saṃskāra*.

अष्टौ रससंस्काराः द्रव्ये च रसायने च समाः ।।९१।।
एते प्रथमं कार्याः पश्चात्सर्वत्र योजयेद्रसराजम्"[२] ।।९२।।
विधिमेनं परित्यज्य योऽन्यथा कुरुते शवः [?] ।
न सिद्धिर्जायते तस्य रसे वाऽथ रसायने ।।९३।।

Eight Saṃskāra-s

The first eight *saṃskāra-s* are equally relevant for *lauha siddhi* (transmutation of the basic metals into noble metals like gold) and *rasāyana* or *deha siddhi* (rejuvenation of the body and curing diseases). These eight *saṃskāra-s* should be performed in the beginning and only thereafter, mercury should be used for all the different purposes.

If an unwise person procedes with the use of mercury ignoring these eight *saṃskāra-s*, then he does not attain *siddhi* (accomplishment of perfection) either in *lauha* (transmutation of basic metals into noble metals) or in *rasāyana* (rejuvenation of the body).

एवं विशोधितः सूतो भवेदष्टांगशोधितः[५३] ।
स्यात्[५४] भृंगशृङ्गवेराभ्यां मार्क्वार्द्रहरिद्रया ।।१४।।
उत्थानाद्यवशिष्टं तु ऊर्ध्वपातनयन्त्रके।
धृतोर्द्धभाण्डसंलग्नं संग्रहेत्पारदं बुधः ।।१५।।

।। इत्यष्टौ संस्कारा[५५]: ।।

In the above mentioned manner, processing of mercury, will make it totally (*aṣṭāṅga*) pure. Thus, mercury, retrieved after *pātana saṃskāra*, etc. should be added with either *bhṛṅgarāja*, and *śṛṅgavera*, or *mārkava*, *ārdraka* and *haridrā*, triturated and made to a paste. The paste, thus obtained, should be processed through *ūrdhva pātana yantra*. The mercury, thus got adhered to the bottom of the upper jar, should be collected.

Thus, ends the description of the [first] eight *saṃskāra-s* of mercury.

अजीर्णं तु अबीजं तु सूतकं यस्तु घातयेत् ।
ब्रह्महा स दुराचारी मम द्वेषी महेश्वरी[५६] ।।१६।।
मूषायामभ्रलिप्तायां चतुःषष्ट्यंशकादिना ।
विधिना गंधकं दत्वा भूधरे तं पुटेल्लघु ।।१७।।

Calcination or Māraṇa of Mercury

If a person does *māraṇa* (calcination) of mercury which is *ajīrṇa* (in which *jāraṇa* has not been done) and *abīja* (in which *bīja* or seed is not added) then he is a scoundrel and he is an enemy of Lord Śiva.

[For the preparation of the *bhasma*], mercury should be placed in a crucible smeared with mica. To this mercury, 1/64th in quantity or in similar other proportions, sulphur should be added. This crucible should be placed in *bhūdhara yantra* and cooked in *laghu puṭa*.

रसराजहंसात्

इत्थं संदीपितः सूतो विद्युत्कोटिसमप्रभः ।
यस्त्वेवं विधिमासाद्य जारणाक्रमवर्जितम्[९७] ।
सूतकं मारयेत्तेन मारितं सकलं जगत् ।।९८।।
न भवेत्तस्य संसिद्धिः रसे वाथ रसायने।
द्रष्टव्यं परिभाषायां जारणाक्रममुत्तमम् ।।९९।।

According to Rasarājahaṃsa

The mercury, after eight *saṃskāra-s,* becomes ignited of its digestive power (*sandīpita*) and it possesses the lusture of crores of lightening. If these processes of eight *saṃskāra-s* and *jāraṇā* are not followed before the *māraṇa* (calcination; lit. killing) of mercury, then with this misdeed, the physician causes death of all the people in the universe. Such a person becomes incapable of attaining perfection in *rasa* (transmutation of basic metals into noble ones) and *rasāyana* (rejuvenating effect of mercury).

In the chapter on *paribhāṣā* (of *Rasarāja-haṃsa*), the process of *jāraṇā* is elaborated.

अथ रससिन्धुः

देव्या रजो भवेद्गन्धो धातु शुक्लमथाभ्रकः ।
आलिङ्गने समर्थौ द्वौ प्रियत्वाच्छिवरेतसः ।।१००।।
आश्लेषादेतयोः सूतो न[९८] वेत्ति मृतिजं भवम् ।
शिवशक्तिसमायोगे प्राप्यते परमं पंदम् ।।१०१।।

Affinity of Mercury with Sulphur and Mercury According to Rasasindhu

The *rajas* (menstrual blood) of the goddess Pārvatī is sulphur and the *śukra* (ovum or secretion of bartholin gland) is mica. Both of them are capable of embracing (binding) the mercury which is the semen of Lord Śiva because of their inherent love for the latter. Because of their embrace (binding effect) the mercury does not experience the pain (undergo deterioration) by the process of *māraṇa*.

Because of the combination of Śiva (mercury) and *Śakti* (sulphur and mica), a person doing the processing of mercury attains liberation.

षड्गुणे गन्धके जीर्णे रसो भवति रोगहा ।
तस्माद् गन्धं सुशुद्धं हि जीर्यते रसरेतसि ।।१०२।।

Ganadhaka Jāraṇa

jāraṇā of mercury with six times of sulphur makes the former capable of curing all diseases. It is the purified sulphur which is useful in the *jāraṇā* of mercury (the semen of Lord Śiva).

'अथाभ्रं, गौरीतेजः परमममृतं वातपित्तं क्षयार्त्तम् ।
प्रज्ञोद्बोधि प्रशमितजरं वृष्यमायुष्यमग्र्यम् ।।१०३।।
बल्यं स्निग्धं रुचिरसकफं दीपनं शीतवीर्यम् ।
तत्तद्योगे सकलगदहृद् व्योमसूतेन्द्रवेधी'[१] ।।१०४।।

Abhraka Jāraṇa

Abhraka is the procreating element (*tejas*) of the goddess Gaurī and it is the ambrosia *par excellence* . It cures the diseases caused by *vāyu* and *pitta* and tuberculosis. It prevents ageing process and promotes virility, longevity and strength. It is unctuous, promoter of wisdom, appetite , *rasa dhātu* and *kapha* and stimulant of digestion. It is cooling in potency . With the addition of appropriate drugs, it cures all diseases. Its addition to mercury makes the latter capable of *vedhana* (transmutation of basic metals into noble ones).

गौरीयन्त्रं प्रवक्ष्यामि सुखदं जारणाविधौ ।
अष्टाङ्गुलोच्छ्रयां कृत्वा चतुरस्त्रं समेष्टकाम् ।।१०५।।
सूतमानात्समुत्कृष्य मध्ये चूर्णेन लेपयेत् ।
श्लक्ष्णवस्त्रावृतां पिष्टीं कृत्वा प्राग्बद्धताम्रजाम् ।।१०६।।
रूप्यजां हेमजो वापि स्वसत्वेनापि निर्मिताम् ।
निवेश्य तत्र चोर्द्धाधो बलेः चूर्णं पिधाय च ।।१०७।।
तस्या पिष्ट्याश्चतुर्थांशं वारं वारं विशोषयेत्[६०] ।
वक्त्रे खर्परचक्रीं तु दत्वा लेप्य विशोष्य च ।।१०८।।

ऊर्ध्वं हयखुराकारं पुटं दद्याल्लघूपलैः ।
शीते[61] पुटे बलौ[62] जीर्णे पुनस्तद्वद्बलिं न्यसेत् ।।१०९।।
रुद्ध्वा[63] पुटं पुनर्दद्याद्यथा स्यात्षट्गुणावधिः ।
यथेष्टविक्रमेणैव[64] जारयेद्वापि गन्धकम् ।।११०।।
बालसूर्यनिभः साक्षात्खोटी भवति सूतकः ।
विचूर्ण्य[65] सर्वरोगेषु मूर्छितं तं प्रयोजयेत् ।।१११।।
जारणादभ्रवज्राणां पातयेत्पातनाविधौ ।
द्रवरूपस्तेन रसः स्यादीषल्लोहितप्रभः ।।११२।।

।। गौरीयन्त्ररसार्णवात्[66] ।।

Gaurī Yantra
According to Rasārṇava

Now will be described the *Gaurī yantra* which is useful in the *jāraṇā* of mercury with sulphur. A pit should be dug on the earth with its boundary wall made of bricks. It should be eight *aṅgula-s* in length , breadth and height. Leaving the space for mercury the remaining part of this pit should be filled with the plaster of lime. Mercury should first of all be made to a paste by triturating with copper, silver, gold or *sattva* of mica and thereafter, wrapped in a silken cloth and tied. This bolus should be placed in the hole with the powder of sulphur below and above it. The quantity of sulphur, thus added, should be one foruth of that of mercury. It should be repeatedly allowed to get dried. A circular piece of *kharpara* (piece of broken jar) should be placed over this bolus of mercury placed in the hole and the joint should be sealed with mud and dried. Above it, in the shape of the hoof of a horse, *puṭa* should be given with the fuel of light cowdung cakes. After the *puṭa* is cooled down and the sulphur is digested, again fresh quality of sulphur should be added, the hole should be sealed and *puṭa* should be given. This process should be continued till the *jāraṇā* is done with six times of sulphur. More of sulphur can also be used for *jāraṇā* if it is intended to make mercury more potent. By this process of *jāraṇā*, mercury becomes solid (*khoṭī*) and looks [pink] like a rising sun. This mercury should be made to a powder and in this powder form (*mūrchita*) it should be used in all types of diseases.

For the purpose of *jāraṇā* with *abhraka* (mica) and *vajra* (diamond) the solidified mercury obtained with the above mentioned process should be distilled (*pātana*) according to the prescribed procedure . Thus, mercury can be retrieved in liquid form but in a slightly pinkish form.

गन्धकस्य क्षयो नास्ति न रसस्य क्षयो भवेत् ।
क्षयोऽयं तमविज्ञाय यन्त्रे विक्रियते[६७] क्रियाम् ॥११३॥
सम्यग्यंत्रपरिज्ञानात्किञ्चित्सूतक्षयो भवेत् ।
वह्निलक्ष्यमविज्ञाय रसस्यार्द्धं क्षयो भवेत्[६८] ।
अथवा सर्वशो हानिर्जायतेति ध्रुवं वचः ॥११४॥

Loss of Mercury and Sulphur

By the above mentioned process neither the sulphur nor the mercury is diminished in quantity. If such diminution takes place and the physician is unable to notice it, then the process becomes defective. If the defect in the *yantra* (instrument) is located in time , then there will be loss of only a small quantity of mercury. If the physician is unable to locate this defect which can be ascertained from the flame then almost half of the mercury gets lost. Ignorance of the physician may even result in complete loss of mercury.

अथ रत्नाकरात्
"वर्तुला गोस्तनाकारा वज्रमूषा प्रकीर्तिता ।
द्वौ भागौ तुषदग्धस्य एकं वल्मीकमृत्तिका ॥११५॥
लोहकिट्टस्य भागैकं श्वेतपाषाणभागकम् ।
नरकेशं समं[६९] किञ्चिच्छागीक्षीरेण पेषयेत् ॥११६॥
यामद्वयं दृढं मर्द्यं तेन मूषाऽथ सम्पुटम् ।
शोषयित्वा रसं क्षिप्त्वा तत्कल्कैः सन्धिः[७०] रुध्यते ॥११७॥
वज्रमूषा हीयं ख्याता सम्यक् सूतस्य[७१] मारणे ।
यावदाकृष्णतां याति तावद्दाह्यं तुषादिकम्[७२]" ॥११८॥

॥ इति वज्रमूषा ॥

[रसकामधेनु : पृष्ट १२ : ८१-८५]

Vajramūṣā
According to Ratnākara

Vajra mūṣā is round and like the teat of a cow in shape. For the preparation of this crucible, ash of paddy husk (2 parts), mud from the ant-hill (one part), *maṇḍūra* or iron-rust (one part), white clay (one part) and ash of human hair (one part) should be strongly triturated by adding a small quantity of goat's milk for two *yāma-s*. Out of this paste, the crucible of the above mentioned shape should be prepared and burnt. Inside this crucible, mercury should be kept and covered with the lid. The joint between the crucible and the lid should be sealed with the above mentioned paste. This is called *vajra mūṣā* and it is used for the *māraṇa* (calcination) of mercury. The paste of the above mentioned ingredients (ash of paddy husk, etc.) should be burnt till the crucible becomes blackish in colour.

खटिका लवणं माषचूर्णं गुडपुरौ तथा ।
अतसी च दृषदचूर्णं मृल्लेपादिषु पूजिताः ।।११९।।
।। इति सन्धिकर्पटलेपनार्थानि ।।

Sealing Clay

For sealing joints of crucible , etc., pieces of cloth should be smeared with the clay prepared of *khaṭikā* (chalk), salt, paste of *māṣa*, jaggery, *guggulu*, *atasī* and powder of stone.

"तुषं वस्त्रसमं दग्धं तत्पादांशां तु मृत्तिकाम्[७३] ।
कुर्यात्पाषाणपादांशं वज्रवल्याः द्रवैर्दिनम् ।
मर्दयेत्कारयेन्मूषां वज्राख्यं रसबन्धने ।।१२०।।

Another Recipe for Vajramūṣā

Ash of paddy husk (one part), ash of cloth (one part), mud (one fourth part) and stone dust (one fourth part) should be triturated for one day by adding the juice of *vajra-vallī*. Out of this clay, *vajra-mūṣā* should be prepared and used for the *bandhana* (solidification) of mercury.

गौरा दग्ध्वा तुषं दग्धं 'दग्धा[७४] वल्मीकमृत्तिका ।
गजाश्वानां मलं दग्धं' यावदाकृष्णतां गतम् ।।१२१।।
षाषाणभेदिपत्राणि कृष्णमृत्सा[७५] समा समम् ।

वज्रवल्याः द्रवैर्मर्द्य दिनं च पेषयेत् दृढम् ।
तेन कोष्टीं वक्रनालीं वज्रमूषां च कारयेत् ।।१२२।।

Another Recipe for Vajramūṣā, etc.

Gaurā (chalk), paddy-husk, mud of ant-hill and stool of elephant and horse should be burnt till they become black. This ash and the leaves of *pāṣāṇabheda* should be taken in equal quantities and strongly triturated by adding the juice of *vajra-vallī* for one day. With this clay *koṣṭhī* (oven), *vakra-nālī* (bent pipe) and *vajra-mūṣā* should be prepared.

कांचकूपी लोहकूपी चतुःपञ्चनवाङ्गुला ।
सप्तधा लेपिता शुष्कं सैव कर्मटमृत्स्नया ।।१२३।।

Wrapping of Glass Bottles

Glass bottles and iron bottles should be four, five or nine *aṅgula-s* in length. These bottles should be wrapped with seven layers of mud-smeared cloth and dried before use.

वल्मीकमृत्तिकांगारचूर्ण[७६] लोहकिट्टकम्[७७] ।
श्वेतपाषाणकं चैव तत्सर्वं चूर्णयेत्समम् ।।१२४।।
सर्वतुल्यं तुषं दग्धं सर्वं तोयैर्विमर्दयेत् ।
मूषादिसम्पुटं कुर्यात्सर्वसन्धिप्रलेपनम्[७८] ।।१२५।।

Recipe of Sealing Clay

Mud of ant-hill, charcoal, *maṇḍūra* (rust of iron) and white clay, all these taken in equal quantities should be made to a powder. To this, equal quantity of the ash of paddy husk should be added. By adding water, these ingredients should be triturated and made to a paste. This paste should be used for sealing the joints of crucibles, etc.

कुलालभाण्डरूपा या दृढा च परिपाचिता ।
पक्वमूषेति सम्प्रोक्ता सा सर्वत्र विपाचने" ।
[रसकामधेनु : पृष्ठ १२-१३ : ८५-९३]
"सैव छिद्रान्विता मन्दा गम्भीरा सारणोचिता" ।।१२६।।
[रसकामधेनु : पृष्ठ १३:९६]

Pakva-mūṣā

A crucible, which is strong and burnt well like a jar, is called *pakva-mūṣā*. It is used for all types of cooking. If this crucible has a small hole at the bottom and is deep inside, it is useful for the *sāraṇa saṃskāra* of mercury.

"अन्धमूषा[७९] च कर्त्तव्या सुरभिस्तनसन्निभा।
पिधानकसमायुक्ता किञ्चिदुन्नतमस्तका" ।।१२७।।
[रसकामधेनु : पृष्ठ १३ : ९५]
निर्दिष्टा मल्लमूषा[८०] सा मल्लद्वितयसम्पुटा ।।१२८।।

Malla-Mūṣā (Andha Mūṣā)

A crucible should be prepared like the teat of a cow. It should have a lid and its head (upper part) should be slightly elevated. It should be burnt after smearing with two layers of *malla* (arsenic).

तिलभस्म द्विभागं स्यादेकांशा च तथेष्टका ।
तत्कृतामस्य [?] मूषैषा[८१] तारसंशोधने हिता[८२] ।।१२९।।

The crucible prepared of the ash of *tila* (two parts) and brick (one part) is useful for the purification of silver. [There are errors in the text.]

अथ शैवालभक्षः
स्वर्णभागं भवेदेकं द्विगुणं मृतभास्करम् ।
रसकं पञ्चभागाश्च षष्टभागानि धौतमृत् ।।१३०।।
आटरूषजले पिष्ट्वा सम्पुटं तेन कारयेत् ।
मूषां च रचयेत्सत्यं रसस्य निगडो[८३] भवेत् ।।१३१।।
वह्निमध्ये न गच्छेत् पक्षच्छेदीव[८४] तिष्ठति ।
काचकूपी द्वितीयस्तु[८५] मृतायोलोहसम्पुटः ।।१३२।।
।। इति रसनिगडयन्त्रम्[८६] ।।

Rasanigaḍa Yantra
According to Śaivālabhakṣa

Gold (one part), *bhasma* of copper(two parts), *rasaka* (five parts) and washed clay (six parts) should be triturated by adding the juice or decoction of *vāsaka*. A crucible should be prepared of this paste which is useful for the *nigaḍa* (a type of processing) of mercury. Mercury kept inside this crucible does not vapourate even if placed over fire and remains stable as if it has lost its power of vapourisation. Alternatively, the *nigaḍa* state of mercury could be attained by putting it in a glass bottle smeared with the *bhasma* of iron.

अथ रसार्णवात्

"स्नुह्यर्कसंभवं क्षीरं ब्रह्मबीजानि गुग्गुलुः ।
सैन्धवं द्विगुणं दत्वा मर्दयित्वा विचक्षणः ॥१३३॥
पिष्टिकावेष्टनं कृत्वा कल्केनानेन सुन्दरी[८७] ।
बिल्वप्रमाणं कृत्वा तु मूषामतिनवां दृढाम् ॥१३४॥
ऊर्द्ध्वाधो लवणं दत्वा मूषामध्ये रसं क्षिपेत् ।
मूषालेपे प्रदातव्यं दग्धं शंखादिचूर्णकम् ॥१३५॥
मूषां तस्य दृढं बद्ध्वा लोणमृत्तिकया पुनः ।
कारयेच्च सुधालेपं छायाशुष्कं च कारयेत् ।
उक्तो निगडबन्धोऽयं[८८] पुत्रस्यापि न कथ्यते" ॥१३६॥

[रसकामधेनु : पृष्ठ १८ : १४७-१५१]

Nigaḍabandha
According to Rasārṇava

One part of each of the latex of *snuhī* and *arka, brahmabīja* and *guggulu* should be added with double the quantity of *saindhava* and triturated. The paste of these durgs should be made to the shape of a *bilva* fruit and a strong crucible is thus prepared . Inside this crucible, mercury should be kept with salt placed below and above the mercury. The opening of the crucible should be sealed with the powder of the burnt conch-shell. The crucible should then be tightly tied with strings and wrapped with the paste of saline clay. Around the clay , the paste of *arka* should be smeared and the bolus, thus prepared, should be allowed to dry in shade. This is called *nigaḍa-bandha*, the secret of which should not be disclosed to [any unworthy person even to an unworthy] son.

चिक्कणा पिच्छिला गुर्वी कृष्णा मृत्सर्वपूजिता ।
पीता वा तद्गुणैर्युक्ता सिक्तादीन् विवर्जयेत् ॥१३७॥

Mud

The mud which is soft, slimy, heavy and black in colour should be used. Yellow clay having similar properties may also b used. The mud or clay should be free from particles of sand, etc.

शैवालभक्षः
तुषं भागद्वयं ग्राह्यं भागैकं वस्त्रखण्डकम् ।
मृदं च त्रिगुणां कृत्वा जलं[८९] दत्वा प्रमर्दयेत् ।।१३८।।
नरकेशसमं किञ्चिदत्वा तावत्प्रकुट्टयेत् ।
यावत्सिक्थसमाभासं मृत्पिण्डं जायते तदा ।।१३९।।
यथा न शुष्कतां यान्ति तथा यत्नं समाचरेत् ।
एवं सप्तदिनादूर्ध्वं मृदायोगे[९०] प्रयोजयेत् ।
कूपिकादिविलेपार्थं[९१] सन्ध्यर्थं चैव शस्यते ।।१४०।।

Recipe for Sealing Mud According to Śaivālabhakṣa

Two parts of paddy-husk, one part of cloth-pieces and three parts of mud should be added with water and pounded. To this, some human hair should be added and further pounded till the paste becomes sticky. Effort should be made to keep this paste wet so that it should not get dried up. After keeping it wet for seven days, the paste should be used for the purpose of wrapping around glass bottles and sealing the joints of crucibles, etc.

द्रष्टव्यं परिभाषायां बीजलक्षणमुत्तमम् ।
शास्त्रेण सम्प्रदायेन जारणा पुनरुच्यते ।।१४१।।

Characteristic features of *bīja* are already described in the chapter dealing with *paribhāṣā* [of the work of Śaivālabhakṣa?]. The process of *jāraṇā,* according to scriptures and traditions will be described later.

कंकुष्टं हरितालं च गन्धकं दरदं शिला ।
माक्षिकं सैन्धवं तुल्यं [?] नवसारं तथाभ्रकम् ।।१४२।।
सौवीरं गैरिकं काचं राजावर्तं विषत्रयम् ।

प्रवालं यावकं पिण्डं सिन्दूरं सरसाञ्जनम् ।।१४३।।
समुद्रफलकर्पूरं पीतकासीसवेतसम् ।
खर्परं किंशुकं रक्तं तापिकां नूतनां नयेत् ।।१४४।।
कृत्वा चूर्णं काकिनीनां रजसा परिभावयेत् ।
जया-दाडिम-बन्धूक-हेमपुष्परसैस्तथा ।।१४५।।
चांगेरिका - हस्तिशुण्डी - धूसरैः स्वरसैस्तथा ।
निशामुनिरसेनापि पञ्च पञ्च च भावना ।।१४६।।
शृङ्गीविषेण च तथा दुग्धिकेक्षुतजेन च ।
कुण्डलीगणिकाजातिपुष्पेणैव च भावना ।।१४७।।
कंकुष्ठादिगणो ह्येष रसचिन्तामणौ स्थितः ।
रक्तिकां दशकं दद्याद्रसे खल्वनिवेशिते ।।१४८।।
कर्मणोऽनन्तरं पूर्वं निम्बूकद्रवमिश्रितम् ।
एवं रागयुतः सम्यक्प्रोज्ज्वलो निश्चलस्तरम्[१२] ।।१४९।।
सर्वकर्मसहः[१३] श्रीमान् वह्निस्थायी स्थिरप्रभः ।
हेमाभ्रसत्वप्रभृतिं ग्रसते निःप्रयासतः ।।१५०।।
यद्यदारभते कर्म तत्तदेव करस्थितम् ।
अनेन सदृशं[१४] नास्ति रसरागकरः परः ।।१५१।।
असौ रक्तगणः साक्षात् क्षुद्बोधोऽतीव शोभितः ।
अवश्यं पीतनं[१५] सः स्याद्वह्निबुद्ध्यनं व्रजेत् ।।१५२।।
।। रसचिन्तामणौ कंकुष्ठादिगणः ।।

Kankuṣṭhādi Gaṇa
According to Rasacintāmaṇi

Kankuṣṭha, haritāla, gandhaka, darada, śilā, mākṣika, saindhava, navasāra, abhraka, sauvīra, gairika, kāca, rājāvarta, three types of poisons , *pravāla, yāvaka, piṇḍa, sindūra, rasāñjana, samudra-phala, karpūra, pīta-kāsīsa, vetasa, kharpara, kiṃśuka* (red variety), *tāpikā* and *nūtanā* should be made to a powder and impregnated with the menstrual blood of *kākinī* type of woman. In addition , this powder should be impregnated with the juice of *jayā, dāḍima, bandhūka*.

hema-puṣpa, *cāṅgerī*, *hasti-śuṇḍī*, *dhūsara*, *haridrā* and *agasti* for five times in each. Similarly, *bhāvanā* (impregnation) should be given with the decotion of *śṛṅgī-viṣa,* latex of *dugdhikā,* the juice of *ikṣu* as well as *taja* and the juice of the flowers of *kuṇḍalī, gaṇikā* and *jāti.* These drugs belong to *Kaṅkuṣṭhādi-gaṇa* as described in the work *Rasacintāmaṇi.*

This paste and mercury should be placed in a mortar and triturated with the juice of lemon. Before and at the end of the trituration, ten seeds of *guñjā* should be added to the paste in the mortar. These seeds should also be soaked in lemon juice. By this process , mercury becomes red in colour, lusturous, stable, tolerant of all types of processes, *śrīmān* (which endows auspiciousness), *vahnisthāyī* (which does not get evaporated when kept over fire) and *sthiraprabha* (which has stability of complexion). This mercury can digest gold, *abhraka sattva*, etc., easily. It is easy to futher process this mercury for any purpose. There is no better process which can impart colour to mercury so effectively . These drugs, mentioned above , are called *Rakta gaṇa* (group of red-drugs). It stimulates the appetite of mercury. This type of mercury [when used in the form of *bīja*] can impart yellow colour to other base metals and can stimulate their power of digestion.

पिष्टी

विलोलिते स्वर्णजले विशुष्के वस्त्रेऽथ दत्त्वा नवनीतगर्भे।
चूर्णे[९६] शिलातालकगन्धकनांसपन्नगानांसमभाजिकनाम्[९७] ।।१५३ ।।
कर्षप्रमाणं[९८] च ततोऽस्य वर्तिः[९९]
प्रज्वालयेत्तद्गलितं हि स[१००] स्यात्।
अनेन कुर्याद्रसनायकस्य सर्वत्र पिष्टी[१०१] बलिजारणाय।।१५४ ।।

Preparation of Piṣṭī for Gadhaka-Jāraṇa

A piece of cloth should be soaked in the juice of *dhustūra (svarṇa)* and dried. This cloth should be smeared with butter. Over this cloth, one *karṣa* of mercury and equal quantities of each of *manaḥ-śilā, haritāla, gandhaka* and *nāga bhasma*, all in powder form, should be placed and wick *(varti)* of this should be prepared by rolling the cloth. This should be ignited and the paste *(piṣṭī)* which comes out of this process should be used for *gandhaka-jāraṇā*.

रसं खर्परके कृत्वा अधो वह्निं प्रतापयते ।
निंबूकं द्रवसंमिश्रं भूनागतनुजं[१०२] द्रवम् ।।१५५।।
प्रदद्यात्सूतकश्चोतं बहुशः सम्प्रदायवित् ।
जायेतारुणपीताभो[१०३] नित्यमेव महौषधात् ।।१५६।।
अतिस्निग्धछवि सूतोऽरुणरूपो महाबली ।
यथा यथा ग्रसेद्ग्रासो भूनागद्रवसंभवः[१०४] ।
तथा तथा भवेत्सूतो दाडिमीकुसुमच्छविः ।।१५७।।
चतुर्गुणेन वस्त्रेण पीडितो यदि निःसरेत् ।
ग्रासं जीर्णं विजानीयादजीर्णस्त्वन्यथा भवेत् ।।१५८।।

Jāraṇa Saṃskāra

Mercury should be placed on a *kharparaka* (piece of broken jar) and fire should be ignited below it. To the mercury, the juice of earth-worm added with lemon juice should be added in large quantity accordings to tradition. This makes the colour of mercury yellowish pink, excessively unctuous in look, like the colour of *Aruṇa* and exceedingly potent. As the mercury consumes more and more of *grāsa* (food) in the form of the juice of earth-worm, it becomes more and more [pink] like the flower of *dāḍima*. If this mercury is tied in four layers of cloth and squeezed and it comes out as such (without any residue left in the cloth), then it should be assumed that *grāsa* (feed) has become digested. If, on the other hand, the residue remains in the cloth then the *grāsa* (feed) is not digested.

अजीर्णे पातयेत्पिष्टीं स्वेदयेन्मर्दयेत्तथा ।
बदराम्लप्रयोगेण जीर्णे ग्रासं प्रदापयेत्[१०५] ।।१५९।।

Treatment of Indigestion

If there is indigestion, then the paste (*piṣṭī*) of mercury should be distilled (*pātana*), given fomentation and triturated. By trituration with *badarāmla* (sour liquid prepared of *badara* fruit) the digestive power of mercury gets stimulated and after the earlier *grāsa* is digested, the second *grāsa* should be given to it.

रसदर्पणात्

आरोटः लोहजीर्णः स्यात्पतंगी पारदेश्वरः ।
तद्विद्धो न[१०६] लभेल्लोहः स्थिरदेहः कदाचन ।
तस्माद्बीजं प्रयुञ्जीत परिभाषोक्तलक्षणम् ।।१६० ।।

Need for Impregnating with Bīja

If the mercury digests metals then it is called *āroṭa.* If a base metal is transmuted into noble metal with the help of such vapourable mercury, then the transmuted noble metal (gold) does not remain stable. Therefore, to make the process of transmutation stable , the physician should process mercury by adding *bīja* as described in *paribhāṣā.*

रसांकुशात्

निर्मुखं सन्मुखं चैव वासनामुखमेव च ।
जारणा[१०७] त्रिविधा ज्ञेया द्रष्टव्या रसशास्त्रके ।।१६१ ।।
समजीर्णो[१०८] भवेद्बालो यौवनश्च चतुर्गुणम् ।
वृद्धः षोडशजीर्णं च तदा कर्म पृथक् पृथक् ।।१६२ ।।
कुमारो रोगरसते[१०९] तरुणो देहरक्षणे ।
वृद्धो विध्यति[११०] लोहानि सर्वं[१११] ज्ञात्वा चरेत्क्रियाम् ।।१६३ ।।
निर्दग्धशंखचूर्णात्तु रविक्षीरशतप्लुतम्[११२] ।
षड्बिन्दुकीटसंयुक्तं विडं देयं सुजारणे ।।१६४ ।।

Different Types of Jāraṇa According to Rasāṅkuśa

According to *Rasaśāstra*, there are three types of *jāraṇa,* viz., *nirmukha jāraṇa, sanmukha jāraṇa* and *vāsanāmukha jāraṇa.*

Jāraṇa of mercury with the same quantity of sulphur is called *bāla jāraṇa* (young), *jāraṇa* with four times of sulphur is *yauvana jāraṇa* (youthful) and *jāraṇa* with sixteen times of sulphur is called *vṛddha jāraṇa* (old). Their actions are of different types.

The young variety cures diseases; the youthful variety protects (rejuvenates) the body and the *vṛddha* variety causes transmutation of all the base metals. One should act accordingly.

While doing *jārana, vida* (a type of catalytic agent), prepared of the unburnt powder of *śaṅkha* soaked (impregnated) with the milky latex of *arka* for one hundred times and added with six drops of *kiṭa*, should be added.

अथ हिंगुलोत्थः[११३]

पारिभद्ररसे पिष्टं हिङ्गुलं[११४] याममात्रकम्[११५] ।
जंबीराणां द्रवैर्वाऽथ पात्यं पातनयन्त्रके ।
तं सूतं योजयेद्योगे सप्तकंचुकवर्जितम् ।।१६५।।

Hiṅgulottha Pārada (Mercury Extracted from Hiṅgula)

Hiṅgula should be soaked for one *yāma* with the juice of *pāribhadra* or *jambīra*. Then this paste should be treated with the process of distillation or sublimation *(pātana)*. The mercury, thus obtained, is free from seven types of *kañcuka doṣa-s* and can be used in recipes.

रसदर्पणात्

दरदस्त्रिविधो[११६] रक्तचर्मारः[११७] शुकतुण्डकः ।
हंसपादस्तृतीयश्च[११८] गुणवानुत्तरोत्तरम् ।।१६६।।

According to Rasadarpaṇa

Hiṅgula (cinnabar) is of three types, viz., *rakta carmāra, śuka tuṇḍaka* and *haṃsa-pāda*. The succeeding ones are better than the former ones i.e. these are progressively better in quality (properties).

शैवालभक्षमतात्

हंसपादं च तत्राद्यं तारकर्मणि योजयेत् ।
तद्धेमकिट्टसदृशं तदन्यत्तीक्ष्णमारणे ।।१६७।।
चर्मरः[११९] कृष्णरूपः स्यात्सुपीतः शुकतुण्डकः[१२०] ।
सत्त्वपाते च तत्प्रोक्तं शोध्यं पौरभ्रदुग्धके[१२१] ।।१६८।।

According to Śaivālabhakṣa

Haṃsapāda which is the best, should be used for processing silver. It is like *hema* (gold)-*kiṭṭa*. It is uncomparable in its effect to reduce *tīkṣṇa* type of iron into *bhasma* form. *Carmāra (rakta carmāra)* is black in colour and *śuka-tuṇḍaka* is exceedingly yellow. This should be used in *sattva pātana* (taking out essence from metals). This may be purified with milky latex of *paurabhra*.

पुरन्दररहस्ये
रसगन्धकसम्भूतं हिंगुलं प्रोच्यते बुधैः ।
तस्मात्सूतं च यद्ग्राह्यं शोध्यं तमपि सूतवत् ।।१११।।

According to Purandara-Rahasya

The compound of mercury and sulphur is called *hiṅgula*. The mercury extracted from it should also be purified like ordinary mercury.

रससारात्
जपाकुसुमसंकाशो हंसपादो महोत्तमः ।
रसायने सर्वलोहमारणे रसरंजने ।।१७०।।

According to Rasasāra

Haṃsapāda type of *hiṅgula* is excellent in property and in colour, it is like the red flower of *japā*. It is useful as a rejuvenating agent, for the *bhasma* (calcination) of metals and for imparting colour to mercury.

शुद्धः स्याद्दरदः सप्तकृत्वः[१२२] लाक्षाम्बुभावितः[१२३] ।
मलदोषादिकं नास्ति सर्वकार्येषु युज्यते[१२४] ।।१७१।।

Purification of Hiṅgula

Hiṅgula impregnated with the solution of *lākṣā* (*lākṣāmbu*) for seven times becomes pure and free from *mala-doṣa*, etc. It can be used for all therapeutic purposes.

कषायतिक्तं कटु हिंगुलं स्यान्नेत्रामयघ्नं[१२५] गलगण्डकुष्ठम् ।
हन्त्यम्लपित्तज्वरशोषशोफशूलातिसारं समुखप्रसेकम् ।।१७२।।

।। इति हिंगुललक्षणशोधनपातनगुणाः ।।

Properties of Hiṅgula

Hiṅgula is astringent, bitter and pungent in taste. It cures eye-diseases, goitre, *kuṣṭha* (obstinate skin diseases including leprosy), *amla pitta* (gastritis), fever, consumption, oedema, colic pain, diarrhoea and excessive salivation from the mouth.

Thus, ends the description, purification, *pātana* (sublimation and distillation) and properties of *hingula*.

अथ रसचिन्तामणि

मल्लिकाव्याघ्रकदलीकाकमाचीरसेन च ।
स्वर्णभण्डीरभृङ्गारारग्वधफलेन च ।।१७३।।
कन्याभल्लातपत्रोत्थरसेन[126] परिमर्दयेत् ।
इष्टिकाकाञ्जिकेनापि त्रिफलाक्वथितेन च ।।१७४
कपिलिका[127] देवदाली वह्निगोक्षुरकेण च ।
वज्रार्कजेन दुग्धेन स तु लाक्षारसेन च ।।१७५।।
त्र्यूषणोत्थकषायेण कीटषड्बिन्दुकेन च ।
चिंचिकालशुनोत्थेन दुग्धिकाया रसेन च ।।१७६।।
सितपर्णी-[128] मूषपर्णी-लांगली-स्वरसेन च ।
हिंगुलालशिलागन्धहिंगुसौवर्चलैः पृथक् ।।१७७।।
कांजिकेन समं पिष्ट्वा यामं यामं पृथक् पृथक् ।
मर्दयेच्च तथा यामं महाशंखेन मर्दयेत् ।।१७८।।
पलषट्कमितं सूतं बहुशो निंबुकेन च ।
रसेन मर्दयेत्तापे भाव्यते च पुनः पुनः ।।१७९।।
नवं[129] तापीद्वयं नीत्वा समं सममुखं[130] ततः ।
अधस्ताद्या भवेत्तापी पर्णचूर्णेन लिप्यते ।।१८०।।
पुनः पञ्चमृदा देया मृन्मध्ये लघुगर्त्तिका ।
तन्मध्ये शिंबिकापत्रधत्तूरदलसंभवाम्[131] ।।१८१।।
विरच्य मूषिकां गाढां तस्मिन्[132] गर्त्ते निवेशयेत् ।
तस्यां रसं विनिक्षिप्य सिंबीपत्ररसं[133] रसे ।।१८२।।
दीयते सेरमात्रेऽस्मिन्सूक्ष्मछिद्रा शराविका ।
तत्पार्श्वे खर्परीर्देया निर्दोषा नूतना[134] ततः ।।१८३।।
तापिकामानयेच्चान्यां कन्यकाद्रवलेपिताम् ।
ततो नौसादरेणाक्तामेकतः[135] कुरुतः द्वयम् ।।१८४।।

सन्धिलेपं दृढं कृत्वा सुशुष्कं चुल्लिसंस्थिताम्[१३६] ।
यथाग्निरुद्भवेच्चातुर्दिक्षु ताप्यो[१३७] समन्ततः ।।१८५।।
यामषोडशकं यावन्मन्दमध्यक्रमेण च ।
तदा निष्पद्यते[१३८] भस्म सूतकं शृणु यादृशम् ।।१८६।।
हीरकद्युतिसंकाशं प्रमाणे[१३९] हीरकाकृतिम् ।
क्वचित्पर्पटिकाभासं गलद्रूप्यनिभं क्वचित् ।।१८७।।
पिण्डरूपमिदं साक्षाद् दृश्यते दृष्टिसौख्यदम् ।
भक्षयेद्रक्तिकामेकां मरीचेन समं रसम् ।।१८८।।
गुडेनाबध्य मतिमान् ज्वरनाशाय तं पुरा ।
मन्देग्नौ चाथ हृद्रोगे दद्याल्लोणीरसेन[१४०] च ।।१८९।।
अम्लपित्ते प्रदातव्यं विमलासत्वसंयुताम् ।
बल्यं वाजीकं मेध्यं मनोत्साहकरं परम् ।।१९०।।
वृद्धानां पुत्रजननं शुक्रायुःश्रीकरं परम् ।
एतस्मान्नापरं भद्रं विद्यते रसभस्मतः[१४१] ।।१९१।।

Bhasma Preparation of Mercury According to Rasacintāmaṇi

Six *pala-s* of mercury should be impregnated and triturated separately for one *yāma* in each of the following :

(1) Juice of *mallikā, vyāghra, kadalī* and *kākamācī*.
(2) Fruit juice of *svarṇa bhaṇḍīra, bhṛṅgāra* and *āragvadha*.
(3) Leaf-juice of *kanyā* and *bhallātaka*.
(4) Powder of brick and *kāñjī* (a soour vinegar).
(5) Decoction of *triphalā*.
(6) Juice or decoction of *kapilikā* (*kaṇṭālikā*), *devadālī, citraka* and *gokṣura*.
(7) Milky latex of *vajra* and *arka*.
(8) *Lākṣā-rasa* (lac mixed with water).
(9) Decoction of *trikaṭu, kīṭa* and *ṣaḍbinduka*.
(10) Juice of *ciñcikā, laśuna* and *dugdhikā*.
(11) Juice of *sita-parṇī, mūṣa-parṇī* and *lāṅgalī*.
(12) *Hiṅgula, haritāla, manaḥśilā, gandhaka, hiṅgu* and *sauvarcala*, separately along with *kāñjī* (sour vinegar).

Thereafter, the mercury should be added with the powder of *mahāśaṅkha* mixed with lemon-juice and triturated for several times. This impregnation and trituration should be done repeatedly.

Two new jars having similar brims should be taken. The inside wall of the lower jar should be smeared with the powder of betel-leaf. Over this, five types of mud should be smeared. In the centre of the mud a small pit should be prepared which is to be covered with the leaves of *śiṃbikā* and *dhattūra*. Inside this pit, a strong crucible (*mūṣā*) should be placed. Inside the crucible, mercury should be placed and covered with the juice of the leaves of *śimbī*, one *sera* in quantity. Over this, an earthen plate having a fine hole should be placed. Over this plate, a new *kharparī* (piece of broken jar) should be placed.

The inside wall of the upper jar should be smeared with the juice of *kumārī*. The brims of these two jars should be smeared with the paste of *navsādara* and put together. The joints of these two brims should be sealed with mud smeared cloth and dried. These jars should then be placed over the oven. Fire should be ignited in such a way that the flame surround the entire jar. Mild, moderate and strong heat should be applied gradually for sixteen *yāma-s*. Thus, the mercury is reduced to *bhasma* form. This *bhasma* looks like a diamond in lustre and shape. At time it appears like a *parpaṭikā* (scale) or like melted silver. In the bolus form the mercury appears pleasing to the eyes.

One *ratti* of this mercury *bhasma* should be added with equal quantity of the powder of *marica* and wrapped with jaggery. Intake of this cures fever. For the treatment of *agnimāndya* (suppression of the power of digestion) and heart diseases, this *bhasma* of mercury should be administered along with the juice of *loṇī*. Along with the *sattva* of *vimalā*, it should be given for the treatment of *amla pitta* (gastritis).

It is an excellent promoter of strength, virility, intellect and enthusiasm. It enables even an old person to procreate progeny. It promotes the quantity of semen, longevity and auspiciousness. Nothing is more *bhadra* (endower of blessings) than this *bhasma* of mercury.

गोरक्षमतात्

खटिका स्फुटिका लवणं च समं।
वनमृद्गलदिष्टरजो गिरिजम् [?]।
तलभाण्डधृतं घटिकोदरगो-

रसराजवरा डमरूर्पिहितः[१४२] ।
तल[१४३] खर्परिकाविहितःपिहितो
निहितः सकलामयनाशकरः ।।१९२।।

Preparation of Mercury-Bhasma According to Gorakṣa

Khaṭikā, *sphuṭikā* and *lavaṇa*, taken in equal quantities should be mixed with the mud collected from the forest and smeared over the inside bottom of the lower jar and over it mercury should be placed. Over it the upper jar of the *ḍamarū yantra* should be kept and the joint should be sealed. The *bhasma* of mercury should be collected after cooking, from the inside wall of the upper jar. This *bhasma* cures many diseases. [There appears to be errors in this verse.]

'द्विपलं'[१४४] शुद्धसूतस्य सूतार्द्धं शुद्धगन्धकम् ।
कृत्वा नीरेण संमर्द्य दिनमेकं निरंबु तत् ।
विदध्यात् भूधरे यन्त्रे दिनैकं मारयेत्पुटात् ।।१९३।।

Another Method of Preparing Mercury Bhasma

Two *pala-s* of purified mercury should be added with one *pala* of purified sulphur and triturated in a mortar by adding water till the water dries up. This powder should be cooked in *bhūdhara yantra* for one day which reduces mercury into *bhasma* form.

अन्यच्च
भुजंगवल्लीनीरेण मर्दितं पारदं दृढम् ।
कर्कोटीकन्देन लिप्तं पुटस्थं पुटयेद्रसम् ।
भवेद्भस्म योगवाहं सर्वकर्मसु योजयेत् ।।१९४।।

Another Method

Mercury should be strongly triturated in the juice of *bhujaṅga vallī* and wrapped with the paste of the root of *karkoṭī*. Then it should be kept in *puṭa yantra* and cooked. The *bhasma*, thus prepared, becomes *yogavāha* (which when added to another drug enhances the potency of the latter) and may be used in all types of recipes.

अन्यमतम्

श्वेताङ्कोठजयावारीसूतो मर्द्यो दिनत्रयम् ।
पुटितश्चांधमूषायां सूतो भस्मत्वमाप्नुयात् ।
प्रत्यहं रक्तिकाः पंच भक्षयेन्मधुसर्पिषा ।।१९५।।

Another Method

Mercury should be triturated for three days with the juice of the white variety of *aṅkoṣṭha* and *jayā*, and then cooked with *andha-mūṣā*. Thus, *bhasma* of mercury is prepared. Five *ratti-s* of this *bhasma* should be taken every day with honey and ghee.

अथ सिन्दूरारणम्

पलमात्रो रसः शुद्धस्तावन्मात्रं तु गंधकम् ।
विधिवत्कज्जलीं कृत्वा न्यग्रोधांकुरवारिभिः ।
भावना त्रितयं दत्वा स्थालीमध्ये निधापयेत्'।
'दद्यात्तस्य[145] च मन्दाग्निं भिषक्यामचतुष्टयम् ।।१९६।।
प्राप्यते रससिंदूरं तनुं णानुं [?] संनिभम् ।
अनुपानविशेषेण निहन्ति विविधान् रोगान् ।।१९७।।

Preparation of Mercury Bhasma According to Sindūrāraṇa

One *pala* of each of purified mercury and purified sulphur should be triturated and made to *kajjalī* (fine black powder like collyrium). This powder should be impregnated and triturated for three days by adding the juice of the stilt-root of banyan tree and kept in a jar. This should be cooked by the physician for four *yāma-s* by applying mild fire as a result of which red coloured *rasa sindūra* is obtained. Administered with different and appropriate *anupāna-s*, it cures various diseases.

अन्यत्

चपलेन समो गन्धो निर्गुण्डीरसमर्दितः ।
पाचितो वालुकायन्त्रे रक्तभस्म प्रजायते ।।१९८।।

Another Method of Preparing Rasasindūra

Mercury (*capala*) and sulphur, taken in equal quantities should be triturated by adding the juice of *nirguṇḍī* and cooked in *vālukā yantra* as a result of which red *bhasma* of mercury (*rasa sindūra*) is prepared.

सूतार्धं गंधकं सूतं माक्षिकोद्भूतसत्वकम् ।
गन्धतुल्यं विमर्द्याथ दिनं निर्गुण्डिकाद्रवैः ।।१९९।।
स्थापयेद्वालुकायन्त्रे काचकूप्यां विपाचयेत् ।
अंधमूषागतवाथ पंचकायंत्रके दिनम् ।
पक्वं पृंगायते [?] भस्म दाडिमीकुसुमोपमम् ।।२००।।

Another Method of Preparing Rasasindūra

Mercury (two parts), sulphur (one part) and *sattva* of *mākṣika* (one part) should be triturated for one day by adding the juice of *nirguṇḍī*. Then it should be kept in a glass bottle and cooked in *vālukā yantra*. The cooking can also be done in *andha-mūṣā* or *pañcakā yantra* (?) for one day. Thus, *rasa sindūra* of pink colour like the flower of *dāḍima* is prepared.

रतिभेया पुरन्दरसुन्दरमन्दिरकंदरियुक् मुदितः' ।
घनसारतुषाररसमुक्तलतामृतशशिशशांककलाधवलः ।।२०१।।
कदलीनवकन्दकलाकुलिको मृगनाभिसचंदनकुंकुमयुक् ।
सममेलालवंगपुरान्विताः सुखयति[१४६] ।
चानुदिनं त्वशिनः रसकर्पूरः ।।२०२।।

Preparation of Rasakarpūra

[The meaning of this text is not clear; hence left untranslated.]

तथा च
[१४७]खष्टीगैरिकवल्मीकमृत्तिका[१४८] सैन्धवसमम्[१४९] ।
भागद्वयमिदं श्लक्ष्णं रसो[१५०] भागद्वयं[१५१] तथा ।।२०३।।
संमर्द्य चैकतः कृत्वा वाढं[१५२] च रसमौषधम् ।
हंडिकायां विनिःक्षिप्य पार्श्वे पार्श्वे च खर्परी ।।२०४।।
अन्यां च हंडिकां कृत्वा[१५३] कुर्यात्सन्धिनिरोधनम् ।
यामषोडशपर्यन्तं[१५४] भक्तिं कुर्यादहर्निशम् ।।२०५।।

अत[155] ऊर्ध्वं रसं तस्माल्लग्नशीतं[156] च मानयेत् ।।२०६।।
कर्पूरपुलककारं बलदं दृष्टिसौख्यदम् ।
ग्रन्थिलं शिथिलं सौम्यं भक्ष्यमाणं निरामयम् ।।२०७।।
पुष्ट्यारोग्यप्रदं[157] तीक्ष्णं कमनीयं सुखावहम् ।
महाप्रमेहशमनं मत्तेभबलकारकम् ।।२०८।।

।। इति द्वितीयरसकर्पूरः ।।

Second Method of Preparing Rasakarpūra

Khaṭikā (chalk clay), *gairika* (red ochre), mud of ant-hill and rock-salt should be taken,one part of each, and made to a fine powder. To this, four parts of mercury should be added and triturated together. This powder should be kept in a jar, and in its sides, *kharparikā* (pieces of broken jar) should be placed. Over this jar, another jar should be placed with its mouth downwards. The joint of these two brims should be sealed and cooked continuously for sixteen *yāma-s*. The mercury attached to the upper jar should be collected after it has cooled down. This stuff appears like a piece of camphor. It promotes strength and is pleasing to the eyes. It is knotty, soft and smooth. When taken, it makes a person free from diseases. It promotes plumpness (nourishment) and health. It is sharp in property. It promotes complexion and happiness. It cures serious types of *prameha* (obstinate urinary disorders including diabetes). By taking this, a person becomes strong like a rogue elephant.

निम्बूरसेन संमिश्रमेकी[158]कुर्याद्रसेन तु ।
पारदं खल्वके कृत्वा सौभाग्यं च तदर्धकम्[159] ।।२०९।।
मर्दयेत्सर्वमेकत्र दिनपञ्चावधिस्तथा[160] ।
माषप्रमाणाः गुटिकाः कर्तव्याः[161] शुष्कतां गताः ।।२१०।।
'[162]काष्ठभाजनमध्यस्था माषचूर्णेन[163] वेष्टिताः' ।
इष्टचूर्णेन वा लोड्याः पुनः शोष्याः सुधीमता ।।२११।।
अधो रक्षां ददात्यादौ पुनरंगारकानथ[164] ।
क्रमेण वटकां क्षिप्त्वा धाम्यमानाः शनैः शनैः ।।२१२।।
अनेन विधिना सूतो ध्मातो रक्षान्तरालगः ।

निःसृत्य वटिकाभ्योऽसौ भवत्यतिसितप्रभः ।।२१३।।
सर्वापि कनकरूपः स्याद्पूर्वो जलयोगतः ।
खोटस्तु जायते ध्मातः पारदः शुक्रसन्निभः ।।२१४।।
अयं मूलिकमाबद्धः[166] पारदो मुखरोगहृत् ।
न जरापि बलं कुर्यान्न कालः कलयत्यमुम्[167] ।।२१५।।

।। इति हरिणखुरीबद्धो रसः ।।

Hariṇakhurī-Baddha-Rasa

One part of mercury should be added with half part of *saubhāgya* (borax) and triturated by adding the lemon-juice for five days. Of this paste, pills of one *māṣa* each should be prepared and dried. These pills should be kept inside a wooden jar and wrapped with the powder of *māṣa* or brick-powder. In another plate kept over fire, these pills should be dropped one after the other and slowly blown by a blower. Mercury coming out of these pills get attached at the bottom of the upper jar. It is very white in colour. When added to water, it looks like gold. When blown, it becomes *khoṭa* (non-volatile) and white. Mixed with herbs, it cures mouth-diseases. A person taking this mercury becomes free from ageing process and [untimely] death.

नागार्जुनीति विख्याता दुग्धिका क्षितिमण्डले ।
तस्मिन्विमर्दितो[168] सूतो दिनमेकं निरन्तरम् ।।२१६।।
काकमाच्यापि कर्त्तव्यं मर्दनं दोषशान्तये ।
पारदं दश टंकं स्याद्दशटंकं च गन्धकम् ।
नौसादरं च कर्षार्धं[169] त्रयमेकत्र मर्दयेत् ।।२१७।।
काचस्य कूपके कृत्वा मुखं तस्य निरुध्यते।
अष्टयामावधिर्यावत्तावत्सूतः प्रपाच्यते[170] ।।२१८।।
'सूतोरुणः[171] प्रजायते' सर्वकार्यार्थसाधकः ।
भक्षयेद्रक्तिका पञ्चमरिचेन समं रसम् ।।२१९।।
क्षुद्बोधकारकः प्रायः सद्यः कामाग्निदीपनः[172] ।
ज्वरं प्रमेहं कासं च नाशयेदनुपानतः ।।२२०।।

Another Recipe of Rasasindūra

A type of *dugdhikā* called *nāgārjunī* is well known. With the juice of this plant, ten *taṅka-s* of mercury should be continuously triturated for one day. For the removal of adverse effects (*doṣa-s*), trituration should also be done with the juice of *kākamācī*. This mercury (ten *ṭaṅka-s*) should be added with ten *ṭaṅka-s* of sulphur and half-*karṣa* of *navasādara* and all the three should be triturated together. This powder should be kept in a glass bottle and its mouth should be sealed. It should be cooked for eight *yāma-s*. Thus, the mercury becomes pink in colour. It is useful for curing all diseases. It should be taken in the dose of five *rattī-s* along with equal quantity of *marica*. It promotes appetite, instantaneously stimulates sex desire and along with appropriate *anupāna-s* (vehicles) it cures fever, *prameha* (obstinate urinary disorders including diabetes) and bronchitis.

अन्यच्च[१७३] रसराजलक्ष्मीतंत्रात्
कोरंटकाम्बुसंयोगादातपे मर्दयेद्रसम् ।
म्रियतेऽसौ ततः सूतः सर्वकर्माणि साधयेत् ।।२२१ ।।

Another Method of Preparing Mercury Bhasma According to Rasarājalakṣmī

Along with the juice of *koranṭaka* mercury should be triturated while exposing it to the sun. Thus, the mercury is reduced to *bhasma* form and it can be used in all recipes.

स्तोकं स्तोकं गन्धकं सूतराजं
दत्वा[१७४] दत्वा ताम्रपात्रे निघृष्टम्[१७५] ।
शीघ्रं पिष्टी जायते सद्विगन्धा-
न्मंदं पक्त्वा भूधरे भस्मं सूतः ।।२२२ ।।

In a copper mortar (vessel) mercury should be triturated by adding sulphur in small quantities. It takes the form of a paste (*piṣṭī*) quickly. This should be cooked in *bhūdhara yantra* by which the *bhasma* of mercury is prepared.

रसालंकारात्
उत्तरावारुणीदुग्धैः सर्पारिजरसैस्तथा ।
हंसपादीरसैस्तद्वत् वज्र्यर्कमयसा[१७६] तथा ।।२२३ ।।

ब्रह्ममूलरसैस्तद्वत्कपिकच्छूशिफारसैः ।
विष्णुक्रान्ताविडङ्गोत्थरसैः पौनर्नवैस्तथा ।।२२४।।
यवचिंचादेवदालीकंचुकीपाठिकावरी-
रसैः प्रमर्दयेत्सूतं भिषक् दशदिनावधिः ।।२२५।।
तं कल्कं गोलकं कृत्वा यन्त्रे सोमानले पचेत् ।
एकविंशद्दिनं यावदग्निं संज्वालयेदधः ।।२२६।।
यन्त्रादुत्तारयेत्सूतं भस्मीभूतं सुपाण्डुरम् ।
तस्मै तत्सारयेल्लोहं सुवर्णाद्यमसंशयम्[७७] ।
लेपेन पुटयोगेन सर्वलोहानि मारयेत् ।।२२७।।

।। इति स्वर्णादिमारणार्थम्[७८] ।।

Processing Mercury for Calcination of Gold, etc., According to Rasālaṅkāra

Mercury should be triturated for ten days with the milky latex of *uttarā-vāruṇī*, juices of *sarpāri* (*sarpagandhā*) and *haṃsapādī*; milky-latex of *vajrī* and *arka* and juices of *brahma-mūla*, root of *kapikachū*, *viṣṇukrāntā*, *viḍaṅga*, *punarnavā*, *yava*, *ciñcā*, *devadālī*, *kañcukī*, *pāṭhikā* and *avarī*. The paste, thus obtained, is made to a bolus form and cooked in *somānala yantra* for twenty one days over fire. Thereafter, mercury should be removed from the *yantra*. It is in *bhasma* form with yellowish brown colour. With this powder of mercury, metals, gold, etc., should be smeared and cooked in *puṭa pāka* which undoubtedly reduces these metals into *bhasma* form.

सुसूक्ष्मं रेतितं कृत्वा सुवर्णं शुक्तिमात्रकम् ।
पारदं शोधितं सम्यक् दद्यात्पलचतुष्टयम् ।।२२८।।
सुशोधितं गन्धकं च देयं[८७] हि कुडवद्वयम् ।
वृषकर्पासपुष्पोत्थरसं मर्द्यं दिनद्वयम् ।।२२९।।
ततः कन्यारसेनैव भावयित्वा विनिक्षिपेत् ।
कर्षार्द्धं रेतितं नागं ततो यन्त्रं प्रकल्पयेत् ।।२३०।।
अष्टादशांगुलोत्सेधं विस्तारेण षडङ्गुलम् ।
सुचिक्कणं सुवृतं च सम्पुटं रचयेत्तथा ।।२३१।।

यथोर्द्धं सम्पुटश्चाधः सम्पुटार्द्धं ग्रसेद् दृढम् ।
सकुलालेन रचितं सुपक्वं ताम्रसन्निभम् ।।२३२।।
मध्ये काचप्रलिप्तं च रसमारणकर्मसु ।
अधःसम्पुटखण्डेषु रसचूर्णं नियोजयेत् ।।२३३।।
किञ्चिदंशं परित्यज्य मुखे[180] देया पिधानिका ।
काचं भस्मसमं कृत्वा भस्मना[181] सह पेषयेत् ।।२३४।।
तेनैव मुद्रयित्वाऽथ सम्पुटं कारयेत्ततः ।
सन्धियुक्तं ततः[182] खंडं मृच्चैलेन प्रयोजयेत् ।।२३५।।
सन्धिं पक्त्वा ऊर्द्धखण्डं[183] जलमुद्रां प्रकल्पयेत्[184] ।
शुद्धांजननिभं किट्टं किट्टार्धं संमितां कुरु[185] ।।२३६।।
स्वर्णपुष्पस्य निर्यासं संमितार्द्धं नियोजयेत् ।
दक्षांडजद्रवेणैव मर्दयित्वा दृढं भिषक् ।।२३७।।
सर्वतोमुखमुद्रेयं पुत्रस्यापि न कथ्यते ।
तथापि रचयेद्यन्त्रं पारं[186]पर्योपदेशतः ।।२३८।।
'सम्पुटस्य[187] यथा सन्धिर्जलमध्येन तिष्ठति ।
विरच्यैवं प्रकारेण भवेद्भैरवसंज्ञकः' ।।२३९।।
यन्त्रः सोमानलो नाम क्वचिदुक्तः सुगोपितः ।
यन्त्रराज इति क्वापि योज्यः[188] परमदुर्लभः ।।२४०।।
रसस्य निगदः साक्षादनेन प्रपचेद्रसम् ।
शनैः शनैर्मन्दवह्निं भिषक्[189] दिनचतुष्टयम् ।।२४१।।
ततः प्रवालसंकाशं रसं ग्राह्यं सुधोपमम् ।
यदि किञ्चिच्च तिष्ठेत् यन्त्रराजेषु गन्धकः ।।२४२।।
ततोर्द्धं गन्धकं दत्त्वा तेनैव विधिना पचेत् ।
अथवा वालुकाख्ये[190] च काचकूप्यां पुनः क्षिपेत् ।।२४३।।
स्वांगशीतं समादाय नवपल्लवसन्निभम्[191] ।
सूक्ष्मचूर्णं रसं कृत्वा रक्षेत्स्वर्णकरण्डके ।।२४४।।
जातीफलं लवंगं च कंक्कोलं जातिपत्रिका ।
मस्तकी कर्षमात्रं स्यात्कस्तूरी कर्षमात्रिका ।।२४५।।

तदर्द्धं पक्वकर्मूरं तथार्कं करहाटकम् ।
समुद्रशोषजफलं समभागं विचूर्णयेत् ।।२४६।।
माषमात्रं[192] रसं नित्यं चूर्णमेतद्विमाषकम्[193] ।
मिश्रयित्वा भक्षयेच्च शृणु पथ्यं अतः परम् ।।२४७।।
प्रथमं मृदुमांसं च सघृतं च सुशीलयेत् ।
अतः परं बहुविधं मांसभक्ष्यं[194] प्रकल्पयेत् ।।२४८।।
मंडकान् वटकांश्चैव पक्वान्नं दुग्धसंयुताम् ।
भोजयेद्रमयेद्बालां कामांचितगतां[195] तथा ।।२४९।।
सर्वधातुक्षयं[196] कासं मन्दाग्निं ग्रहणीगदम् ।
श्लेष्मामयान्बहुविधान्प्रमेहान्विंशतिं जयेत् ।।२५०।।
अपस्मारं तथा ग्रन्थिं[197] हृद्रोगं पाण्डुदुर्जयम् ।
अरुचिशोफरोगांश्च[198] प्रमेहपिडकाञ्जयेत्[199] ।।२५१।।
जीर्णज्वरं प्रलेपाख्यं सामवातं गुदामयम् ।
जयेत् शूलं गरं श्वासं जयेदाशु उरःक्षतम् ।।२५२।।
बालानां च प्रदातव्यं मात्राभेदेन सर्वथा ।
कृशानां[200] च परां पुष्टिं वीर्याढ्यं कुरुते भृशम् ।।२५३।।
तिमिरं च जयेदाशु रसायनमनुत्तमम् ।
स्त्रीणां प्रकान्तिजननं वलीपलितनाशनम् ।।२५४।।
रक्तं पीतं सितं नीलं मेचकं जलसन्निभम् ।
शुक्रस्रावं कटिशूलं[201] नाशयेच्च[202] किमद्भुतम् ।।२५५।।
कक्षापुटिमते प्रोक्तो[203] रसः परमदुर्लभः ।
सानुभूतश्चात्र मया लेखितः[204] सम्प्रदायतः ।।२५६।।

।। इति श्री[205]कक्षापुटिमतात् परमदुर्लभो पारदभस्म[206] रसः ।।

Bhasma of Mercury
According to Kakṣāpuṭimata

One *śukti* of the fine filed powder of gold should be added with four *pala-s* of purified mercury and two *kuḍava-s* of purified sulphur. This should be triturated by adding the juice of *vāsaka* and flower of cotton tree for two days. Then it should be impregnated with the juice of *kumārī* and added with half of *karṣa* of filed powder of lead.

Then a *yantra* of eighteen *aṅgula-s* height and six *aṅgula-s* breadth should be prepared. It should be smooth and round.

For the preparation of the *bhasma* of mercury, *puṭa yantra* should be prepared in two pieces with well cooked and copper like pieces of jar and the inside wall of this *puṭa yantra* should be smeared with glass powder. In the lower piece, mercury powder mentioned above should be kept. After leaving some space, the lid should be covered. Fine powder of glass and ash should be made to a paste by trituration. The joint of *puṭa yantra* should be sealed with this paste. Then the whole *yantra* should be wrapped with mud smeared cloth. After the joint is dried up, the upper part of the *yantra* should be smeared with *jala mudrā* (water-proof seal).

Kiṭṭa of the colour of pure collyrium should be mixed with half the quantity of *sammitā* (fine wheat flour) and one fourth in quantity of the juice of *svarṇa-puṣpa*. This should be strongly triturated by adding the yolk and sap of egg. This paste is called *Sarvatomukha mudrā* (water-proof seal) and this recipe should not be disclosed even to a son if not worthy of it.

The outer *yantra* should be prepared according to traditional method. The *puṭa yantra* (inner one) should be kept in it with its joint submerged in water (kept inside the outer *yantra*). This is called *bhairava yantra*. Sometime, this secret instrument is called *somānala yantra*. This is the king among the pharmaceutical instruments and it is rare. Mercury cooked in this instrument makes an excellent recipe. Mild fire should be applied below this *yantra* for four days. Thereafter, coral like mercury should be collected from it which is like an ambrosia.

If there is a residue of uncooked sulphur [and mercury] remains inside this instrument, then half the quantity of sulphur should be added to it again and cooked in the same *somānala yantra*. Alternatively, this powder can be kept in a glass bottle and cooked in *vālukā yantra*. When the instrument becomes cool of its own, the mercury [of pink colour] like the colour of a new leaf should be collected, made to a fine powder and kept in a gold jar.

One *karṣa* of each of *jātīphala*, *lavaṅga*, *kaṅkola*, *jātipatra*, *mastakī* and *kastūrī*; half *karṣa* of each of camphor, copper *bhasma* and gold *bhasma* and one *karṣa* of the fruit of *samudra śoṣa* should be made to a powder.

One *māṣa* of the mercury *bhasma* and two *māṣa-s* of the above mentioned powder should be mixed together and taken.

The patient taking this recipe should first of all use soft meat mixed with ghee. Thereafter, he can take different types of meat preparations including *maṇḍaka*, *vaṭaka* and *pakvānna* (sweets prepared by frying with ghee) along with milk. He should indulge in sex with young and excited girls.

It cures diminution of all the tissues, bronchitis, suppression of the power of digestion, sprue syndrome, many different diseases caused by *kapha*, twenty types of *prameha* (obstinate urinary disorders including diabetes), epilepsy, tumour, heart diseases, serious type of anemia, anorexia, oedema, diabetic carbuncles, chronic fever, *pralepa* type of fever, rheumatism, anal diseases, colic pain, poisoning, asthma and phthisis.

To children, this medicine should always be administered in reduced dose.

It provides excellent nourishment to emaciated persons and promotes their semen. It immediately cures cataract and it is an excellent recipe for rejuvenation. It promotes the complextion of women. It prevents wrinkling and graying of hair. It cures seminal discharge of red, yellow, white, blue or black colour or like water. It cures lumbago and there is nothing to be surprised about its therapeutic effects. This excellent recipe is described in the text called *Kakṣāpuṭi-mata* and I [the original author] have written it on the basis of my own experience and also on the basis of tradition.

धान्याभ्रकं सूततुल्यं भावयेन्मार्कवद्रवैः ।
दिनैकं तेन कल्केन पटं लिप्त्वाथ वर्तिकाम् ॥२५७॥
कृत्वैरण्डस्य तैलेन लिलेप्य[२०७] च पुनः पुनः ।
प्रज्वाल्य तामधःपात्रे सतैलः पारदः पतेत् ॥२५८॥
स दिनं भूधरे पक्त्वा भस्मीभवति नान्यथा ।
योजितो रसयोगेन तत्तद्रोगहरो भवेत् ।
विशेषान्मेहपाण्डुर्तिक्षयकासादिकाञ्जयेत् ॥२५९॥

Another Method of Preparing Mercury Bhasma

Dhānyābhraka and mercury taken in equal quantities should be impregnated by adding the juice of *bhṛṅgarāja* and triturated for one day. A piece of cloth should be smeared with this paste and a wick of it should be prepared by rolling the cloth. This wick should be smeared with castor oil again and again. This should then be ignited. The mercury along with castor oil will thus fall down. This should then be cooked in *bhūdhara yantra* for one day to obtain *bhasma* of mercury. Appropriately use of this cures several diseases. It specially cures *meha* (obstinate urinary disorders including diabetes), anemia, tuberculosis, bronchitis, etc.

पञ्चांगं वर्वरी-लिंगीद्रवैश्च वासरं त्रयम् ।
मर्दितः पुटितो भस्म स्वर्णवर्णं प्रजायते ।।२६०।।

Preparation of Yellow Bhasma of Mercury

Mercury triturated with the juice of all the five parts of *varvarī* and *liṅgī* should be cooked in *puṭa*. Thus, the golden colour *bhasma* of mercury is produced.

रसरहस्यात्[२०८]

'रामठं[२०९] मुशलीकन्दं लांगलं रक्तचित्रकम् ।
मूषालेपनमात्रेण रसो भवति कुङ्कुमम्' ।।२६१।।

According to Rasarahasya

The crucible should be smeared with the paste of *rāmaṭha*, *muśalī-kanda*, *lāṅgalī* and *rakta-citraka*. Mercury kept in this crucible and cooked in *puṭa* produces saffron-coloured *bhasma*.

अथ शिवागमात्

सुवर्णस्य सुवर्णस्य तोलैकं रेतितस्य च ।
कर्षं च शुद्धवैक्रान्तं रसं षोडशकार्षिकम् ।।२६२।।
शरावमात्रं गन्धस्य खल्वमध्ये[२१०] विचूर्णयेत् ।
हस्तिकर्ण्याश्च पर्णोत्थं[२११] रसं दत्त्वाऽथ तोलकम् ।।२६३।।
कुमारीस्वरसेनैव मर्दयेच्च दिनद्वयम् ।
सप्तमृच्चैलसंलिप्ते काचकुम्भे क्षिपेद्रसम् ।।२६४।।
तन्मुखे खटिकां[२१२] दत्त्वा लेपयेत्सप्तधा मृदा ।

मृतूर्क्मटपिधानं च परिभाषां विलोक्येत् ।।२६५।।
संस्थाप्य वालुकायन्त्रे पचेद्दिनं चतुष्टयम् ।
शनैः शनैः प्रदातव्यो वीतिहोत्रो[२१३] भिषक्तमैः ।।२६६।।
स्वांगशीतो रसो ग्राह्यो यथारोगानुपानतः ।
दापयेत्सर्वरोगाणां विनिहंता न संशयः[२१४] ।।२६७।।

अथ अनुपानम्[२१५]
जातीफलं जातिपत्री कुंकुमं सलवङ्गकम् ।
कंकोलार्कक्करंभं च स्वस्थे स्यादनुपानकम् ।।२६८।।

अस्य[२१६] गुणम्
अतीव कान्तिजननमतीवोत्साहवर्धनम् ।
अतीव कामवृद्धिं च वह्निवृद्धिं करोति[२१७] च ।।२६९।।
शोषं क्षयं राजरोगं प्रमेहं विषमज्वरम् ।
प्रलेपकं च जीर्णं च तथा मन्दज्वरं जयेत् ।।२७०।।
वृद्धानां कान्तिजननं पुत्रदं श्रीकरं परम् ।
ओजोवृद्धिकरं श्रेष्टं महावातविनाशनम् ।।२७१।।
श्लेष्मामयप्रशमनं कर्मजव्याधिनाशनम् ।
वैक्रान्तबद्धसूतोऽयं बृंहणः परमो मतः ।।२७२।।

।। इति वैक्रान्तबद्धसूतः ।।

Vaikrāntabaddha Sūta
According to Śivāgama

One *tolā* of the gold having radiant beauty should be filed and made to a powder. To this, one *karṣa* of purified *vaikrānta*, sixteen *karṣa-s* of mercury and one *śarāva* of sulphur should be added and triturated in a mortar by adding one *tolā* of the juice of the leaf of *hasti-karṇa-palāśa* and the juice of *kumārī* for two days. This powder should be kept in a glass bottle and its mouth should be corcked with chalk clay. This is to be smeared with seven layers of mud smeared cloth as described in *paribhāṣā* section [*Śiva rahasya*]. The bottle should be kept in *vālukā yantra* and cooked for four days over mild fire. Thereafter, when the bottle becomes cool of its own, *bhasma* of mercury should be collected. With appropriate *anupāna-s*, this *bhasma* of mercury undoubtedly cures all types of diseases.

Anupāna or Vehicle

A healthy person should take the *bhasma* of mercury along with *jāti phala*, *jāti-patrī*, *kuṅkuma*, *lavaṅga*, *kaṅkola*, *arka* and *karambha* as *anupāna* (vehicle).

Properties

Bhasma of mercury is an excellent promoter of complexion, enthusiasm, viritity and power of digestion. It cures consumption, phthisis, tuberculosis, *prameha* (obstinate urinary diseases including diabetes), *viṣama jvara* (irregular fever), *pralepaka* (hectic fever), chronic fever and slow fever (continuous). It promotes lustre of an old person, makes him capable of procreating progeny and endows him with auspiciousness. It promotes *ojas* (vital essence) and it is an excellent drug for curing serious types of *vātika* diseases. It cures diseases caused by *kapha* and *karman* (effect of the evil acts in the past life). It is an excellent *bṛṃhaṇa* (nourishing agent). It is called *Vaikrānta-baddha-sūta*.

इष्टिकायां[२१८] तु पक्वायां सुरवातं चतुरङ्गुलम् ।
कृत्वा काचेन संलिप्तं तस्यान्तः पिष्टिकां क्षिपेत् ।।२७३ ।।
निंबूद्रवार्द्रो गन्धः[२१९] स्याद्देयो मूर्ध्नि[२२०] च कार्षिकः ।
मुखं[२२१] संरुध्य शुष्केऽथ दद्याल्लघुपुटं[२२२] ततः ।।२७४ ।।
शीते तस्योपरि पुनः पुटं देयं ततोऽधिकम् ।
एवं द्वित्रिचतुःकुर्याद्यावज्जीर्यति षड्गुणः ।।२७५ ।।
मूर्च्छितो विधिना तेन भवेद्रोगहरं किल ।
प्रमेहक्षयपाण्ड्वर्तिशूलकार्श्यहरोऽग्निदः ।।२७६ ।।

Ṣaḍguṇa-Bali-Jārita Bhasma

In a well cooked brick, a hole of four *aṅgula-s* diameter should be made and the inside wall of this hole should be smeared with the paste of glass. Inside this hole, the paste of mercury should be kept and covered with sulphur triturated by adding lemon-juice. Then the opening of the hole should be sealed. After it is dried up, the brick should be cooked by *laghu puṭa*. After it cools down, the seal should be removed and more sulphur should be added in the hole. Thereafter, the hole should be sealed again and cooked. This process should be repeated for two, three or four times till six times of sulphur (of the quantity of mercury) is digested (used). By this process of *mūrcchanā* the *bhasma* of mercury becomes capable of curing diseases. It cures *prameha* (obstinate urinary diseases including diabetes), consumption, anemia, colic pain and emaciation. It also promotes the power of digestion.

पृथक् पृथक् समं कृत्वा पारदं[२२३] गन्धकं तथा ।
नवसारं स्फटिकीं च सनागं याममात्रकम् ।।२७७।।
निम्बूरसेन संमर्द्य काचकूप्यां विनिक्षिपेत् ।
पूर्ववद्वालुकायन्त्रे यामद्वादशकं पचेत् ।।२७८।।
स्फोटयित्वोपयुक्तं[२२४] च ऊर्ध्वलग्नं वलिं त्यजेत् ।
अधः[२२५]स्थं रससिन्दूरं योजयेद्रसकर्मणि[२२६] ।।२७९।।

Another Method of Preparing Rasasindūra

Mercury, sulphur, *navasādara*, alum and the lead-*bhasma* should be taken in equal quantities and each of these ingredients should be separately triturated by adding lemon-juice. All these powders should be kept in a glass bottle and as before cooked in *vālukā yantra* for twelve *yāma-s*. After breaking the bottle, the sulphur adhered to the upper part should be rejected and the *rasa sindūra* attached to the lower part should be collected. It should be used in remedies.

रसदर्पणात्
औषधीघातितः[२२७] सूतो यदा भूयो न जीवति ।
न तु क्रामति लोहेषु न च कुर्याद्रसायनम् ।।२८०।।
तस्मात्सुवर्णादियुतं[२२८] मारयेद्रसभैरवम् ।
कज्जलाभो यदा सूतो विहाय घनचापलम् ।
दृश्यतेऽसौ तदा ज्ञेयो मूर्च्छितः सुतरां बुधैः ।।२८१।।

According to Rasadarpaṇa

If mercury reduced to *bhasma* form (killed) by processing with other drugs is not envigorated (returned to life) again, then does not help in the transmutation of base metals and in rejuvenation of the body. Therefore, *bhasma* of mercury should be prepared by adding gold, etc.

When mercury abandoning its compactness and fickleness, looks like collyrium, then it should be considered as *mūrcchita* (fainted).

रसार्णवात्

रसस्तु पादांशसुवर्णयुक्तः[२२९] पिष्टीकृतो गोघृतगंधयोगात् ।
तुल्यो सुगन्धपुटितः क्रमेण निर्वीर्यनामा खलु रोगहन्ता ।।२८२ ।।
बीजीकृतैरभ्रकसत्वहेममाक्षिकक्रान्तैः[२३०] सह साधितो यः ।
पुनस्ततः षड्गुणगन्धजीर्णः[२३१] सवीर्यनामा ह्यधिकप्रभावः ।।२८३ ।।

Nirvīrya and Savīrya Mercury According to Rasārṇava

Mercury mixed with one fourth in quantity of gold should be made to a paste by adding cow's ghee and sulphur .Then it is to be cooked by *puṭa-pāka*. The *bhasma*, thus prepared, is called *nirvīrya* and it is useful in curing diseases.

If mercury is processed with *bīja-s* (seeds) like *sattva* of *abhraka*, *svarṇa mākṣika* and *kānta lauha* and again given *jāraṇā* with six times of sulphur, then it is called *savīrya* which is therapeutically more effective.

दुतकज्जलिका[२३२] मोचापत्रेषु चिपिटीकृता ।
सपाद्[?] पर्पटश्चैव शिशूनामतिशस्यते ।।२८४।।

Rasa Parpaṭī (Scale Preparation of Mercury)

Melted *kajjalī* (fine black powder prepared by triturating mercury with sulphur) should be pressed between two banana-leaves. This is called *parpaṭī* (scale preparation) and it is specially useful for the treatment of children.

रसदर्पणात्

क्लिास-हल्लास-बलास-कास-श्वास-त्रिदोषादि गदाः पलादाः ।

तावद्दलं यातु[२३३] न यावदेव वैद्याधिराजो रसचक्रपाणिः[२३४] ।।२८५।।

According to Rasadarpaṇa

[The meaning of this verse is not clear; hence left untranslated.]

प्रथमं मारयेत्ताम्रं शास्त्रोक्तं सुपरीक्षितम् ।
पश्चात्तं योजयेद्देहे सूतकं तदनन्तरम् ।।२८६।।
गुंजाद्वयं समारभ्य यावन्माषद्वयं भवेत् ।
क्षेत्रमेतत् भवेद्देहं सूतवीर्यं प्रसाधकम् ।
अक्षेत्रे योजितः सूतो न प्ररोहेत्कदाचन ।।२८७।।

।। इति क्षेत्रीकरणम् ।।

Kṣetrīkaraṇa (Preparation of the Body)

First of all, *bhasma* of copper should be prepared according to methods prescribed in scriptures and it should be administered to the patient in the beginning. Thereafter, *bhasma* of mercury should be administered to him started from a dose of two *rattī-s* and gradually increased till the dose is two *māṣa-s*. By the administration of the *bhasma* of copper, the body becomes suitable to accept the *bhasma* of mercury and the latter becomes more potent therapeutically. Administration of the *bhasma* of mercury to a person whose body is not suitable does not produce the desired (prescribed) therapeutic effects.

रसार्णवात्

प्रभाते भक्षयेत्सूतं पथ्यं यामद्वयाधिके ।
नो लंघयेत्त्रियामं तु मध्याह्नेनैव भोजयेत् ।।२८८।।
कुंकुमागुरुलेपं च तथा कर्पूरभक्षणम् ।
भूमिशय्यातिपानं च अध्वानं परिवर्जयेत् ।।२८९।।
कूष्माण्डं कर्कटी 'चैव[२३५] कालिंगं कारवेल्लकम् ।
कुसुंभिकां च कर्कोटीं' कदलीं काकमाचिकाम् ।।२९०।।
ककाराष्टकमेतद्धि वर्जयेद्रससेवकः ।
कुलत्थाश्चातसीतैलं तिलान्माषान्मसूरकान् ।।२९१।।
कपोतं कांजिकान्नं च तक्रभक्तं तथैव च ।

वार्ताकं राजिकं[२३६] बिल्वं वातलानि च वर्जयेत् ।।२९२।।
तिलतैलं दधि क्षारं द्राक्षाक्षौद्रपरूषकम् ।
बदरं नारिकेलं[२३७] च सहकारं सुवर्चलाम् ।।२९३।।
नारंगं कांचनारं च सौभांजनमपि त्यजेत् ।
वर्ज्यं चैवातिमधुरमत्यम्लं कटुतिक्तकम् ।।२९४।।
वर्ज्या वृद्धा विरूपा स्त्री वर्जयेल्लवणं ततः ।
सूतस्रावः[२३८] प्रजायेत ज्वरश्चैव प्रजायते ।।२९५।।
उद्भिन्नचूचुका श्यामा सुभोगा सुभगा[२३९] शुभा ।
दिव्याभरणसंयुक्ता कामभोगविवर्जिता[२४०] ।
सन्निधानेषु कर्तव्या वृद्धैश्च परिरक्षिता ।।२९६।।
अतिपानमपानं च जलक्रीडां च वर्जयेत् ।।२९७।।
कुंचिताग्रास्तु ये केशा[२४१] ये श्यामा पद्मलोचना ।
विस्तीर्णजघनं तस्या संकीर्णहृदयं भवेत् ।।२९८।।
कृष्णपक्षे भवेद्यस्याः युवत्याः पुष्पदर्शनम् ।
काकिनी सा समाख्याता उत्तमा च रसायने ।।२९९।।
आलिंगने स्पर्शने च मैथुनालापयोरपि ।
सर्वरोगविनिर्मुक्तो वलीपलितवर्जितः ।।३००।।

Method of Administration of Mercury Bhasma According to Rasārṇava

Mercury should be administered to the patient early in the morning and wholesome food should be given to him after two *yāma-s* during the noon time. He should never be kept fasting for more than three *yāmā-s*. His body should be anointed with *kuṅkuma* and *aguru* and he should be given camphor to eat. He should avoid sleeping on the ground, excessively drinking alcohol and walking a long distance.

Prohibitions

Kūṣmāṇḍa, *karkaṭī*, *kāliṅga*, *kāravellaka*, *kusumbhikā*, *karkkoṭī*, *kadalī* and *kākamācikā*- these vegetables taken together are called *Kakārāṣṭaka* (eight names beginning with the alphabet '*ka*'). A person using mercury should avoid eating these ingredients.

He should aviod eating *kulattha*, oil of *atasī*, *tila*, *māṣa*, *masūra*, *kapota*, food mixed with *kāñjī* or butter-milk, *vārtāka*, *rājikā*, *bilva* and such other ingredients which aggravate *vāyu*.

He should also avoid oil of sesame, yoghurt, alkalies, *drākṣā*, honey, *parūṣaka*, *badara*, *nārikela*, *sahakāra*, *suvarcalā*, *nāraṅga*, *kāñcanāra*, *sobhāñjana*, excessively sweet or sour ingredients, pungent or bitter spices, sexual intercourse with old women and ladies with unpleasing appearance and salt.

If a person uses these unwholesome ingredients and regimens, then the mercury does not remain in the body and gets excreted. He suffers from fever.

Attendants

The patient or healthy person taking the *bhasma* of mercury should be closely attended by women having plumpy nipples and of *śyāmā* type (having bluish complexion), who are enjoyable, who are without any blemish in their genital organs, who are auspicious, who are wearing beautiful ornaments and who are not exposed to sexual intercourse by other persons. These women should be protected from outsiders by old people. They should not indulge in excessive drinking of alcohol nor should they be teetotallers. They should avoid aquatic games.

Kākinī Type of Women

Women having hair curlled at the end, having bluish complexion, having plumpy thighs and narrow chest and having menstruation during the black fortnight of the lunar month are called *kākinī* . They are excellent for the purpose of rejuvenation therapy. Embracing and touching them, having sexual intercourse with them and having pleasant talks with them make a person free from all diseases including wrinkling and graying of hair.

रसार्णवात्

एको हि दोषः सूक्ष्मो यः[२४२] भक्षिते भस्मसूतके ।
त्रिसप्ताहाद्वरारोहे कामान्धो जायते नरः ॥३०१॥
मैथुनाच्छुक्रमेहस्य त्रिसप्ताहादधः कृतात् ।
जायते प्राणसन्देहस्तावत्तन्मैथुनं त्यजेत् ॥३०२॥
युवत्या जल्पनं कार्यं युवत्या चांगमर्दनम् ।
तस्याः स्पर्शनमात्रेण रसः क्राम्यति विग्रहे ॥३०३॥

यथा यथा ह्लादयते सुस्त्रीरूपनिरीक्षणात् ।
तथा क्रामति दैवेशि सूतकोऽसौ ततः क्रमात् ।।३०४।।
कस्तूरीसंयुतं नित्यं ताम्बूलं भक्षयेद्वरम् ।
सुरभीणि च पुष्पाणि चन्दनागुरुलेपनम् ।
लवणादिक्रियां याति स्त्रीसंगान्म्रियते[२४३] नरः ।।३०५।।

According to Rasārṇava

Intake of the *bhasma* of mercury has a subtle blemish inasmuch as by taking it for three weeks, a person becomes mad with sex desire. Within these three weeks, if the person indulges in sex, then the gets *śukra meha* (ejaculation of semen while urinating) and his life becomes in danger. Therefore, he should aviod sexual intercourse [for these three weeks]. [Thereafter], the person taking mercurty should have pleasant talks with youthful women and these women should be employed to give massage to his body. By the touch of these women, mercury permeates through all the tissues of the body. As the person gets pleausre in watching these youthful women, the mercury permeats through the tissues of the body in succession.

Other Regimens

A person taking mercury should regulary take betel-leaf along with musk, wear garlands of fragrant flowers and anoinet his body with the paste of sandal-wood and *aguru*.

Prohibitions

Intake of salt creates several morbidities and sexual intercourse with women causes death.

सूताजीर्णाज्ज्वरस्तन्द्री नाभिमूलेऽतिगौरवम् ।
अन्तर्दाहो जडत्वं च वह्निनाशः प्रजायते ।।३०६।।
तथा च
मूर्छा शोके भ्रमः कंमश्छर्दिमोहो ज्वरस्तथा ।
'हिक्का[२४४] वेपथु शूलानि निद्रालस्यमरोचकम् ।।३०७।।
लिंगस्तम्भो ह्यतीसारः कासश्वासविजृम्भकाः' ।
कर्णादिचक्षुकुक्षेश्च चरणोदरमूर्धनि ।।३०८।।

मेढ्रदाहोऽग्निबन्धश्च भवेत्सर्वाङ्गवेदना ।
ये चान्ये च महारोगाः रसाजीर्णे भवन्ति हि ॥३०९॥
चविका स्वर्जिकाक्षारं कारवल्लीरसप्लुतम् ।
गोमूत्रसैन्धवयुतं रससंस्राविनं पिबेत् ॥३१०॥
मोचकस्य रसं देवि राजकोशातकीरसम् ।
रसाजीर्णे तु जीर्येत नियतं[२४५] नात्र संशयः ॥३११॥
लंघनं[२४६] त्रिदिनं कुर्याद्रसं चैव विवर्जयेत् ।
कर्कोट्याः हि[२४७] कषायं च पाययेद्दिवसत्रयम् ॥३१२॥
सौवर्चलं गोजलेन पिबेद्वा सुखवाञ्छया ।
विश्वसैन्धवचूर्णं च मातुलुंगाम्लवारिणा ।
रसाजीर्णविनाशार्थं पिबेद्रोगी दिनत्रयम् ॥३१३॥

॥ रसेऽजीर्णे[२४८] ॥

Indigestion of Mercury

If the *bhasma* of mercury does not get digested, then the person suffers from fever, drowsiness, excessive heaviness in the umbilical region, burning sensation inside the body, numbness and suppression of the power of digestion.

In addition, the person suffers from fainting, grief, giddiness, shivering, vomiting, unconsciousness, fever, hiccup, trembling, colic pain, excessive sleep, laziness, anorexia, stiffness of phallus, diarrhoea, cough, asthma, yawning, burning sensation in ears, eyes, pelvic region, legs, abdomen, head and phallus, loss of appetite, pain all over the body and such other serious diseases because of the indigestion of the *bhasma* of mercury.

Treatment of Mercury-Indigestion

If the mercury is not digested and gets excreted, then the patient should be given *cavya* and *svarjikṣāra* mixed with the juice of *kāravellaka*, cow's urine and *saindhava*.

Intake of the juice of *mocaka* and *rāja kośātakī*, undoubtedly helps in the digestion of undigested mercury.

The person having indigetion of mercury should regularly keep fast for three days abstaine from taking mercury further and take the decoction of *karkoṭī* for three days.

For getting cured of mercury indigestion, the patient should take either *sauvarcala* mixed with cow's urine, or the powders of *śuṇṭhī* and *saindhava* mixed with the sour juice of *mātuluṅga* for three days.

पाठायुक्तं पिबेन्मूलं कारवल्लीभवं तदा ।
नागदोषः शमं याति पारदस्य न संशयः ।।३१४।।

।। नागदोषनाशनम्[२४९] ।।

Treatment of Nāga Doṣa

Intake of the decoction of *pāṭhā* along with the root of *kāravallī* cures the adverse poisoning effects caused by the association of *nāga doṣa* (lead poisoning) in mercury.

वंगदोषप्रशान्त्यर्थं शरपुंखां[२५०] हि भक्षयेत्[२५१] ।।३१५।।

।। वंगदोषनाशनम्[२५२] ।।

Treatment of Vaṅga Doṣa

For correcting the adverse poisoning effects of *vaṅga doṣa* (tin-poisoning) associated with mercury, the patient should take *śarapuṅkhā*.

अनुलोमगतिर्वायुः स्वस्थता[२५३] सुमनस्कृता ।
क्षुत्तृष्णेन्द्रियवैमल्यं रसपाकस्य लक्षणम् ।।३१६।।

Signs of Proper Digestion of Mercury

Downward movement of flatus in the abdomen, feeling of good health, happiness, proper appetite and thirst and clarity of senses, these are the signs of proper digestion of the *bhasma* of mercury.

अथ कक्षापुटिमतात्

वसति गिरिगुहायां नैव सिंहो न नागः ।
न च भवति खगेन्द्रो जातपक्षद्वयो न ।।३१७।।
अरुणकिरणवर्णो दृश्यते चाम्बरस्थः[२५४] ।
सकलजनप्रसिद्धस्तेन बद्धो रसेन्द्रः ।।३१८।।

Description of Hiṅgula According to Kakṣāpuṭi

A substance, which is located in the caves of mountains but it is neither lion nor elephant nor the chief of birds nor the ordinary birds and it looks pink like the rising sun in the sky, is the abode of mercury. This is popularly known [as *hingula*].

रसार्णवात्

निर्जीवत्वं गतः सूतः कथं जीवं ददाति सः ।
निर्जीवेन तु निर्जीवः कथं जीवति शंकरः ।।३१९।।
परस्य हरते कालं कालिकारहितो[२५५] रसः ।
अष्टानां चैव लोहानां मलं शमयति क्षणात् ।।३२०।।
महामूर्च्छागतं सूतं को वापि[२५६] कथयेन्मृतम् ।
दिव्यौषध्या रसेनैव जायते नष्टचेतनः ।
कालिकारहितश्चापि आधिव्याधिं च नाशयेत् ।।३२१।।

।। इति पारदशोधन-अष्टसंस्कार-जारण-मारणविधिः ।।

According to Rasārṇava

Mercury *bhasma* which itself is lifeless, how can it give life to others ? How can a lifeless person become alive by this lifeless substance? [This is a dialogue between Lord Śiva and Goddess Pārvatī]. When mercury is free from blemishes (*kālikā*), it takes away the life (*kāla*) of the opponents (diseases). It instantaneously makes the eight types of metals free from any impurity. Processed mercury remains in great swoon (*mahā mūrcchā*) and it is never dead. It is because of the combination with celestial herbs (*divyauṣadhi-s*) that the mercury becomes unconscious. If it becomes free from *kālikā* (blemishes), the mercury cures diseases.

Thus, ends the description of purification, eight *saṃskāra-s*, *jāraṇa* and *māraṇa* of mercury.

GANDHAKA (SULPHUR)

श्वेतद्वीपे पुरा[२५७] देव्याः क्रीडन्त्याः प्रसृतं रजः ।
क्षीरार्णवे[२५८] तु स्नाताया दुकूलं रजसान्वितम् ।
धौतं यन्मथिता[२५९] वस्त्रं गन्धवद्गन्धकं स्मृतम् ।।३२२।।

Sulphur

Mythological Origin

In the days of yore, while the goddess Pārvatī was playing in *Śveta-dvīpa, rajas* (menstrual blood) came out. She went to wash her blood-smeared cloth in the *kṣīrārṇava* (ocean of milk). While she was washing and squeezing her cloth, the foul smelling sulphur took its origin.

चतुर्धा गन्धकः प्रोक्तो रक्तः पीतः सितोऽसितः ।
रक्तो हेमक्रियासूक्तः पीतश्चैव रसायने ।
व्रणादिलेपने श्वेतः श्रेष्ठः कृष्णं[२६०] सुदुर्लभः ॥३२३॥

Varieties

Sulphur is of four types, viz., red, yellow, white and black. Red variety of sulphur is useful in the [preparation of *bīja* of mercury] for the transmutation of base metals into gold (*hemakriyā*). Yellow variety of sulphur is useful in rejuvenation therapy. White variety of sulphur is useful in the preparation of ointments for the treatment of ulcers. The black variety of sulphur which is the best in properties is extremely rare.

क्षीरेण भाण्डमापूर्य वस्त्रमावेष्ट्य तन्मुखम् ।
वस्त्रमध्ये क्षिपेद्गन्धं मुखं यत्नात् पिधापयेत् ॥३२४॥

Purification of Sulphur

An earthen vessel should be filled with milk and its mouth should be tied with a piece of cloth. Over this cloth, [melted] sulphur should be poured. While doing so, the face should be carefully covered.

'कंगुणीसर्षपैरण्डं[२६१] तैलं वाऽथ कुसुम्भजम् ।
मेषीक्षीरं घृतं वाऽथ गोक्षीरं वाऽऽरनालकम् ॥३२५॥
एतेष्वेकं तु भांडान्तं किंचिदूनं प्रपूरयेत् ।
बद्ध्वा वस्त्रेण तत्र तु गन्धचूर्णं ततोपरि ॥३२६॥
लोहपात्रे निनुध्याथ पृष्ठे स्थाप्यं च खर्प्परम् ।
साग्निमुपलकैः पूर्णमिदं द्रव्यं समुद्धरेत् ॥३२७॥

तं धत्तूरद्रवैः पिष्ट्वा शोष्यं द्राव्यं च पूर्ववत् ।
पुनरेवं प्रकर्त्तव्यं शुक्रदो गन्धको भवेत् ।।३२८।।

।। रसरत्नाकरात्' ।।

Detailed Method of Sulphur Purification According to Rasaratnākara

A vessel should be filled up with either of the following liquids:

(1) oil of *kaṅguṇi*
(2) oil of *sarṣapa*
(3) oil of *eraṇḍa*
(4) oil of *kusumbha*
(5) sheep-milk
(6) cow's ghee
(7) cow's milk
(8) *āranāla* (sour vinegar)

With any of these liquids the vessel should be filled leaving some space at the top. The mouth of the vessel should be tied with a piece of cloth. The powder of sulphur should be melted by keeping in an iron spoon over the fire of cowdung cake. It should be poured into the liquid kept in the vessel through a piece of *kharpara* (broken jar). From the liquid, the solidified sulphur should be collected. It should be made to a paste by triturating with the juice of *dhattūra* and dried. This powder should again be melted and processed as before. This purified sulphur enhances the production of semen.

अन्यच्च
शरावेण ततो वह्निं[२६२] प्रज्वाल्योर्द्धमवस्थितम् ।
भाण्डके निपतेद्यावद्गन्धस्तावत्समिन्धयेत्[२६३] ।
कृशानौ तु स्वयं शीते गन्धकं तु समुद्धरेत् ।।३२९।।

Another Method of Sulphur Purification

Sulphur should be kept inside two earthern plates with their joint sealed. The lower plate should have a hole at the bottom and it should be kept over a vessel containing milk. Fire should be applied over the upper jar and the melted sulphur then drops down into the liquid kept in the vessel below. When the fire cools down sulphur should be collected.

अन्यच्च

एवमेरण्डभृङ्गारधत्तूरस्य रसेन वै ।।३३०।।

Another Method

In the place of milk, the juice of *eranda*, *bhṛṅgarāja* and *dhattūra* can be used in the vessel and the sulphur should be processed as before.

अन्यच्च

स्निग्धां दर्वीं वह्निसंस्थां गन्धं तेन द्रवीकृतम् ।
क्षीरभाण्डे विनिक्षिप्तं शुद्धं भवति तत्क्षणात्[२६४] ।।३३१।।

Another Method

An iron spoon should be smeared with ghee and kept over fire. In the spoon, sulphur powder should be kept and melted. The melted sulphur should be poured into a vessel containing milk. Thus, sulphur is purified.

गन्धकः कृमिकुष्टघ्नः विषनेत्रामयापहः ।
रसायनश्चातिबल्यो विषमज्वरनाशनः ।।३३२।।

Properties of Sulphur

Purified sulphur cures *kṛmi* (parasitic infestation), *kuṣṭha* (obstinate skin diseases including leprosy), poisoning and eye-diseases. It rejuvenates the body and promotes strength in excess. It also cures *viṣama jvara* (irregular fever).

"[२६५]देवदाल्यम्लपर्ण्याः वा नारंगं वाऽथ दाडिमम् ।
मातुलुंगं यथालाभं द्रवमेकस्य चाहरेत् ।।३३३।।

For the purification of sulphur, the juice of *devadālī*, *amlaparṇī*, *nāraṅga*, *dāḍima* or *mātuluṅga*, whatever is available, [can be used in the place of milk].

गंधकस्य तु पादांशं टंकणद्रवसंयुतम् ।
यताभ्यां गंधकं भागं त्रिभिर्वारं ततः पुनः ।।३४४।।

[The meaning of this verse is not clear, hence left untranslated.]

"धत्तूरस्तुलसी कृष्णा लशुनं देवदालिका ।
शिग्रुमूलं काकमाची कर्पूरं शंखिनीद्वयम् ।।३३५।।
कृष्णागुरु च कस्तूरी बंध्याकर्कोटिकी समम् ।
मातुलुंगरसैः पिष्ट्वा लोहपात्रस्थं[२६६] भावयेत्"।
[रसकामधेनु : पृष्ठ २८१ : ४७-५०]
पूर्वगंधकं त्रिवारं क्षौद्रतुल्यं तु जायते ।।३३६।।

Preparation of Liquid Gandhaka

Sulphur should be made to a paste by triturating with the juice of *mātuluṅga*. This paste should be impregnated with the juice or decoction of *dhattūra*, *tulasī*, *kṛṣṇā*, *laśuna*, *devadālī*, root of *śigru*, *kākamācī*, *karpūra*, both the varieties of *śaṅkhinī*, *kṛṣṇāguru*, *kastūrī* and *vandhyā-karkkoṭikī* three times in each in an iron vessel.

This produces sulphur in a liquid form and looks like honey.

गंधकवर्जितं एवं गन्धकतैलं स्यात् तत् योगेषु योजयेत्' ।।३३७।।

The above mentioned recipe of sulphur is free from bad odour and it is called *Gandhaka taila*. This may be used in recipes.

अशुद्धगन्धः[२६७] कुरुते तु कुष्ठतापरुजं पित्तरुजं तनोति ।
रूपंसुखंवीर्यबलंनिहन्ति तस्मात्सुशुद्धं विनियोजनीयम् ।।३३८।।

Adverse Effects of Impure Sulphur

Impure sulphur causes *kuṣṭha* (obstinate skin diseases including leprosy), burning sensation and *paittika* diseases. It reduces complexion, happiness, potency, and strength. Therefore, only purified sulphur should be used.

रससिन्धुः
गन्धकस्य[२६८] च पादांशं दद्याद् टंकणकं पुनः ।
मर्दयेन्मातुलुंगाम्लैरुष्णतैलेन भावयेत् ।।३३९।।
पुनः खर्परके कृत्वा दीपाग्निं ज्वालयेदधः ।

न्यसेत्तत्र जलं कोष्णं मानाधिक्यं च यत्नतः ।
जलेन युक्तं यत्तैलं तत्तैलं रससाधकम् ।।३४०।।

Preparation of Gandhaka Taila
According to Rasasindhu

One part of sulphur and 1/4th part of *ṭaṅkaṇa* should be triturated by adding the sour juice of *mātuluṅga*. This should then be added with warm oil and kept in a *kharparaka* with strong fire below it. After sometime, more warm water should be added. This oil mixed with water helps in processing mercury.

"[२६९]अर्कक्षीरैः स्नुहीक्षीरैर्वस्त्रलेपं तु सप्तधा ।
गंधकं नवनीतेन पिष्ट्वा वस्त्रं लिपेत्तु[२७०] तम् ।।३४१।।
तद्वर्तिर्ज्वलिता दण्डे[२७१] धृत्वा धार्यमधोमुखः ।
तैलं पतेदधो[२७२] भाण्डे ग्राह्यं योगेषु योजयेत्" ।।३४२।।
[रसकामधेनु : पृष्ठ २८२ : ५४ - ५५]

।।इति गन्धकोत्पत्ति - जाति- शोधन-गुण-तैलपाननञ्च ।।

Another Method of Preparing Gandhaka Taila

A piece of cloth should be smeared with the milky latex of *arka* and *snuhī* for seven times in each. Sulphur should be made to a paste by triturating with butter. The above mentioned cloth should be smeared with this paste and made to a wick by rolling. Holding this wick with a stick [at the top], the lower end should be ignited. Thus, the oil of sulphur comes down and it should be collected by keeping a jar below. This sulphur oil should be used in different recipes.

Thus, ends the description of the origin, varieties, purification, properties and oil preparation of sulphur.

शिवस्य तेजः प्रथितं रसोऽयं देवीभवं गन्धमथाभ्रकाख्यम् ।
शुल्वं च सूर्यस्य सहरश्मेश्चन्द्रस्य रौप्यं परमेश्वरस्य ।।३४३।।
स्वर्णं तु विष्णुप्रभवं[२७३] वदन्ति सीसं तु नागस्य च[२७४] वासुकेश्च ।
लोहं यमस्यैवं तु कालमूर्तेर्वंगं च शुक्रस्य पुराविदो बुधाः ।।३४४।।

Mythological Origin of Different Metals

Mercury is the product of the semen of Lord Śiva. From the goddess Pārvatī, sulphur and mica originated. Copper is the potency of Sun. Silver originated from moon, the Parameśvara. Gold originated from Lord Viṣṇu. Lead took its origin from the serpent god Vāsuki. Iron originated from Yama, the god of time. Tin took its origin from Śukra. This is the opinion of wise people who are well versed in mythology.

मृत्यूपमृत्युनाशार्थं पारदं शिवदं भवेत् ।
ये गुणाः पारदे देवि गन्धकाभ्रे च ते गुणाः ।।३४५।।

Death and untimely death can be prevented by mercury . The properties of sulphur and mica are similar to those of mercury.

आरोग्यं भास्करादिच्छेत्सोमो धातुसमृद्धये ।
रोगाणां शान्तये सेव्यं देवदेवेशमुत्तमम् ।।३४६।।

A person desirous of good health should offer prayer to Sun. Offering prayer to Moon promotes nourishment of tissue elements. For the cure of diseases, prayer should be offered to Lord Śiva.

ABHRAKA (MICA)

कदाचिद्गिरिजा देवि हरं दृष्ट्वा मनोहरम् ।
मुमोच[२७५] यत्तदा वीर्यं तज्जातं शुभ्रमभ्रकम् ।।३४७।।

Mythology About Origin of Mica

Once upon a time the goddess Pārvatī being passionately attracted by the handsome Lord Śiva, ejaculated *vīrya* (ovum or bartholin secretion). From out of this secretion, pure mica originated.

श्वेतं पीतं तथा कृष्णं रक्तं तद्भूमिसंगमात् ।
पीतं हेम्नि सितं तारे रक्तं चैव रसायने ।
कृष्णाभ्रकं च रोगेषु द्रुतिपाते तथा तथैव च ।।३४८।।

Varieties of Mica

Mica, because of its contact with different types of soil, becomes white, yellow, black or red in colour.

Yellow type of mica is useful for processing gold, white type of mica for silver; red type of mica for rejuvenation therapy; and black type of mica is useful for treatment of diseases and for the extraction of *sattva* (essence).

"पिनाकं[७६] दर्दुरं नागं वज्रं चेति चतुर्थकम् ।"३४९ ।।
[रसकामधेनु : पृष्ठ २४१ : ७४]

Mica, on the basis of its attributes is also divided into four types, viz, *pināka*, *dardura*, *nāga* and *vajra*. [This classfication, according to some physicians, relates to black variety of mica].

मुञ्चत्यग्नौ विनिक्षिप्तः पिनाको दलसंचयम् ।
अज्ञानाद्भक्षणात्तस्य महाकुष्टं प्रजायते ।।३५० ।।

***Pināka* Type of Mica**

When placed over the flame of fire, the different layers of *pināka* type of mica get separated. If because of ignorance, the *bhasma* of such type of mica is taken in, then the person suffers from *mahā kuṣṭha* (obstinate types of skin diseases including leprosy).

दर्दुरोऽग्निगतोऽत्यर्थः[७७] कुरुते दर्दुरध्वनिम्[७८] ।
तस्य देहं प्रविष्टस्य भगन्दरभयं भवेत् ।।३५१ ।।

***Dardura* Type of Mica**

Dardura type of mica, when placed over fire produces sound like that of a frog. If taken in it causes fistula-in-ano.

वह्निप्रविष्टो नागस्तु फूत्कारं प्रविमुञ्चति ।
स तूदरं प्रमेहं च प्रकरोति नपुंसकम् ।।३५२ ।।

***Nāga* Type of Mica**

Nāga type of mica, when placed over fire, produces hissing sound like a cobra. If taken in, it causes *udara* (obstinate abdominal diseases including ascites), *prameha* (obstinate urinary disorders including diabetes) and impotency.

वज्रस्तु वज्रवत्तिष्ठेद्वयाधिवार्धक्यमृत्युहा ।।३५३।।

Vajra Type of Mica

Vajra type of mica, when placed over fire , remains stable like a thunder-bolt. It cures diseases, prevents aeging and death.

अथ मतान्तरात्[२७९]

पुरा वधाय वृत्रस्य[२८०] वज्रिणा वज्रमुद्धृतम् ।
विस्फुल्लिंगास्ततस्तस्य गगनं परिसर्पतः[२८१] ।।३५४।।
निपेतुर्मेघनिर्घोषाच्छिखरेषु महीभृताम् ।
तेभ्य एव समुत्पन्नं तद्गिरिषु चाभ्रकम् ।।३५५।।
तद्वज्रं वज्रजातत्वादभ्रमभ्ररवोद्भवात् ।
गगनच्युतिजातत्वाद्वचिरे गगनं[२८२] सुराः ।।३५६।।

Another Mythological Story

In the days of yore, when Lord Indra raised his *vajra* (thunder-bolt) to kill the demon Vṛtra, the sparklings from this thunder-bolt moved around the sky and along with the roaring rain fell on the top of mountains. From out of these sparklings, mica originated in those mountains. It is called *vajra* because of its origine from *vajra* (thunder-bolt) and it is called *abhra* because it was produced from the roaring sound in the *abhra* (cloud) since it fell down from *gagana* (sky) it is also called *gagana.*

तद्विप्रक्षत्रं विट् शूद्रभेदाच्चैव चतुर्विधम् ।
क्रमेणैव सितं रक्तं पीतं कृष्णं च वर्णतः ।।३५७।।

Varieties

It is of four types , viz., *brāhmaṇa, kṣatriya, vaiśya* and *śūdra* which are white, red, yellow and black in colour respectively.

तत्र दक्षिणशैलेर्क्शोषादल्पगुणं हि तत् ।
अल्पसत्त्वं तदाधत्ते अभ्रे सत्त्वं गुणप्रदम् ।।३५८।।
अतश्चोत्तरशैलोत्थं बहुसत्त्वगुणोत्तमम ।
शंसन्ति मुनयः सर्वे प्रयोगे कृष्णमभ्रकम् ।।३५९।।

Relative Merits

In the southern mountains, because of drying effect of the sun, mica is less effective and it has less of *sattva* (mineral essence). In mica, it is actually this *sattva* which is responsible for its therapeutic efficacy. Therefore, mica collected from the northern mountains is the most effective because it contains more of *sattva* (mineral essence). For therapeutic purposes, physicians prefer to use black variety of mica (*kṛṣṇābhra*).

आदौ सुतापितं कृत्वा गगनं सप्तधा क्षिपेत् ।
'निर्गुण्डी[२८३]स्वरसे सम्यक् गिरिदोषप्रशान्तये ।।३६०।।

Purification of Mica

Black variety of mica heated over fire should be immersed in the juice of *nirguṇḍī*. This process should be repeated for seven times which makes mica free from *giri-doṣa*.

अंगारोपरि विन्यस्तं ध्मातमेकदलीकृतम्' ।
निक्षिपेत्काञ्जिके कृष्णमभ्रकं विह्निसन्निभम् ।।३६१।।
ततोऽस्य काञ्जिकस्यास्य वरं घर्मविधारणम् ।
शोषणं[२८४] च विधातव्यं पौनः पौन्येन पण्डितैः ।।३६२।।
चांगेरी[२८५]स्वांगनिर्यासैरप्येवं विधिमाचरेत् ।
तण्डुलीयकमूलस्य रसेनापि ततः परम् ।।३६३।।
ततो[२८६]ऽस्मिन् बदराङ्गारैर्नीते नीतेऽग्निवर्णताम् ।
क्षिपेत्पुनः पुनः क्षीरं यथाग्निश्चन्द्रिकं भवेत् ।।३६४।।

Thereafter, mica should be placed over burning charcoal by whicl different layers of it get separated. Then this should be placed in *kāñjī* (vinegar) and dried in the sun. This process should be repeated several times.

Then the process should be repeated along with the juice of *cāṅgerī* and the root of *taṇḍulīyaka*. After that, mica should be made red hot by placing over the fire of the charcoal of *badara*. Over this red hot mica, milk should repeatedly be sprinkled till the fire becomes white in colour like a moon.

अन्यच्च
क्षिप्त्वा क्षिप्त्वारनालेन तप्तं कुर्याच्च खर्परम् [?]।
त्रिःसप्तधा पुटं वा[२८७] तु दत्वा शुध्यति चाभ्रकम् ।।३६५।।

Another Method of Mica Purification

Pieces of mica should be made red-hot and immersed in *āranāla* (a type of vinegar). This process should be repeated for several times. Then it should be cooked in *puṭa* for 21 times which purifies mica.

चूर्णाभ्रं शालिसंयुतं[२८८] बद्धा कम्बलिके श्लथम् ।
त्रिरात्रं काञ्जिके स्थाप्यं तत्क्लिन्नं मर्दयेद् दृढम् ।
कंबलाद्गलितं श्लक्ष्णं मारणादौ प्रशस्यते[२८९] ।।३६६।।

Preparation of Dhānyābhra

Powder of mica mixed with *śāli* type of paddy should be loosely tied in a piece of woolen cloth and immersed in *kāñjī* (vinegar) for three nights. Thereafter, it should be strongly squeezed as a result of which mica powder comes out of the woolen cloth. This smooth mica powder is useful for the preparation of its *bhasma* (calcination).

अशुद्धाभ्रं निहन्त्यायुर्वर्धयेन्मारुतं कफम् ।
अहतं छेदयेदन्त्रं मन्दाग्निकृमिवृद्धिकृत् ।।३६७।।

Effect of Impure Mica

Use of impure mica takes away the sapn of life and aggravates *vāyu* and *kapha*. Similarly, use of mica which is not reduced to *bhasma* form leads to rupture of intestines, suppresses the power of digestion and gives rise to parasitic infestation.

धान्याभ्रं गुडतुल्यं च श्रेष्टं[२९०] [?] क्षीरेण[२९१] मर्दितम् ।
कुर्यात्सुचक्रिकां शुष्कां समयग्गजपुटे पचेत् ।।३६८।।
ततो धत्तूर-पत्तूर[२९२]-कुमारी-शशिवाटिका ।
प्रत्येकं स्वरसेनैव पुटेदाशु[२९३] मृतिं व्रजेत् ।।३६९।।

Preparation of Mica-Bhasma

Dhānyābhra mixed with equal quantity of jaggery should be

triturated with milk. From out of this, *cakrikā-s* (round & flat tablets) should be prepared , dried (in sun) and cooked in *gaja puṭa*. Thereafter, it should be given *puṭa* separately by triturating with the juices of *dhattūra*, *pattūra*, *kumārī* and *śaśivāṭikā*. This immediately reduces mica into *bhasma* form.

अन्यच्च

केनाप्यस्य तृणस्यापि रसेनाथ[२१४] प्रमर्दितम् ।
पुटितं दशधा भस्म निश्चन्द्रं जायते ध्रुवम् ।।३७० ।।

Second Method of Preparing Mica-Bhasma

Mica should be triturated with the juice of any [?] grass and cooked in *puṭa* for ten times which reduces it to *bhasma* form without any glaze particles.

रससिन्धु

तथा च

"धान्याभ्रकस्य भागैकं भागार्द्धं टङ्कणस्य च ।
पिष्ट्वा तदन्धमूषायां रुद्ध्वा तीव्राग्निना पचेत्" ।
[रसकामधेनु : पृष्ठ २४५ : ११२]
विचूर्ण्य योजयेद्योगे भेषजानामसंशयम् ।।३७१ ।।

Third Method of Preparing Mica-Bhasma According to Rasasindhu

One part of *dhānyābhraka* and half part of *ṭaṅkaṇa* should be triturated and made to a psate. Keeping this paste in *andha-mūṣā*, it should be cooked with strong fire. Then it should be made to a powder and used in recipes.

तथा च रसराजहंसात्

सपादटंकणं धान्यं गगनं धामितं दृढम् ।
निश्चन्द्रं जायते शीघ्रं बालभृङ्गरसप्लुतम् ।।३७२ ।।

Fourth Method of Preparing Mica-Bhasma According to Rasarājahaṃsa

Dhānyābhraka mixed with one fourth in quantity of *ṭaṅkaṇa* should be impregnated and triturated by adding the juice of tender variety of *bhṛṅgarāja*. This should be kept in a crucible and cooked over fire by blowing strongly which quickly reduces it to *bhasma* form without any glaze particles.

देवदालीरसे वापि[९५] धान्याभ्रं शतधा धमेत्[९६] ।
कर्पूरधवलं सूक्ष्मं निश्चन्द्रं जायते ध्रुवम् ।।३७३।।

Fifth Method of Preparing Mica-Bhasma

Dhānyābhra, triturated with the juice of *devadālī* should be cooked by *puṭa* for one hundred times which produces white and fine *bhasma* of mica without any glaze particles.

तथा च
ज्वालामुखीपुटैर्घर्मो धर्मेण परिकीर्तितः ।
कर्पूरपुलकाकारं निर्विकारं सुधोपमम् ।।३७४।।

[The meaning of this verse is not clear; hence left untranslated.]

"धान्याभ्रकं[९७] समादाय मुस्ताक्वाथैः पुटत्रयम् ।
तद्वत्पुनर्नवानीरैः कासमर्दरसैस्तथा ।।३७५।।
नागवल्लीदलैस्त्वर्क्क[९८]क्षीरैर्दद्यात्पृथक् पृथक् ।
दिनं दिनं मर्द्दयित्वा क्वाथैर्वटजटोद्भवैः ।।३७६।।
दत्वा पुटत्रयं पश्चात् त्रिपुटेन्मुशलीजलैः ।
त्रिर्गोक्षुरकषायेण त्रिः पुटेद्वानरीरसैः ।।३७७।।
मोचाकन्दरसैः पाच्यं त्रिवारं कोकिलाक्षकैः ।
रसैः पुटेत् ततो[९९] देयं क्षीरादेकं पुटं पुनः ।।३७८।।
दध्ना घृतेन मधुना स्वच्छया सितया तथा ।
एकमेकं पुटं दद्यादभ्रमेवं[१००] मृतं भवेत् ।।३७९।।

Sixth Method of Preparing Mica-Bhasma

Dhānyābhraka should be processed as follows :

(1) Triturating with the decoction of *mustā*, three *puṭa-s* should be given.

(2) One *puṭa* should be given after triturating with the juices of each of *punarnavā*, *kāsamarda*, leaf of *nāgavallī* and milky latex of *arka*.

(3) Three *puṭa-s* should be given after triturating with each of decoctions of the stilt root *vaṭa*, of *muśalī* and *gokṣura*, and juices of *vānarī*, *kadalī-kanda* and *kokilākṣa*.

(4) One *puṭa* should be given after triturating with milk.

(5) One *puṭa* should be given after triturating with each of curd, ghee, honey and solution of pure sugar.

सर्वरोगहरं व्योम जायते योगवाहकम् ।
कामिनीमददर्पघ्नं शस्तं पुंस्त्वोपघातिनाम् ।
वृष्यमायुष्करं शुक्रवृद्धिसंतानकारकम्' ।।३८० ।।

Therapeutic Properties of Mica-Bhasma

Thus, the *bhasma* of mica is prepared which cures all diseases and which works as *yogavāha* (which enhances the effect of drug to which it is added). It helps a person to satisfy the sex-desire of passionate women. It is useful for the treatment of impotency. It promotes virility, longevity and semen. It also helps a person to procreate children.

धान्याभ्रकस्य भागौ द्वौ भागैकं शुद्धगन्धकम्[३०१] ।
[रसकामधेनु : पृष्ठ : २४५ : १०६ - ११२]
वटक्षीरेण संमर्द्य अंधमूषां निरोधयेत् ।
पचेद्गजपुटेनैव वारमेकं मृतो भवेत् ।।३८१ ।।

Quick Method of Preparing Mica-Bhasma

Two parts of *dhānyābhraka* and one part of purified sulphur should be triturated by the milky latex of *vaṭa*, and keeping inside an *andha mūṣā*, it should be cooked in *gaja puṭa*. Processing like this even once reduces mica into *bhasma* form.

स्वच्छन्दात्
पुनर्नवां कुमारीं च चपलां वानरीं[३०२] तथा ।
मुशलीं चेक्षुवल्लीं च तथार्द्रामलकीरसैः ।।३८२ ।।

प्रत्येकैक्केन पुटयेत्सप्तवारं पुनः पुनः ।
अर्क्सेहुण्डदुग्धेन प्रदेया सप्तभावना ।
एवं संम्रियते वज्रं सर्वरोगहरं परम् ।।३८३।।

Another Method of Preparing Mica- Bhasma

Vajra type of mica should be repeatedly cooked in *puṭa* for seven times in each of the decoctions or juices of *punarnavā*, *kumārī*, *capalā* (?), *vānarī*, *muśalī*, *ikṣuvallī*, *ārdraka* and *āmalakī*. Thereafter, it should be impregnated for seven times in each of the milky latex of *arka* and *sehuṇḍa*. Thus, mica is reduced to *bhasma* form which cures all diseases.

रसालामुशलीवारि-पुटितं च मुहुर्मुहुः ।
निश्चन्द्रं मृतिमायाति कर्मयोग्यं भवेत्ततः ।।३८४।।

Another Method of Preparing Mica-Bhasma

Mica should be repeatedly cooked by the decoctions of *rasālā* and *muśalī* which reduces it to *bhasma* form without any glaze particles. This *bhasma* can be used in recipes.

अथ अमृतीकरणम्

रसरत्नाकरात्

"त्रिफलायाः[२०३] कषायस्य पलान्यादाय षोडश ।
गोघृतस्य पलान्यष्टौ मृताभ्रस्य पलान्दश[२०४] ।।३८५।।
एकीकृते लोहपात्रे विपचेन्मृदुवह्निना ।
द्रवे जीर्णे समादाय योगवाहे प्रयोजयेत्" ।
[रसकामधेनु : पृष्ठ २५६ : २११ - २१२]
अन्येषामपि धातूनाममृतीकरणं ह्ययम् ।।३८६।।

Amṛtikaraṇa of Mica
According to Rasaratnākara

In an iron pot, sixteen *pala-s* of the decoction of *triphalā*, eight *pala-s* of cow's ghee and ten *pala-s* of mica *bhasma* should be put together and cooked over mild fire till the liquid gets dried up. This should be used for the purpose of *yogavāha* (which enhances the properties of other added drugs). Same process should be followed for the *amṛtīkaraṇa* (inculcating the effect of ambrosia) of other metals also.

रोगान्हत्वा दृढ़बलवयं वीर्यवृद्धिं विधत्ते ।
तारुण्याढ्यो रमयति शतं योषितां नित्यमेव ।।३८७।।
दीर्घायुष्मान् जनयति सुतान् सिंहतुल्यप्रभावान् ।
मृत्योर्भीतिं हरति रुचिरं सेव्यमानं मृताभ्रम् ।।३८८।।

Therapeutic Efficacy

Mica *bhasma* [which has undergone the process of *amṛtīkaraṇa*] while curing diseases, promotes strength, longevity and seminal power. A person taking this *bhasma* can have sexual intercourse daily with hundred of women and can procreate children with long span of life and great strength like that of a lion. It prevents the fear of [untimely] death and promotes the desire to live.

क्षयकुष्टज्वरहरं प्रमेहव्याधिनाशनम् ।
जरामरणभीतिघ्नं वातपित्तकफापहम् ।
अभ्रकं सेवितं नित्यं कासश्वासहरं परम् ।।३८९।।

Regular use of mica *bhasma* cures consumption, *kuṣṭha* (obstinate skin diseases including leprosy), fever and *prameha* (obstinate urinary disorders including diabetes). It annihilates the fear of ageing and death. It alleviates *vāyu*, *pitta* and *kapha*. It also cures bronchitis and asthma.

रक्तिकैकात्समारभ्य यावट्टंकमितं भवेत् ।।३९०।।

Dose of Mica-Bhasma

It should be administered in the dose of one *ratti* and gradually increased by one *ratti* till the dose becomes one *ṭaṅka*.

चूर्णीकृतं गगनपत्रमथारनाले
धृत्वा निशामथ प्रपीड्य च सूरणस्य ।
भाव्यं रसैस्तदनुमूलरसैः कदल्याः

पादांशटंकणयुतं शफरीसमेतम् ।।३९१।।
पिंडीकृतं तु बहुधा महिषीमलेन
संशोष्य कोष्ठगतमाशु धमेद्धि वह्नौ ।
सत्वं पतेच्च सुरसायनमारणेषु[305]
योग्यं भवेत्सकलरोगचयं निहन्ति ।।३९२।।

Preparation of Mica-Sattva

Mica sheets should be made to powder and soaked in *āranāla* (vinegar) for one night. Then it should be squeezed and impregnated with the juice of *sūraṇa* and thereafter, with the juice of the rhizome of *kadalī*. Then one fourth in the quantity of *ṭaṅkaṇa* and *śapharī* (a small fish) should be added . This paste should be made to a bolus form, wrapped with buffalo dung and dried. Keeping this in a *koṣṭhī*, the fire should be blown by which the *sattva* (metallic essence) comes out. This *sattva* is useful in rejuvenation therapy and for preparing *bhasma* of other metals . It cures all diseases.

अन्यच्च
ऊर्णासर्जरसं चैव क्षुद्रमीनसमन्वितम् ।
एतत्सर्वं तु संचूर्ण्य छागदुग्धेन पिण्डिका ।।३९३।।
कृत्वाध्माता खराङ्गारैः सर्वसत्त्वान्निपातयेत् ।
उमादंडविमर्देन गगनं द्रवति स्फुटम् ।।३९४।।

Second Method of Preparing Mica-Sattva

Ūrṇā, *sarjarasa* and small variety of fish, all should be made to powder. By triturating with goat's milk this powder should be made to a paste. This should be kept over ignited charcoal and blown through a blower. Thus, the *sattva* of mica comes out.

By the trituration with the stick of *umā*, mica melts quickly.

क्षयान्तकरसः[306]
कांकचण्डेश्वरात्
सूततुल्यं व्योमसत्त्वं तयोस्तुल्यं च गन्धकम् ।
कुमारीस्वरसैर्मर्द्य यन्त्रे सैकतके पचेत् ।।३९५।।

दिनद्वयान्ते संगृह्य भक्षयेन्माषमात्रकम् ।
क्षयं शोफं तथा कासं प्रमेहं चापि दुष्करम् ।
पाण्डुरोगं च कार्श्यं च जयेच्छीघ्रं न संशयः ।।३९६ ।।

। इत्यभ्रकोत्पत्तिलक्षण शोधन-मारण-सत्वपातन-सत्त्वमारणम् ।।

।।रसः ।।

Kṣayāntaka Rasa
According to Kākacaṇḍeśvara

One part of mercury, one part of the *sattva* of mica and two parts of sulphur should be triturated with the juice of *kumārī*. This should be cooked in *sikatā yantra* for two days after which the recipe should be collected. It should be taken in the dose of one *māṣā* which immediately cures comsumption, oedema, bronchitis, serious type of *prameha* (obstinate urinary diseases including diabetes), anemia and emaciation.

Thus, ends the description of the origin, characteristics, purification, calcination, *sattva pātana* (extraction of metallic essence) and the calcination of *sattva*.

अथ क्षीरसिंधुः
अभ्रस्त्वष्टादशपुटाद्वातहा द्विगुणेन च ।
पित्तघ्नस्त्रिगुणेनैव कफहा मेहशोफहा ।
अम्लपित्तामवातादिरोगे स्याद्गजकेसरी ।।३९७।।

According to Kṣīrasindhu

Bhasma of mica prepared by eighteen *puṭa-s* cures *vātika* diseases; by thiry six *puṭa-s* cures *paittika* diseases and by seventy two *puṭa-s* cures *kaphaja* diseases including *meha* (obstinate urinary diseases including diabetes), oedema, *amla pitta* (hyper acidity) and *āma vāta* (rheumatic arthritis). These diseases are overcome by mica *bhasma* as an elephant is subdued by a lion.

अभ्रं शतपुटादूर्द्ध्वं[३०७] बीजसंज्ञां ध्रुवं लभेत् ।
वीर्यौजःकान्तिमूलश्च स बीजो देहधारकः ।।३९८।।

After one hundred *puṭa-s*, mica *bhasma* is called *bīja* (seed). This *bīja* promotes *ojas* (vital essence) and complexion and it sustains the physique of the individual.

सुवर्णं रजतं ताम्रं तीक्ष्णं कुटिलपन्नगौ ।
अकृत्रिमाः इमे ख्याता षट्लोहरसकर्मणि ।।३९९।।

Gold, silver, copper, *tīkṣṇa lauha* (a type of iron), tin and lead are the six natural (*akṛtrima*=not artificially prepared) metals which are used in processing mercury.

इति श्रीमहाराजाधिराजटोडरमल्लविरचिते टोडरानन्दे आयुर्वेदसौख्ये रसदोषशोधनाष्टसंस्कार-गौरीयन्त्र-वज्रमूषा-मृत्तिकासाधन-क्षुद्बोधकरण-सोमानल[308] यन्त्र-निगडद्रवजारण-दरदोत्थरसग्रहणोपाय - रसमारण - भक्षण - रसदोष - मृतसूतजदोषोपशमन - गन्धकोत्पत्ति-जाति-लक्षण-शोधनाभ्रकोत्पत्ति-जाति-शोधन-मारण-सत्वपातन-सत्वमारणकथनंनाम नवमोहर्षः ।।४००।।

Thus, ends the ninth chapter of *Āyurveda-saukhya* in *Ṭodarānanda* by the great king Ṭodaramalla dealing with the following topics :

(1) *Doṣa-s* (faults) of mercury, their purification & eight *saṃskāra-s* of mercury.

(2) *Gaurī yantra*, *vajra mūṣā* and preparation of clay.

(3) Increasing the digestive power of mercury, *Somānala yantra* and *nigaḍa drava jāraṇa.*

(4) Extraction of mercury from cinnabar.

(5) Method of preparing *bhasma* of mercury, its mode of use, adverse effects and correcting the defects in the *bhasma* of mercury.

(6) Origin of sulphur and its varieties, characteristics and purification.

(7) Origin of mica and its varieties, purification, calcination, extraction of *sattva* (metallic essence) and preparation of *bhasma* of the *sattva*.

NOTES AND REFERENCES

(1) This is the beginning of the ninth chapter of *Āyurveda-saukhya* in *Ṭodarānanda* and the invocation reads as follows :

गोपाङ्गनादत्तसुभक्तभोक्ता पीयूषमब्धेर्न हि संगृहाणा।
शान्तं स दद्यान्नृपटोडरेन्द्रे पितामहो यः सनकादिकनाम्।।

२. रसस्य इति चतुर्थपंचमपुस्तकयोः पाठः।

३. पाठोऽयं द्वितीयषष्ठपुस्तकयोः नोपलभ्यते।

४. कपाली इति पंचमपुस्तके पाठः।

५ तद्रूपी स्यात् इति प्रथमपंचमपुस्तकयोः पाठः।

६. कुर्यादसंशयः इति प्रथमपुस्तके पाठः।

७. तान्निचारयेत् इति चतुर्थपुस्तके पाठः।

८. धूर्म्मा च इति प्रथमपुस्तके पाठः।

९. भूदोषात्त्वोजनाशनम् इति पंचमपुस्तके पाठः।

१०. हन्यादुमेश्वरम् इति चतुर्थपुस्तके पाठः।

११. कृष्णरीतिका इति प्रथमपंचमपुस्तकयोः पाठः।

१२. रसेन्द्रं सान्निपातकम् इति पंचमपुस्तके पाठः।

१३. मृयन्ते इति प्रथमचतुर्थपंचमपुस्तकेषु पाठः।

१४. 'सप्तकंचुकः .... शृगाली' पाठोऽयं चतुर्थपुस्तकेनोपलभ्यते।

१५. अथ रसराजलक्ष्मीतन्त्रः इति पंचमपुस्तके पाठः।

१६. वज्रच्छेदि इति प्रथमपुस्तके पाठः।

१७. सूतकः इति प्रथमपंचमपुस्तकयोः पाठः।

१८. संशोधितः इति प्रथमपुस्तके पाठः।

१९. स्वेदनार्थे इति द्वितीयपुस्तके पाठः।

२०. क्षीरैस्तथा कषायेन प्रमद्योष्णारनालेन च इति
प्रथमपंचमपुस्तकयोः पाठः।

२१. षण्ढ्याद्या इति पंचमपुस्तके पाठः।

२२. चतुर्गुणम् इति पंचमपुस्तके पाठः।

२३. श्लक्ष्णेन इति द्वितीयपुस्तके पाठः।

२४. क मर्दनं इति द्वितीयपुस्तके पाठः।
ख. मूत्रेनमत्हये इति चतुर्थपुस्तके पाठः।

२५. क्षीराम्ल० इति द्वितीयपुस्तके पाठः।

२६. त्वक्या इति पंचमपुस्तके पाठः।

२७. अथ रसदर्पणात् इति चतुर्थपुस्तके पाठः।

२८. रसे इति पंचमपुस्तके पाठः।

२९. च ज्वालयित्वा भुवि क्षिपेत् इति आकरे पाठः।

३०. क. तत्रोक्तं मर्दयेद्रसम् इति आकरे पाठः।
ख. विनिर्दिशेत् तप्तखल्वं इति पंचमपुस्तके पाठः।

३१. भाम्यां स्यात् इति चतुर्थपुस्तके पाठः।

३२. सर्वत्रा इति पंचमपुस्तके पाठः।

३३. सन्धिर्लेपयेत्सुदृढं इति पंचमपुस्तके पाठः।

३४. सुन्वं इति चतुर्थपुस्तके पाठः।

३५. क. श्रुत्वा इति चतुर्थपुस्तके पाठः।
ख. 'शुल्वाद्रसो....यन्त्रके' पाठोऽयं आकरे नोपलभ्यते।

३६. जन्त्रके इति प्रथमपंचमपुस्तकयोः पाठः।

३७. तक्रं संयुतम् इति पंचमपुस्तके पाठः।

३८. न रोधयेत् इति प्रथमपंचमपुस्तकयोः पाठः।

३९. रंगवंगसंज्ञौ इति प्रथमपंचमपुस्तकयोः पाठः।

४०. 'रसार्णवात्.... सिद्धैर्नागार्जुनादिभिः' पाठोऽयं द्वितीयपुस्तके नोपलभ्यते।

४१. जीवत्सूतो इति चतुर्थपुस्तके पाठः।

४२. विस्तारत्र्यस्य इति चतुर्थपुस्तके पाठः।

४३. तन्मध्यं इति द्वितीयपुस्तके पाठः।

४४. नवं दृढम् इति द्वितीयपुस्तके पाठः।

४५. क्षिपेद्व्राजभूजं इति पंचमपुस्तके पाठः।

४६. गंध्ये इति चतुर्थपुस्तके पाठः।

४७. ०सादिनम् इति चतुर्थपुस्तके पाठः।

४८. विराजिनः इति चतुर्थपुस्तके पाठः।

४९. कथितो इति प्रथमचतुर्थपंचमपुस्तकेषु पाठः।

५०. हितशयं इति चतुर्थपुस्तके पाठः।

५१. पटुकाम्लकैः इति प्रथमपंचमपुस्तकयोः पाठः।

५२. योजयेद्रसराट् इति प्रथमपंचमपुस्तकयोः पाठः।

५३. भवेदष्टांगांशशोधितः इति प्रथमचतुर्थपुस्तकयोः पाठः।

५४. तस्य शृंङ्गवेराभ्यां इति चतुर्थपुस्तके पाठः।

५५. इत्यष्टसंस्काराः इति पंचमपुस्तके पाठः।

५६. महेश्वरि इति पंचमपुस्तके पाठः।

५७. ०क्रमवर्जितः इति द्वितीयपुस्तके पाठः।

५८. भवेत्तिमृत्युभयम् इति प्रथमपंचमपुस्तकयोः पाठः।

५९. व्योमसूतेन्द्रवेधि इति पंचमपुस्तके पाठः।

६०. विशोधयेत् इति पंचमपुस्तके पाठः।

६१. शांते इति प्रथमपंचमपुस्तकयोः पाठः।

६२. पुटे जीर्णे इति पंचमपुस्तके पाठः।

६३. रुंद्धा इति प्रथमपुस्तके पाठः।

६४. विक्रमेनैव इति चतुर्थपुस्तके पाठः।

६५. विचूर्णं इति प्रथमपंचमपुस्तकयोः पाठः।

६६. गौरीयन्त्रं इति पंचमपुस्तके पाठः।

६७. विकृयते इति पंचमपुस्तके पाठः।

६८. 'यन्त्रालक्षे विधिज्ञस्य चतुर्थांशक्षयो भवेत्' पाठोऽयं चतुर्थपुस्तके अधिकमुपलभ्यते।

६९. शमं इति पंचमपुस्तके पाठः।

७०. संधिमुद्रणा इति आकरे पाठः।

७१. भूतस्य इति चतुर्थपुस्तके पाठः।

७२. तुषादिकैः इति पंचमपुस्तके पाठः।

७३. मृत्तिका इति चतुर्थपुस्तके पाठः।

७४. 'दग्धा......दग्धं' पाठोऽयं द्वितीयपुस्तके नोपलभ्यते।

७५. कृष्णमृत्तत् इति पंचमपुस्तके पाठः।
७६. चूर्णं इति पंचमपुस्तके पाठः।
७७. क्रिद्रकं इति प्रथमपंचमपुस्तकयोः पाठः।
७८. सन्धिप्रलेपनैः इति प्रथमपंचमपुस्तकयोः पाठः।
७९. अन्धमूखा इति प्रथमचतुर्थपंचमपुस्तकेषु पाठः।
८०. मल्लमूखाजा इति प्रथमचतुर्थपंचमपुस्तकेषु पाठः।
८१. मुखैषा इति चतुर्थपंचमपुस्तकयोः पाठः।
८२. हितः इति पंचमपुस्तके पाठः।
८३. निगदो भवेत् इति पंचमपुस्तके पाठः।
८४. ०छेदी च इति पंचमपुस्तके पाठः।
८५. द्वितीयश्च तृतीयो इति प्रथमचतुर्थपंचमपुस्तकेषु पाठः।
८६. रसनिगडत्रयम् इति प्रथमपंचमपुस्तकयोः पाठः।
८७. सुन्दरि इति पंचमपुस्तके पाठः।
८८. निगदबन्धोऽयं इति पंचमपुस्तके पाठः।
८९. नलं इति द्वितीयचतुर्थपुस्तकयोः पाठः।
९०. मृदां इति प्रथमपंचमपुस्तकयोः पाठः।
९१. विलोपार्थं सन्चार्थं च भिषक्तमः इति प्रथमपंचमपुस्तकयोः पाठः।
९२. निश्चलोस्मरै इति चतुर्थपुस्तके पाठः।
९३. सर्वकर्मसिद्धः इति पंचमपुस्तके पाठः।
९४. सदृशो इति पंचमपुस्तके पाठः।
९५. पतिवशा इति प्रथमचतुर्थपंचमपुस्तकेषु पाठः।
९६. चूर्णं इति प्रथमपंचमपुस्तकयोः पाठः।
९७. क समभागिकनाम् इति प्रथमपुस्तके पाठः।
ख. समभाविकनाम् इति पंचमपुस्तके पाठः।
९८. च कर्षप्रमाणं इति चतुर्थपुस्तके पाठः।
९९. वर्ति इति चतुर्थपुस्तके पाठः।
१००. घृतस्यात् इति प्रथमपंचमपुस्तकयोः पाठः।

१०१. पिष्टीं वलि जारणाया इति पंचमपुस्तके पाठः।

१०२. भूनागतनुजद्रवा इति प्रथमपंचमपुस्तकयोः पाठः।

१०३. जघतोरुणपीताभो इति चतुर्थपुस्तके पाठः।

१०४. संभंव इति चतुर्थपुस्तके पाठः।

१०५. प्रदीपयेत् इति प्रथमपुस्तके पाठः।

१०६. नभवेल्लोहः इति प्रथमपंचमपुस्तकयोः पाठः।

१०७. तस्माद्वीजं प्रयुंजीत परिभाषोक्तलक्षणं इति चतुर्थपुस्तके अधिके पाठः।

१०८. समजीर्णं इति प्रथमपुस्तके पाठः।

१०९. रोगसंरभेतरुणो इति पंचमपुस्तके पाठः।

११०. विद्धति इति प्रथमपंचमपुस्तकयोः पाठः।

१११. स च ज्ञात्वा इति पंचमपुस्तके पाठः।

११२. शतमुत्तम् इति चतुर्थपुस्तके पाठः।

११३. हिंगुलोत्थं इति प्रथमपंचमपुस्तकयोः पाठः।

११४. हिंगुले इति चतुर्थपुस्तके पाठः।

११५. जाममात्रकम् इति प्रथमपंचमपुस्तकयोः पाठः।

११६. ०विधः प्रोक्तश्चर्मारः इति चतुर्थपुस्तके पाठः।

११७. जयश्चर्मारः इति प्रथमपंचमपुस्तकयोः पाठः।

११८. स्त्रिजीयश्च इति चतुर्थपुस्तके पाठः।

११९. चर्म्मारः इति चतुर्थपुस्तके पाठः।

१२०. सुकतुण्डकः इति प्रथमपंचमपुस्तकयोः पाठः।

१२१. क. शोध्यं सौरभ्रदुग्धके इति चतुर्थपुस्तके पाठः।
ख. सोध्यऽभ्रौडरभ्रदुग्धके इति प्रथमपंचमपुस्तकयोः पाठः।

१२२. सप्तकृत्वो इति चतुर्थपुस्तके पाठः।

१२३. स्थापितः इति चतुर्थपुस्तके पाठः।

१२४. युज्यतो इति चतुर्थपुस्तके पाठः।

१२५. स्यान्नेत्रामयस्त इति चतुर्थपुस्तके पाठः।

१२६. कृत्यासल्लातपत्रोत्थ० इति चतुर्थपुस्तके पाठः।
१२७. कंटालिका इति प्रथमपंचमपुस्तकयोः पाठः।
१२८. सितपर्णीलांगली इति चतुर्थपुस्तके पाठः।
१२९. दृढं इति प्रथमचतुर्थपंचमपुस्तकेषु पाठः।
१३०. समां सममुखां इति प्रथमचतुर्थपंचमपुस्तकेषु पाठः।
१३१. सिंबिका० इति प्रथमचतुर्थपंचमपुस्तकेषु पाठः।
१३२. तस्मिनार्त्ते इति द्वितीयपुस्तके पाठः।
१३३. शिंबीपत्ररसं इति द्वितीयपुस्तके पाठः।
१३४. नूनतास्ततः इति प्रथमपंचमपुस्तकयोः पाठः।
१३५. सादरेताक्ता इति चतुर्थपुस्तके पाठः।
१३६. चुल्लिसंस्थिताम् इति प्रथमपंचमपुस्तकयोः पाठः।
१३७. ताप्योः इति प्रथमपुस्तके पाठः।
१३८. निःपद्यते इति प्रथमचतुर्थपंचमपुस्तकेषु पाठः।
१३९. प्रमाणं इति प्रथमचतुर्थपंचमपुस्तकेषु पाठः।
१४०. दद्यान्सौण्डी इति प्रथमचतुर्थपंचमपुस्तकेषु पाठः।
१४१. क. भस्मढत् इति प्रथमपुस्तके पाठः।
ख. भस्मतुतः इति पंचमपुस्तके पाठः।
१४२. ०बटो० इति चतुर्थपुस्तके पाठः।
१४३. तरल इति प्रथमचतुर्थपंचमपुस्तकेषु पाठः।
१४४. 'द्विपलं...निधापयेत्' पाठोऽयं चतुर्थपुस्तके अधिकमुपलभ्यते।
१४५. 'दद्यात्तस्य .....मुदितः' पाठोऽयं चतुर्थपुस्तके अधिकमुपलभ्यते।
१४६. सममेललवंगपुरान्वितः कुरंगषुरान्वितः सुखयति इति प्रथमपंचमपुस्तकयो पाठः।
१४७. षटीष्टा इति प्रथमचतुर्थपुस्तकयोः पाठः।
१४८. बल्मिकमृतिका इति पंचमपुस्तके पाठः।

१४९. सैन्धसमांश इति चतुर्थपुस्तके पाठः।
१५०. रसभागं द्वयं इति पंचमपुस्तके पाठः।
१५१. द्वये इति चतुर्थपुस्तके पाठः।
१५२. दाढं इति पंचमपुस्तके पाठः।
१५३. दत्वा इति प्रथमपंचमपुस्तक्योः पाठः।
१५४. ०पर्यन्तमग्निं कुर्यादहर्निशम् इति प्रथमपंचमपुस्तक्योः पाठः।
१५५. अध उर्द्धं रसं इति प्रथमचतुर्थपंचमपुस्तकेषु पाठः।
१५६. लग्नं शीतं तमानयेत् इति प्रथमपंचमपुस्तक्योः पाठः।
१५७. पुष्टारोग्यप्रदं तन्द्री कमनीयं इति प्रथमपुस्तके पाठः।
१५८. संमिश्रमेनी षुर्यारसनतं इति प्रथमपंचमपुस्तक्योः पाठः।
१५९. तदद्वैकम् इति प्रथमपंचमपुस्तक्योः पाठः।
१६०. ०स्तदा इति प्रथमचतुर्थपंचमपुस्तकेषु पाठः।
१६१. कर्त्तव्या इति चतुर्थपंचमपुस्तक्योः पाठः।
१६२. 'काष्ठभाजन ..... वेष्टिताः' पाठोऽयं प्रथमचतुर्थपुस्तक्योः अधिकमुपलभ्यते।
१६३. चूर्णिन वेष्टिताः इति चतुर्थपुस्तके पाठः।
१६४. पुररंगारकनथ इति प्रथमपंचमपुस्तक्योः पाठः।
१६५. पूर्वा इति द्वितीयपुस्तके पाठः।
१६६. मूलिकाबद्धं इति प्रथमपुस्तके पाठः।
१६७. कलयत्यमः इति प्रथमपंचमपुस्तक्योः पाठः।
१६८. तया विमर्द्दयेत्सूतं इति प्रथमचतुर्थपंचमपुस्तकेषु पाठः।
१६९. कर्षार्द्धं इति चतुर्थपंचमपुस्तक्योः पाठः।
१७०. प्रपाच्यतो इति चतुर्थपुस्तके पाठः।
१७१. पाठोऽयं द्वितीयपुस्तके नोपलभ्यते।
१७२. कमाग्निवर्द्धनः इति चतुर्थपुस्तके पाठः।
१७३. पाठोऽयं प्रथमपंचमपुस्तक्योः नोपलभ्यते।
१७४. पाठोऽयं चतुर्थपुस्तके नोपलभ्यते।

१७५. निघृष्टो इति द्वितीयचतुर्थपुस्तक्योः पाठः।

१७६. वज्रार्क इति द्वितीयपुस्तके पाठः।

१७७. सुवर्णाद्याम इति पंचमपुस्तके पाठः।

१७८. सुवर्णादिमारणार्थम् इति प्रथमपुस्तके पाठः।

१७९. प्रदेयं इति प्रथमचतुर्थपंचमपुस्तकेषु पाठः।

१८०. सुखे इति चतुर्थपुस्तके पाठः।

१८१. भक्तेन इति प्रथमपुस्तके पाठः।

१८२. मधः इति प्रथमपंचमपुस्तक्योः पाठः।

१८३. नुर्द्ध० इति पंचमपुस्तके पाठः।

१८४. प्रलेपयेत् इति प्रथमचतुर्थपंचमपुस्तकेषु पाठः।

१८५. कुनु इति चतुर्थपुस्तके पाठः।

१८६. पांरपथोपदेशतः इति पंचमपुस्तके पाठः।

१८७. 'संपुटस्य...संज्ञक' पाठोऽयं पंचमपुस्तके नोपलभ्यते।

१८८. क. प्रोक्ताः इति प्रथमपंचमपुस्तक्योः पाठः।
ख. योगपरमदुर्लभः इति चतुर्थपुस्तके पाठः।

१८९. भिषग् दिनचतुष्टयम् इति पंचमपुस्तके पाठः।

१९०. बालुकाख्येन काचकुप्यां इति प्रथमपंचमपुस्तक्योः पाठ।

१९१. जातिपत्रिकम् इति प्रथमपुस्तके पाठः।

१९२. मासमात्रं इति द्वितीयपुस्तके पाठः।

१९३. चूर्णमेतद्विमासकम् इति द्वितीयपुस्तके पाठः।

१९४. मांसं भक्षं इति प्रथमपंचमपुस्तक्योः पाठः।

१९५. गत्ते राप्तं तथा इति पंचमपुस्तके पाठः।

१९६. सप्तधातुक्षयं इति प्रथमपंचमपुस्तक्योः पाठः।

१९७. गुल्महृद्रोगं इति प्रथमपंचमपुस्तक्योः पाठः।

१९८. अरुचिः शोथ इति प्रथमपंचमपुस्तक्योः पाठः।

१९९. पिडकाक्षयेत् इति प्रथमपंचमपुस्तक्योः पाठः।

२००. वृद्धानां इति प्रथमचतुर्थपंचमपुस्तकेषु पाठः।

२०१. क्टीशूलं इति चतुर्थपंचमपुस्तक्योः पाठः।

२०२. नाशयेत्तु इति प्रथमपंचमपुस्तक्योः पाठः।

२०३. प्रक्तो इति पंचमपुस्तके पाठः।

२०४. लिखितः सम्प्रदायतम् इति पंचमपुस्तके पाठः।

२०५. पाठोऽयं द्वितीयपुस्तके नोपलभ्यते।

२०६. पाठोऽयं चतुर्थपंचमपुस्तक्योः नोपलभ्यते।

२०७. विलेप्य इति प्रथमचतुर्थपंचमपुस्तकेषु पाठः।

२०८. रसरणात् इति चतुर्थपुस्तके पाठः।

२०९. 'रामठं...कुङ्कुमम्' पाठोऽयं पंचमपुस्तके ४२ पृष्ठे नोपलभ्यते।

२१०. खल्लमध्ये इति प्रथमपुस्तके पाठः।

२११. गन्धोत्थं इति प्रथमचतुर्थपंचमपुस्तकेषु पाठः।

२१२. खलिकं इति प्रथमचतुर्थपंचमपुस्तकेषु पाठः।

२१३. प्रदातव्यो वीतिहोत्रे भिषक्तमैः इति पंचमपुस्तके पाठः।

२१४. शंप्तं यः इति चतुर्थपुस्तके पाठः।

२१५. पाठोऽयं पंचमपुस्तके अधिकमुपलभ्यते।

२१६. पाठोऽयं पंचमपुस्तके अधिकमुपलभ्यते।

२१७. क्रोत्यसा इति प्रथमचतुर्थपंचमपुस्तकेषु पाठः।

२१८. इष्टकयां इति पंचमपुस्तके पाठः।

२१९. गन्धो इति पंचमपुस्तके पाठः।

२२०. द्विकार्षिक इति पंचमपुस्तके पाठः।

२२१. सुखं इति चतुर्थपुस्तके पाठः।

२२२. दद्याल्लावपुटं इति प्रथमपंचमपुस्तक्योः पाठः।

२२३. सरोगं इति चतुर्थपुस्तके पाठः।

२२४. स्फोटयित्वा प्रयुक्ता इति चतुर्थपुस्तके पाठः।

२२५. अधःस्थ इति द्वितीयपुस्तके पाठः।

२२६. सिंदूररसः पाठोऽयं चतुर्थपुस्तके अधिकमुपलभ्यते।

२२७. यातितः इति चतुर्थपुस्तके पाठः।

२२८. तस्मात्सुवर्णा हि युतं इति चतुर्थपुस्तके पाठः।

२२९. सुवर्णयुक्तः पिष्टीकृतो गंधकयोगतश्च
इति प्रथमचतुर्थपंचमपुस्तकेषु पाठः।

२३०. सत्वहेमपरीक्षकान्तैः इति चतुर्थपुस्तके पाठः।

२३१. ०जीर्णे इति चतुर्थपुस्तके पाठः।

२३२. द्रुताकज्जलिका इति चतुर्थपुस्तके पाठः।

२३३. यान्तु इति प्रथमचतुर्थपंचमपुस्तकेषु पाठः।

२३४. वैद्याधिराजो चक्रपाणिः इति चतुर्थपुस्तके पाठः।

२३५. 'चैव...कर्कोटीं' पाठोऽयं द्वितीयपुस्तके नोपलभ्यते।

२३६. राजिका बिल्ववातलानि इति द्वितीयपुस्तके पाठः।

२३७. नालिकेरं इति चतुर्थपंचमपुस्तकयोः पाठः।

२३८. भूतस्रावः इति द्वितीयपुस्तके पाठः।

२३९. सुलभा इति द्वितीयपुस्तके पाठः।

२४०. कामशक्तिविवर्जिता इति प्रथमपंचमपुस्तकयोः पाठः।

२४१. क केशाः इति प्रथमपुस्तके पाठः।
ख. कुंचिताग्री ये केशायाः या श्यामा इति पंचमपुस्तके पाठः।

२४२. सूक्ष्मोयं इति प्रथमपुस्तके पाठः।

२४३. स्त्रीसंगान्मृयते इति चतुर्थपुस्तके पाठः।

२४४. 'हिक्का...०जृम्भकः' पाठोऽयं द्वितीयपुस्तके नोपलभ्यते।

२४५. नियते इति प्रथमपुस्तके पाठः।

२४६. संघनं इति चतुर्थपुस्तके पाठः।

२४७. ह्नि इति प्रथमचतुर्थपुस्तकयोः पाठः।

२४८. पाठोऽयं प्रथमद्वितीयपुस्तकयोः नोपलभ्यते।

२४९. पाठोऽयं द्वितीयपुस्तके नोपलभ्यते।

२५०. शरपुंखांघ्रि इति द्वितीयपुस्तके पाठः।

२५१. भक्षयनम् इति चतुर्थपुस्तके पाठः।

२५२ पाठोऽयं प्रथमपुस्तके अधिकमुपलभ्यते।

२५३. स्वस्था इति पंचमपुस्तके पाठः।

२५४. चाम्बरश्च इति पंचमपुस्तके पाठः।

२५५. रहिते कथं जीवनदा इति चतुर्थपुस्तके पाठः।

२५६. वारि इति पंचमपुस्तके पाठः।

२५७. पुरे इति प्रथमचतुर्थपंचमपुस्तकेषु पाठः।

२५८. क क्षीरार्णवेषु स्नातायां इति प्रथमपुस्तके पाठः।
ख. क्षीरार्णवे तु इति पंचमपुस्तके पाठः।

२५९. यन्मथितवस्त्रं इति प्रथमचतुर्थपंचमपुस्तकेषु पाठः।

२६०. कृष्णः इति प्रथमचतुर्थपंचमपुस्तकेषु पाठः।

२६१. 'कंगुणी...रसरत्नाकरात्' पाठोऽयं चतुर्थपुस्तके अधिकमुपलभ्यते।

२६२. वन्हिं इति पंचमपुस्तके पाठः।

२६३. तावत्समींधयते् इति पंचमपुस्तके पाठः।

२६४. "शोधितो रमएजस्याज्जएमृत्पुरुजा पटः।
अग्निसंदीपनः श्रेष्ठो वीर्यवृद्धिकरस्त्वयम्।।"
पाठोऽयं चतुर्थपुस्तके अधिकमुपलभ्यते।

२६५. 'देवदाल्य...योजयेत्' पाठोऽयं चतुर्थपुस्तके अधिकमुपलभ्यते।

२६६. क क्षिपेदेरण्डतैलके इति आकरे पाठः।
ख. क्षिपेदे तलके अनेन इति आदर्शपुस्तकेषु अधिको पाठः।

२६७. अशुद्धगन्धं कुरुते तु कुष्ठं तापं भ्रमं पित्तरुजं इति प्रथमपंचमपुस्तकयोः पाठः।

२६८. गन्धस्य इति पंचमपुस्तके पाठः।

२६९. 'अर्कक्षीरैः..योजयेत्' पाठोऽयं चतुर्थपुस्तके अधिकमुपलभ्यते।

२७०. प्रलेपयेत् इति आकरे पाठः।

२७१. मध्ये इति आदर्शपुस्तकेषु पाठः।

२७२. पतत्यधो इति आकरे पाठः।

२७३. विष्णोः प्रभवं इति प्रथमपुस्तके पाठः।

२७४. तु इति प्रथमपुस्तके पाठः।

२७५. सुमोच इति पंचमपुस्तके पाठः।

२७६. पीनाकं इति पंचमपुस्तके पाठः।

२७७. ०त्यार्थां इति चतुर्थपुस्तके पाठः।

२७८. दर्दुरं इति पंचमपुस्तके पाठः।

२७९. मतान्तरात् लोहपक्षतितः इति प्रथमचतुर्थपुस्तकयोः पाठः।

२८०. वृत्तस्य इति द्वितीयपुस्तके पाठः।

२८१. पर्रिसर्प्पितः इति चतुर्थपुस्तके पाठः।

२८२. जातत्वाद्रचिरेगगनं इति द्वितीयचतुर्थपंचमपुस्तकेषु पाठः।

२८३. 'निर्गुण्डी...कृतम्' पाठोऽयं चतुर्थपुस्तके नोपलभ्यते।

२८४. प्रेषणं इति प्रथमचतुर्थपंचमपुस्तकेषु पाठः।

२८५. 'अप्स्वावदरी क्वाथे ध्मातम् भुवि निःक्षिपेत्।
मर्दितं पाणिना शुप्पुं धान्याभ्रहतिरिच्यते।।'
पाठोऽयं चतुर्थपुस्तके अधिकमुपलभ्यते।

२८६. 'अथवाभ्रस्य भागौ द्वौ मुस्तस्यैकं जलैः।
महद्विदिनं स्यापयैन्यपारित्रे ततः सूक्ष्मं प्रपेषयेत्।।
वध्वाध्वान्यपुतं वस्त्रैर्मरयेत्कांजिकै सह।
आदौ पात्रगतं शुद्धं धान्याभ्रकं भवेत्।।'
पाठोऽयं चतुर्थपुस्तके अधिकमुपलभ्यते।

२८७. वाथ इति प्रथमपंचमपुस्तकयोः पाठः।

२८८. संयुक्तं बद्ध्वा कम्बलिके श्लथम् इति पंचमपुस्तके पाठः।

२८९. प्रशस्यति इति चतुर्थपुस्तके पाठः।

२९०. श्रेष्ठां इति प्रथमपुस्तके पाठः।

२९१. नीरेण इति चतुर्थपुस्तके पाठः।

२९२. पत्तर इति चतुर्थपुस्तके पाठः।

२९३. पुटादाशु इति प्रथमपंचमपुस्तकयोः पाठः।

२९४. रसेनापिऽर्द्धं इति प्रथमपंचमपुस्तकयोः पाठः।

२९५. रसवाढं इति प्रथमचतुर्थपंचमपुस्तकेषु पाठः।

२९६. पुटेत् इति प्रथमपंचमपुस्तकयोः पाठः।

२९७. 'धान्याभ्रकं..०कारकम्' पाठोऽयं चतुर्थपुस्तके अधिकमुपलभ्यते।

२९८. नागवल्लीरसैस्तद्वत्सूर्यक्षीरैः पृथक्पृथक्इति आकरे पाठः।

२९९. रोध्रेस्तु इति आकरे पाठः।

३००. देयमभ्रस्यैवं मृतिर्भवेत् इति आकरे पाठः।

३०१. टङ्कणस्य च इति आकरे पाठः।

३०२. वानसं इति द्वितीयपुस्तके पाठः।

३०३. त्रिफलोत्थकषायस्य इति आकरे पाठः।

३०४. पलान्नव इति आकरे पाठः।

३०५. सुरसाजमजारणेषु इति प्रथमपंचमपुस्तकयोः पाठः।

३०६. पाठोऽयं प्रथमपंचमपुस्तकयोः नोपलभ्यते।

३०७. स्वष्टादशपुटादूर्द्ध्वं इति पंचमपुस्तके पाठः।

३०८. पाठोऽयं प्रथमपंचमपुस्तकयोः नोपलभ्यते।

CHAPTER-III

PROCESSING OF METALS & MINERALS

अथ[1] रससिन्धुः

स्वर्णं तारं ताम्रनागौ वंगं[2] कान्तं च तीक्ष्णकम् ।
मुण्डान्तमष्टकं लोहं देहसिद्धौ[3] प्रयोजयेत् ॥१॥
घोषश्च रीतिकावर्तलोहाः स्युः कृत्रिमास्त्रयः ।
उपलोहं समाख्यातं मण्डूरं मुण्डकिट्टकम्[4] ॥२॥
महालोहं तु साम्बूकं विद्युत्संभूतमुत्तमम् ।
द्रावकोद्भूतमाकाशगलितभूतं[5] भूतले ॥३॥
वेतालादिवराल्लब्धं[6] दुर्लभं[7] स्पर्शसम्भवम् ।
शालग्रामशिलोद्भूतं न भूतं न भविष्यति ।
स्फाटिकं स्फटिकोद्भूतं काश्मीरं विरलं क्वचित् ॥४॥

Metals Used for Rejuvenation According to Rasasindhu

Gold, silver, copper, lead, tin, *kānta* (magnetic iron), *tīkṣṇa* (another type of iron) and *muṇḍa* (ordinary iron)--these eight metals are to be used for *deha siddhi* (rejuvenation).

Artificially Prepared Metals

Ghoṣa (bronze), *rītikā* (bell-metal) and *āvarta*--these are the three artificial metals.

Upaloha

Maṇḍūra (rust of iron) is called *upaloha* (subsidiary metal). It is the waste product of *muṇḍa* type of iron.

Mahāloha

Sāmbūka (meteoric iron) is the *mahāloha* (important iron). It is the product of lightening (*vidyut*) and excellent in property. Getting melted by the melting agents in the sky, it falls down upon the earth. Such type of metal is obtained as a result of boons bestowed by *vetāla* (vampire), etc. and these can be touched.

The iron obtained from the stone of *śālagrāma* is extremely rare.

The *sphāṭika* type of iron is extracted from *sphaṭika* (rock crystal) found in Kashmir and it is rare.

नन्दिकाचार्यतन्त्रे

स्वर्णं[७] तारं ताम्रं नागो बंगः सकान्तविद्युज्जम् ।

स्फटिकोद्भूतं च तथा इति लोहं चाष्टधा ज्ञेयम् ॥५॥

According to Nandikācārya Tantra

The eight types of *loha* (metals) are gold, silver, copper, lead, tin, *kānta lauha* (magnetic iron), *vidyujja* (iron from meteoric stone) and *sphaṭiodkbhūtu* (iron from the rock-crystal).

SVARṆA (GOLD)

वह्निवीर्यसमुद्भूतं सुवर्णं पञ्चधा मतम् ॥६॥

Mythological Origin of Gold

Gold originated from the *vīrya* (potency, semen) of the god Vahni (Fire). It is of five types.

स्वर्णं पञ्चविधं प्रोक्तं प्राकृतं सहजाग्निकम् ।

एतत्स्वर्णं त्रयं दिव्यं वर्णे[८] षोडशव्यंजकम् ।

धारणादेव तत्कुर्यात्पापालक्ष्मीनिवारणम् ॥७॥

रसेन्द्रवेधसंभूतं[९] गिरीणां खनिसंभवम्[१०] ।।८।।

Varieties

Gold is of five types as follows :

(1) *Prākṛta* or natural;

(2) *Sahaja* or in combination with other metals;

(3) *Agnika* or which is obtained from fire or vulcanic eruptions;

These three types of gold are celestial and full of lustre (full of all the sixteen parts). Wearing such gold in the form of ornaments removes sins and inauspiciousness.

(4) Gold prepared by the transmutation of mercury;

(5) Gold obtained from the mines in mountains.

तच्चतुर्दशवर्णाढ्यं श्रेष्ठं सर्वरुजापहम् ।
मध्यं त्रयोदशं वर्णं द्वादशं तु कनिष्ठकम् ।।९।।

Relative Merits

Gold with 14/16th part of lustre is excellent in curing all diseases. Gold with 13/16th of lustre is mediocre and gold with 12/16th of lustre is inferior.

श्वेतांगं कठिनं रूक्षं विवर्णं समलं दलम् ।
दाहे छेदेऽसितं श्वेतं कट्टे स्फुटं लघुं त्यजेत् ।
दशदोषान्वितं स्वर्णं न रसेषु प्रयोजयेत् ।।१०।।

Ten Defects in Gold

(1) Whiteness in colour, (2) hardness, (3) ununctuousness, (4) variegated colour, (5) association of impurities, (6) appearance of scales when placed over the fire, (7), (8) appearance of blackness or whiteness in cut surfaces, (9) cracking while pressed, and (10) lightness--these are the ten defects in gold. Such types of gold should not be used in *rasa-s* (recipes containing metals).

बलं च वीर्यं हरते नराणां ददाति मन्दानलमुग्ररूपम् ।
प्रोत्साहकान्तिं हरते सुखं च शुद्धो मृतश्चामृतरूपहेमः ।।११।।

Adverse Effects of Impure Gold

Gold which is not purified, if taken in, reduces the strength and potency, seriously suppresses the power of digestion, and diminishes enthusiasm, complexion and happiness. After purification, gold works like ambrosia.

अथ शोधनम्
वल्मीकमृत्तिका धूमं गैरिका चेष्टिका पटुः[११] ।
इत्येता मृत्तिकाः[१२] पञ्च जंबीरैरारनालकैः ।
पिष्ट्वा लेप्यं[१३] स्वर्णपत्रं शुध्यते सप्तभिः पुटैः ॥१२॥

Purification of Gold

Mud from ant-hills, house-soot, red-ochre, brick and salt--these five taken together are called *pañca mṛttikā* (five clays). These clays should be triturated with the juice of *jambīra* and *āranāla* (vinegar). The paste, thus prepared, should be smeared over gold-leaves and cooked in *puṭa*. Repeating this process for seven times purifies gold.

अन्यच्च
मृत्तिकां मातुलुंगाम्लैः पंचवासरभावितम्[१४] ।
सभस्मलवणैर्हेम शोधयेत्पुटपाकतः ॥१३॥

Second Method of Gold Purification

Mud should be impregnated with the juice of *mātuluṅga* for five days. Gold smeared with the paste of this mud, ash and salt should be cooked in *puṭa* which purifies gold.

अथ मारणम्
शुद्धसूतसमं स्वर्णं खल्वे कृत्वाथ[१५] गोलकम् ।
अधोर्द्ध्वं[१६] गन्धकं दत्त्वा 'सर्वतुल्यं[१७] निरुध्य च ॥१४॥
त्रिंशद्वन्योपलैर्देयं[१८] पुटान्येवं चतुर्दश ।
निरुत्थं जायते हेम गन्धो[१९] देयः पुनः पुनः ॥१५॥

Preparation of Gold-Bhasma

Purified mercury and purified gold, taken in equal quantities, should be triturated in a mortar and make to a bolus. Equal quantity of sulphur should be placed below and above to this bolus and it should be wrapped on all sides. With thirty cow-dung cakes collected from the forest, it should be cooked in *puṭa*. This process should be repeated for fourteen times. By doing so, gold becomes *niruttha* (which cannot be retrieved). For every *puṭa* fresh quantity of sulphur should be added repeatedly.

अन्यच्च

शुद्धमाक्षिकं भागैकं, भागं च रौप्यमाक्षिकम् ।
द्विभागं सूतकं क्षिप्त्वा त्रयमम्लेन मर्दयेत् ।।१६।।
भागैकं हेमपत्रं च क्षिप्त्वा चाम्लेन मर्दयेत् ।
तदा सम्पातनायन्त्रे हटाद्यामत्रयं पचेत् ।
इत्येवं म्रियते स्वर्णं निरुत्थं नात्र संशयः ।।१७।।

Second Method of Preparing Gold Bhasma

One part of purified *mākṣika*, one part of *raupya mākṣika* and two parts of mercury—all these three should be triturated by adding sour juice. To this, one part of gold-leaf should be added and triturated by adding sour juice. The paste, thus prepared, should be cooked for three *yāma-s* in a *sampātanā yantra*. Thus, the *bhasma* of gold is prepared which is *niruttha* (non-retrievable).

अथ रससिन्धुतः

कांचनारजटातोयैर्भावयेत् हेममाक्षिकम् ।
तेन सर्वेण तल्लिप्तं हेमपत्रं पुनः पुनः ।।१८।।
सुपत्रलंकृतं [?] सम्यक् शोषयित्वा च तत्पुटेत् ।
अरण्यगोमयैः पत्रं सप्तवारं च युज्यते ।
तेन तन्म्रियते पत्रं सौवर्णं वर्णसन्निभम् ।।१९।।

Third Method of Preparing Gold-Bhasma According to Rasasindhu

Suvarṇa mākṣika should be impregnated with the root of *kāñcanāra*. With this paste, gold leaves should be smeared repeatedly, dried properly and cooked in *puṭa* with the help of cowdung-cakes collected from the forest. This process should be repeated for seven times. Thus, the *bhasma* of gold is prepared and the colour of this *bhasma* is golden.

रसचिन्तामणितः

हिंगु[२०] हिंगुलसिन्दूरशिलां पिष्ट्वा द्रवेण च ।
एरण्डवह्नि[२१]भवेनैवं[२२] भस्म स्यात्सूक्ष्मपत्रकम् ॥२०॥
मर्दितं पुटितं चैकवारं सिन्दूरं हानयेत्[२३] ।
पुनः पुटानि देयानि त्रीणि हिंगुलकेन च ॥२१॥

Fourth Method of Preparing Gold-Bhasma According to Rasacintāmaṇi

Hiṅgu, hiṅgula, sindūra and *manaḥśilā* should be made to a paste by triturating with the decoction of *eraṇḍa* and *citraka*. Thin leaves of gold should be smeared with this paste and cooked which makes gold into *bhasma* form. After trituration and one *puṭa pāka*, *sindūra* should be omitted. Thereafter, three *puṭa-s* should be given by adding and triturating with *hiṅgula*.

हेमपत्राणि सूक्ष्माणि जंभांभो नागभस्मतः ।
लेपनः पुटयोगेन त्रिवारं [तत्[२४] मलेच्छतो]
नागहानयेत्[२५] ।
निरुत्थं जायते स्वर्णं सर्वकार्येषु योजयेत् ॥२२॥

Fifth Method of Preparing Gold-Bhasma

Bhasma of lead should be triturated with the juice of *jambīra* and made to a paste. This paste should be applied over fine gold leaves and cooked in *puṭa* for three times. Then the lead should be removed by giving a *puṭa* with *hiṅgula*. Thus, *niruttha* (unretrievable) *bhasma* of gold is prepared which may be used in all recipes.

अन्यच्च

विषरसमरिचानां बिल्वकल्केन गन्धः ।
सलिलवरजपित्तक्षालितस्तेन लेपात् ॥२३॥
मरति तरति तोये लोहवद्हेमभस्म ।
प्रकटितमिहसिद्धैः सिद्धसारस्वतं हि ॥२४॥

Sixth Method of Preparing Gold-Bhasma

Sulphur should first of all be washed with the solution of the *pit* (bile) of *rohi* fish and by triturating with aconite, mercury, *marica* and *bilva* should be made to a paste. By the application of this paste over gold leaves [and cooking in *puṭa*] *bhasma* of gold is prepared. This *bhasma* floats over water. This perfect method of preparing gold *bhasma* is propounded by *Siddha-s.*

सर्वौषधिप्रयोगैर्ये व्याधयो न विनिर्जिताः[२६] ।
कर्मभिः पञ्चभिश्चैव सुवर्णं तत्र योजयेत् ।
तत्तथा संस्कृतं कृत्वा यथा भूरिफलं भवेत् ।।२५।।

Therapeutic Excellence of Gold

Patients whose diseases are not cured by ordinary treatment should be cleansed by the administration of *pañca karma* therapy and then administered gold *bhasma*. To obtain maximum therapeutic effect, the gold *bhasma* should be suitably processed by adding appropriate ingredients.

पारदस्य पलं चैकं गन्धकस्य पलद्वयम् ।
तद्वन्माक्षिकधातोश्च कुर्यात्कज्जलिकां ततः ।
मर्दयेत्तां प्रयत्नेन रसे कन्यासमुद्भवे ।।२६।।
कृत्वा हेममयीं मूषां चतुष्पलमितां शुभाम् ।
नात्युच्चां नाति विपुलां न गम्भीरां न चोन्नताम् ।
मूषामेवंविधौ[२७] कुर्यात्प्रयत्नाद् बुद्धिमान्नरः ।।२७।।
ततः कज्जलिकापिंडं स्थाप्य खर्परकोटके ।
मूषां तदुपरि स्थाप्य मृन्मयीं च तथोपरि[२८] ।।२८।।
विधाय निखिलां तां तु तत्पार्श्वं लेपयेन्मृदा ।
शुष्कां तत्तु सिकतया पूरयित्वा समंततः ।।२९।।
अच्छाद्यापरपात्रेण[२९] संपुटं लेपयेत्ततः ।
तन्मूर्ध्नि दापयेद्यलाज्जलाशां [?] मेखलान्वितताम् ।।३०।।
मंदं मंदमहोरात्रं ज्वालयेद्वह्निमाहतः ।
स्वभावशीतलं ज्ञात्वा समुद्धृत्य च बुद्धिमान् ।।३१।।
आकृष्य पेषणं कुर्यान्मुशलेन शिलातले ।

क्षालयेदिति सर्वेषु पुटेष्वेवं[30] यथाविधिम् ॥३२॥
हस्तमात्रं भवेद्गर्भं सर्वतः परिमण्डलम् ।
अरण्यगोमयैः शुष्कैस्तद्भागद्वयपूरणम् ॥३३॥
मृन्मये त्वनतिस्थूले हेमपात्रानुकारिणः ।
तत्पात्रे स्थापयेद् हेम स्थगयेत्तादृशीं तथा ।
अन्तर्भवति तद् हेम काकमाचीरसेन तु ॥३४॥

Seventh Method of Preparing Gold-Bhasma

One *pala* of mercury, two *pala-s* of sulphur and two *pala-s* of *mākṣika* should be added with the juice of *kumārī* and triturated to make *kajjalī* (fine black powder like collyrium).

A *mūṣā* (crucible) coated with gold should be prepared. It should be of four *pala-s* in capacity. It should be neither very high, very bulky, very deep nor very elevated. This type of *mūṣā* should be prepared by a wise physician.

The above mentioned bolus of *kajjalī* should be kept inside a *kharpara* (piece of broken jar) which is to be kept inside the *mūṣā*. This *mūṣā* should be wrapped with mud. Then the sides of this bolus should be smeared with mud and dried. Thereafter, it should be kept in a jar filled all around with sand and covered with another jar. The joint between these two jars should be sealed with mud. In the upper jar a ring of mud and straw should be placed and poured with water. The lower jar should be given mild fire for one day and night. After it has cooled down of its own, the recipe should be taken out and triturated strongly over a stone slab with the help of a pestle. Then the powder should be washed.

Thereafter, it should be given *puṭa* as follows : A round pit of one cubit diameter should be dug on the earth. Two third of this pit should be filled with the cow-dung cakes collected from the forest and in the center of this, an earthen jar of suitable size and shape should be placed. Inside this jar, the gold-*bhasma* should be kept and covered with the juice of *kākumācī*. By igniting the cow-dung-cake, *puṭa* should be given.

पुनः

त्रिफलायाः विशेषेण जंबीरार्द्रकवारिभिः ।
ऐकमण्यश्चि[31] तोयेन[32] राजकर्णरसेन च ॥३५॥

शतावर्याश्च तोयेन दशमूलीरसेन तु ।
पुनर्नवारसेनापि पुटं दद्याद्विचक्षणः ।।३६।।
देशकालवयोवस्थादोषभेदानुसारतः ।
इत्थं निरुत्थं विज्ञेयं चूर्णं सौवर्णमुत्तमम् ।।३७।।

Eighth Method of Preparing Gold-Bhasma

Gold should be given *puṭa pāka* by impregnating with the decoction of *triphalā*, juices of *jambīra*, *ārdraka* and *ekaparṇī*, *rājakarṇa* and *śatāvarī*, decoction of *daśamūla* and juice of *punarnavā* depending upon the location, time, age, condition of the disease and *doṣa-s* aggravated. Thus, the excellent *niruttha* (unretrievable) *bhasma* of gold is prepared.

स्थापयेन्मृन्मये भाण्डे विमले काञ्चनेऽथवा ।
स्फटिकादिकृते वापि नारिकेलफलेऽथवा ।।३८।।

Storage of Gold-Bhasma

Gold-*bhasma* should be stored is a clean earthen jar or jar prepared of gold, crystal etc. or outer shell of coconut.

तत्प्रातर्मधुसर्पिर्भ्यां लिह्यान्मात्रासमन्वितम् ।
अनुपानं तु तोयेन काञ्चनाररसेन[33] च ।।३९।।

Mode of Administration of Gold Bhasma

Gold-*bhasma* should be licked in the morning along with honey and ghee in appropriate dose. The *anupāna* (post-prandial drink) should be water or the juice of *kāñcanāra*.

ततोऽस्ति लोहमातङ्गो यत्र गन्धककेसरी[34] ।
निहन्याद्गन्धमात्रेण किं वा माक्षिककेसरी[35] ।।४०।।

Metals are redduced to *bhasma* form (killed) by the smell of sulphur or by *mākṣika* (copper pyrite) as an elephant is killed by a lion.

रुक्मं हिमं स्वादुकषायलेखनं रसायनं बृंहणवर्णकृद्गुरु ।
शोषज्वरघ्नं विषवातपित्तहृत्तेजोबलायुःसुखकान्तिबुद्धिम् ।।४१।।

Properties of Gold

Gold is cooling in potency and sweet as well as astringent in taste. It is *lekhana* (which scrapes out tissues), *rasāyana* (causes rejuvenation), *bṛṃhaṇa* (causing nourishment of tissues), promoter of complexion and heavy. It cures consumption, fever and poisoning. It alleviates *vāyu* and *pitta*. It promotes complexion, strength, span of life, happiness, lustre and intellect.

स्वर्णं तिक्तं कषायं मधुरमतिवयःकान्तिधीदं च बल्यम् ।
दृश्यं हृद्यं ज्वरघ्नं शुचिकरमनिशं वाग्विशुद्धिप्रदं च ।।४२।।

Second Description of Gold-Properties

Gold is bitter, astringent and sweet in taste. It prevents ageing process. It exceedingly promotes complexion, intellect and strength. It promotes eye-sight and it is cardio-tonic. It cures fever, produces cleanliness and helps in making perfect speech.

'आयुर्वृद्धिं[३६] वलीनां हरणमचिरतो दुष्टमेहामवातम् ।
शोषोन्माद-क्षयघ्नं सुखमनुभवते धातुनाथ तनोति' ।।४३।।

Third Description of Gold-Properties

Gold promotes longevity and cures wrinkling of the skin quickly, serious types of *meha* (obstinate urinary disorders including diabetes), *āmavāta* (rheumatism), consumption, insanity and phthisis. It produces happiness and nourishes the tissues.

आयुर्लक्ष्मीप्रजाधीस्मृतिकरमखिलव्याधिविध्वंसि पुण्यम् ।
भूतावेशप्रशान्तिं[३७] स्मरभरसुखदं पुष्टिप्रकाशिका च ।।४४।।

Fourth Description of Gold-Properties

Gold promotes longevity, auspiciousness, progeny, intellect and memory. It cures all diseases and bestows virtues. It cures affliction by evil spirits and promotes virility as well as nourishment of tissues.

गांगेयं शुद्धसिद्धं गदहरमजराकारिमेहापहारि ।
क्षीणानां पुष्टिकारि स्फुटमतिकरणं कारणं वीर्यवृद्धेः ।।४५।।

।। इति स्वर्णमारणं[३८] गुणदोषकीर्त्तनं च ।।

Fifth Description of Gold-Properties

The *bhasma* of purified gold cures diseases, prevents ageing process and cures *meha* (obstinate urinary diseases including diabetes). It nourishes emaciated persons, promotes the sharpness of the mind and the quantity of semen.

Thus, ends the description of *bhasma* preparation of gold and its good and adverse effects.

RAUPYA (SILVER)

रजतं त्रिविधं प्रोक्तं सहजं खनिजं कृतम् ।
कैलासोत्थं च सहजं खनिजं तु हिमाचले ।
कृत्रिमं रसजातं च वङ्गादौ रूप्यतां गतम् ।।४६।।

Varieties of Silver

Silver is of three types as follows :

(1) *Sahaja* (natural associated with other metals).

(2) *Khanija* (obtained from mines).

(3) *Kṛtrima* (artificial).

Sahaja type of silver is available in the Mount *Kailāsa*; *khanija* type of silver is obtained from the mines of *Himācala* and *kṛtrima* type of silver is prepared with mercury by the transmutation of tin, etc.

'[३९]रसदर्पणात्
श्रीरामपादुकान्यस्तं वंगं यद्रूप्यतां गतम् ।
तत्पादरूपमित्युक्तं कृत्रिमं सर्वरोगनुत्' ।।४७।।

Mythology About Origin of Silver According to Rasadarpaṇa

When the wooden sandals of Lord Rāma were placed on tin, the latter was changed to silver. This artificial silver is like the foot of Lord Rāma and it cures all diseases.

दाहे रक्तं च पीतं च कृष्णं रूक्षं स्फुटं लघु ।
स्थूलांगं कर्कशांगं च रजतं त्याज्यमष्टधा ।।४८।।

Unusable Silver

If the silver placed over fire becomes (1) red, (2) yellow or (3) black, (4) if it is ununctuouss, (5) if it cracks, (6) if it is light, (7) bulky or (8) slims then such silver, (having eight bad features) should be rejected.

गुरुस्निग्धं मृदुश्वेतं छेददाहघनैः सह[४०] ।
शंखाभं स्फोटरहितं ग्राह्यं चन्द्रायुधं शुभम् ।।४९।।

Silver of Good Quality

Silver which is heavy, unctuous, soft, white and compact even after cutting and burning, which is free from cracks, and which looks like conch-shell should be accepted. It is auspicious.

भागेन क्षारराजेन द्रावितं शुद्धिमृच्छति[४१] ।
तारं त्रिवारं निक्षिप्तं [४२]पिशाचीतैलमध्यतः ।।५०।।

Purification of Silver

Mixed with equal quantity of *yavakṣāra*, silver should be melted for its purification. Immersion of heated silver in the oil of *piśācī* for three times also purifies silver.

रसालंकारात्
रजतं दोषनिर्मुक्तं नागोत्तीर्णं [?] समाहरेत् ।
श्वेतागस्तिरसेनापि ढालयेत्सप्तवारकान् ।।५१।।

।। तारशोधनम् ।।

Second Method of Silver Purification According to Rasālaṅkāra

Silver free from *doṣa-s* (defects) and without mixture of lead (?) should be heated and immersed in the juice of the white variety of *agasti* for its purification.

तारं च देहस्य करोति तापं विड्बंधतां चेच्छति शुक्रनाशनम् ।
अवपाटवं वीर्यबलप्रहानिं महागदान्पोषयति ह्यशुद्धम् ।।५२।।

Adverse Effects of Impure Silver

Impure silver produces burning sensation in the body, causes constipation, reduces semen, causes laziness, diminishes potency & strength and gives rise to serious diseases.

तालकेन मृतं वंगं[४३] केनाप्यम्लेन पेषयेत् ।
तारपत्राणि संलिप्य पुटित्वा भस्मतां नयेत् ।।५३।।

Preparation of Silver-Bhasma

Bhasma of tin prepared by cooking with *haritāla* (orpiment) should be triturated by any sour juice. Leaves of silver should be smeared with this paste and cooked in *puṭa* which reduces silver into *bhasma* form.

जृंभाम्भसा हिंगुलेन तारपत्राणि लेपयेत् ।
मुनिसं[४४]पुटयोगेन खर्जूरं म्रियते ध्रुवम् ।।५४।।

Second Method of Preparing Silver Bhasma

Cinnabar should be triturated by adding the juice of *jambīra*. This paste should be smeared over silver-leaves and cooked in *muni* [?]*samputa* which reduces silver into *bhasma* form.

अन्यच्च
भागैकं रसराजस्य गन्धकं पञ्चभागकम् ।
चन्द्रभागं[४५] तयोस्तुल्यमीषन्माक्षिकसंयुतम् ।।५५।।
विरच्य क्वचीयन्त्रं पचेद्यामचतुष्टयम् ।
स्वांगशीते[४६] यथायोगे योजयेन्मतिमान्भिषक् ।।५६।।

Third Method of Preparing Silver-Bhasma

One part of mercury, five parts of sulphur and six parts of silver should be added with small quantity of *mākṣika* (copper pyrite). This powder should be kept in *kav(p)acī yantra* and cooked for four *yāma-s*. When it becomes cool, the *bhasma* of silver should be collected and used in appropriate recipes.

अथवा ताम्रवत्तारं मारयेन्न विचारयेत् ।।५७।।

Fourth Method of Preparing Silver-Bhasma

Alternatively, silver-*bhasma* should be prepared on lines prescribed for the preparation of copper-*bhasma*.

स्निग्धमल्पमपि सारकं हितं पाक्तोऽपि मधुरं च कुथितम्[४७] ।
वातपित्तहरणं प्रमेहजिल्लेखनं गदचयापहारकम् ।।५८।।

Properties of Silver

Silver-*bhasma* is unctuous, slightly laxative and sweet in *vipāka* (the taste that emerges after digestion). It alleviates *vāyu* and *pitta*. It cures *prameha* (obstinate urinary diseases including diabetes). It causes *lekhana* (scraping of tissue elements). It cures several other diseases.

प्रमेहारुचिविष्टम्भप्रमेहपिडिकान् अपि ।
चन्द्रायुधस्तु शमयेद्विकारान्वायुजानपि ।।५९।।

।। इति रजतोत्पत्तिभेदगुणदोषशोधनमारणगुणाः ।।

Another Description of the Properties of Silver

Bhasma of silver cures *prameha* (obstinate urinary disorders including diabetes), anorexia, tympanitis, diabetic carbuncles and diseases caused by *vāyu*.

Thus, ends the description of the origin, varieties, good and bad qualities, purification, calcination and properties of silver.

TĀMRA (COPPER)

शुक्रं[४८] यत्कार्तिकेयस्य पतितं धरणीतले ।
तस्मादेव समुद्भूतं ताम्रमाहुः पुराविदः ।।६०।।

Mythology About Origin of Copper

The semen of Kārtikeya which fell down upon earth gave rise to copper according to scholars of ancient history.

नेपाल-बंगाल-सुदेश-जातं केदारजं[४९] वापि महापवित्रम् ।
संगृह्य ताम्रं त्रिगुणाहि[५०] [?] ताम्रं संशोधयेद्भूमिजदोषशान्तये ।।६१ ।।

Varieties

Copper which is collected from Nepāla, Baṅgāla and Sudeśa or Kedāra is sacred. This copper, after collection, should be purified to remove impurities which have accrued because of its contact with the earth.

सुस्निग्धं मधुरं रक्तं नेपालं निर्विकारकम् ।
बंगाल म्लेच्छजं वापि कृष्णं श्वेतं कठोरकम् ।।६२।।
हीनं, केदारकं श्रेष्टं सर्वलक्षणसम्प्लुतम्[1] ।
घनघातसहं स्निग्धं. रक्तवदमलं[2] मृदुः ।
शुद्धाकारं तु नेपालं 'ताम्रं'[3] शुभकरं मतम् ।।६३।।

Properties of Different Types of Copper

Nepāla type of copper is exceedingly unctuous, sweet in taste and red in colour. It does not produce any adverse effect.

The copper of Baṅgāla or the copper which is from Mleccha deśa is black or white in colour and hard. It is of inferior quality.

The Kedāra type of copper is the best and it possesses all the good qualities.

The Nepāla type of copper can tolerate hard beatings and it is unctuous, reddish, without any impurity, soft and pure in shape. It bestows auspiciousness.

भूशैलाकरजं कृष्णं रूक्षं स्तब्धघनासहम् ।
लोहनागयुतं श्वेतं' दोषाः शुल्वे दश स्मृताः ।।६४।।
भ्रमो मूर्च्छा विदाहश्च स्वेदक्लेदनवान्तयः।
अरुचिश्चित्तसंताप इति दोषाः विषोपमाः ।।६५।।

Impurities and Adverse Effects

Because of the impurities acquired from its association with earth or stone in the mine, copper becomes black, ununctuous, stiff and intolerant of hard impact. Because of its association with iron and lead, copper becomes white in colour.

The ten[?] *doṣa-s* (adverse effects) of copper are giddiness, fainting, burning sensation, sweating, production of stickiness, emesis, anorexia and mental disturbances. [The number of *doṣa-s* enumerated here is eight only.] These adverse effects are similar to those of poisons.

लवणैर्वज्रदुग्धेन ताम्रपत्रं विलेपयेत् ।
वह्नौ तप्तं च निर्गुण्डीरसे सिक्तं च सप्तधा ।
स्नुगर्कस्य रसेप्येवं शुल्वशुद्धिर्भविष्यति ।।६६।।

Purification of Copper

Copper sheets should be smeared with the paste of salt and milky latex of *snuhī*. These sheets should then be heated over fire and immersed in the juice of *nirgundī* for seven times. [Each time sheets are to be smeared and heated.] Similarly, these heated sheets of copper should be immersed in the milky latex of *snuhī* and *arka*. Thus, copper becomes pure.

अथवा महिषीतक्रे सप्तवारं विमज्जयेत्[५४] ।।६७।।

Second Method of Purifying Copper

Hot copper sheets may alternatively be immersed in buffalo-butter-milk for purification.

कालिकासहितं शुल्वं[५५] कोटकुष्टादिकारकम् ।।६८।।

Adverse Effects of Kālikā (Rust)

Copper associated with black rust causes urticaria, *kuṣṭha* (obstinate skin diseases including leprosy), etc.

शतार्द्धं सिन्धुवारस्य रसमध्ये[५६] तु ढालयेत् ।
कूष्माण्डस्वरसे पश्चान्निषेकान्सप्त दापयेत् ।।६९।।
ततस्तक्रे निशाशुक्ते पुनस्तत्रैव दापयेत् ।
शुल्वस्य कालिका ह्येवं प्रणश्यति न संशयः ।।७०।।

Procedure for Removing Kālikā

Heated copper should be immersed in the juice of *sindhuvāra* for fifty times. Thereafter, the heated copper should be immersed in the juice of *kūṣmāṇḍa* for seven times. Then such immersion should be done in butter-milk, in decoction of *haridrā* and in *śukta* (vinegar). Thus, the *kālikā doṣa* (appearance of black rust) of copper is undoubtedly destroyed.

रसार्णवात्
शुल्ववर्गेण संमिश्रा शुल्ववर्गपरिप्लुता ।
शुल्ववर्गकृता लेपा शुल्वशुद्धिषु शोभना ।।७१।।

Śulva-Varga
According to Rasārṇava

Mixed with the drugs belonging to *śulva-varga*, copper should be heated and immersed in the decoction of drugs belonging to *śulva varga* and the paste of drugs belonging to *śulva varga* should be applied over the copper sheets which purifies copper.

दर्शने[५७] शुक्तुण्डाभं छेदने दरदोपमम् ।
ध्मातं तु कालिकाहीनं शुल्वं निःकालिकं मतम् ।।७२।।

Characteristics of Copper Free From Kālikā

The copper which is pink like a parrot's beak, which when cut looks red like cinnabar and which when blown by keeping over fire does not produce any rust is called free from *kālikā*.

स्थूलं वा पत्तलं वापि ताम्रपत्रं पलद्वयम् ।
रसं किञ्चिद्गन्धकं च दद्यात्पलचतुष्टयम् ।।७३।।
विरच्य कवचीयंत्रं[५८] सिक्तापूरितं कुरु ।
प्रोष्णतां सिक्ता यान्ति तावद्वह्निं प्रदापयेत् ।
ततोत्तार्य[५९] विशिष्टोऽयं रोच्यताममृतोपमम्[६०] ।।७४।।

Purification of Copper

Thin or thick sheets of copper (two *pala-s*) should be added with a small quantity of mercury and four *pala-s* of sulphur. This should be kept in *kavacī yantra* in which latter should be filled with sand and heated till the sand becomes hot. The copper should then be removed and used. It is like ambrosia.

स्वच्छन्दो
भ्रमोत्क्लेदादिरहितमम्लपित्तगजाङ्कुशम् ।
कफमवातशमनं संप्रदायात्प्रदर्शितम्[६१] ।।७५।।
महागुणं महाकान्तं महाव्याधिविनाशनम् ।
महत्कौतूहलं लोके मारणस्य गुणस्य च ।।७६।।

Properties of Purified Copper
According to Svacchanda

The above mentioned preparation of copper does not cause giddiness and stickiness. It cures *amlapitta* (hyper acidity) and diseases caused by *kapha*, *vāta* and *āma* as known traditionally. It has many useful properties. It is an excellent promoter of complexion and it cures serious diseases. The properties of copper *bhasma* create considerable interest among the people.

ताम्रं सूरणकन्दगर्भनिहितं कृत्वा[६२] मृदावेष्टितम् ।
तीव्रगोमयवह्निना[६३] प्रपुटितं भस्मीभवत्याशु तत् ।।७७।।

Method of Preparing Copper-Bhasma

Copper should be kept inside a rhizome of *sūraṇa* and wrapped with mud. This should be cooked in strong fire which instantaneously reduces copper into *bhasma* form.

कासश्वासनिवर्हणं क्षयकफाष्ठीलादिरोगापहम् ।
योज्यं कुष्ठविषामशूलमलनुत् जीर्णज्वरं नाशयेत् ।
पाण्ड्वर्शःकृमिपित्तशोफमरुचिं छर्दीं जयेदाशु[६४] च ।।७८।।

Properties of Copper-Bhasma

Bhasma of copper cures bronchitis, asthma, consumption, diseases of *kapha*, *aṣṭhīlā* (hard tumour), *kuṣṭha* (obstinate skin diseases including leprosy), poisoning, *āma-doṣa* (diseases caused by the product of improper digestion and metabolism), colic pain, diseases caused by the accumulation of waste-products, chronic fever, anemia, piles, parasitic infestation, diseases caused by *pitta*, oedema, anorexia and vomiting.

रसदर्पणात्
शुल्वस्य पिष्टिकां कृत्वा सममाक्षिकसत्त्वयुक्।
त्रिदिनं चक्रमर्दस्य रसेन परिमर्दितम् ।।७९।।
गर्भयन्त्रेण पुटितं ताम्रं च श्वेततां व्रजेत् ।
क्षयामशूलशमनं ज्वरश्वयथुनाशनम् ।।८०।।

Second Method of Preparing Copper-Bhasma According to Rasadarpaṇa

Copper should be added with equal quantity of *mākṣika* and triturated for three days by adding the juice of *cakramarda*. This paste should be cooked in *garbha yantra* which produces white type of copper-*bhasma*. This cures consumption, colic pain, fever and oedema.

अन्यच्च राजहंसमतात्

सूताच्च त्रिगुणं गन्धं सूतार्द्धं ताप्यसत्त्वकम् ।
तयोः समं ताम्रपत्रं निर्गुण्डीरसमर्दितम् ॥८१॥
आम्रवल्करसेनापि कुमारीदलजेन च ।
त्रिदिनं भावयित्वाऽथ काचकुंभे विनिक्षिपेत् ॥८२॥
प्ररुध्य वालुकायन्त्रे अहोरात्रं विपाचयेत् ।
अवश्यं म्रियते कृष्ण[६५]वर्णं ताम्रं प्रजायते ।
शोषप्रमेहशूलामकुष्ठज्वरगदापहम्[६६] ॥८३॥

Third Method of Preparing Copper-Bhasma According to Rājahaṃsa

One part of mercury, three parts of sulphur, half part of the *sattva* of *mākṣika* and three and half parts of copper-sheets should be impregnated and triturated in the juices of *nirguṇḍī*, bark of *āmra* and leaves of *kumārī* for three days. This should then be kept in a glass bottle and cooked *in vālukā yantra* for one day and night. This reduces copper into *bhasma* form which is black in colour.

It cures consumption, *prameha* (obstinate urinary diseases including diabetes), colic pain, *āma* (diseases caused by the product of improper digestion and metabolism), *kuṣṭha* (obstinate skin diseases including leprosy) and fever.

अन्यच्च

ताम्रपादांशतः सूतं ताम्रतुल्यं तु गन्धकम् ।
जंबीराम्लेन संपिष्ट्वा ताम्रपत्राणि लेपयेत् ।
निक्षिप्य हंडिकामध्ये शरावेण निरोधयेत् ॥८४॥
हंडिकां[६७] पटुनापूर्य पचेद्यामद्वयं भिषक् ।

स्वांगशीतं विचूर्ण्याथ वान्तिदाहादिवर्जितम् ।।८५।।

Fourth Method of Preparing Copper-Bhasma

One part of mercury and four parts of sulphur should be triturated by adding the juice of *jambīra*. With this paste, four parts of copper-sheets should be smeared. It should be kept in a jar whose remaining empty parts should be filled with salt. The jar should be covered with an earthen lid and sealed. This should be cooked for two *yāma-s*. After it is cooled, the copper should be made to a powder form which does not cause vomiting, burning sensation, etc.

'उदकराराचूर्ण[६८] दत्वा सटंकणं ताम्रं धमेद् शीघ्रं द्रवति' ।।८६ ।।

Melting Copper

Copper mixed with the powder of *udakarārā* (?) and *ṭaṅkaṇa* should be blown by keeping over fire. Thus, copper melts quickly.

सूक्ष्मं शुल्वदलं विलिप्य वलिना दुग्धेन वह्नौ धृतम् ।
सद्योमुक्तकलंक्तिवलिपुटैः स्याद्भस्म दुग्धाग्निभिः ।।८७ ।।
अम्ले वासरयुग्ममेव सुदृढं संस्वेदितं दोलया ।
वान्त्यादीन् सहसा जहाति पुटितं पञ्चामृतैः संप्लुतम्[६९] ।।८८ ।।

Fifth Method of Preparing Copper-Bhasma

Thin sheets of copper should be smeared with the paste of sulphur, and after heating over fire it should be immersed in milk. This process removes the *kālikā-doṣa* (rust) of copper. Mixed with sulphur, copper should be cooked in *puṭa* which reduces it to *bhasma* form. This *bhasma* should be cooked in a *dolā yantra* with milk and sour juice for two days. Strong-heat should be applied. Thereafter, this *bhasma* should be triturated with *pañcāmṛta* and cooked in *puṭa*. The *bhasma*, thus processed, does not cause vomiting, etc.

रसराजलक्ष्मीतः
सगरलं वत्सनाभं च नागिनीकन्दमुत्तमम् ।
लांगली माहिषं पित्तं पञ्चामृतमितीरितम् ।।८९ ।।
दद्यात्पञ्चपुटं पश्चाद्भिषक् पंचामृतेन च ।

दधि मधु दुग्ध - सिता घृतं चैव पञ्चामृतम् ।।९०।।

Pañcāmṛta (Five Nectars)
According to Rasarāja Lakṣmī

Garala (snake venom), *vatsanābha* (aconite), rhizome of *nāginī*, *lāṅgalī* and bile of buffalo—these five taken together are called *pañcāmṛta* (five nectars). With this *pañcāmṛta*, five *puṭa-s* should be given to copper-*bhasma*.

According to some physicians, curd, honey, milk, sugar and ghee taken together are called *pañcāmṛta* (five nectars) and with these ingredients *puṭa* should be given to copper-*bhasma*.

वान्तिं विरेकं कुरुते 'च[70] तापं मूर्च्छां विधत्ते हरते च शुक्रम् ।
नानारुजानां कुरुते' प्रक्षेपं अपक्वशुल्वं न च जीवहारि ।।९१ ।।

Adverse Effects of Uncooked Copper

Uncooked copper causes vomiting, purgation, burning sensation, faintinng, diminution of semen and different types of pain. It does not cause death.

सामान्यशुल्वं न योज्यं गुटिकायां विचक्षणैः ।
कालिका[71]रहितं कृत्वा गुटिकायां च योजयेत् ।।९२।।

Ordinary copper should not be used in the recipes of pills. Copper free from *kālikā* (rust) should only be used in such recipes.

कुष्ठं च गुल्मं च गुदामयं च शूलं च शोफोदरपाण्डुमेहान् ।
उत्क्लेदभेदभ्रमदाहहीनं निहन्ति सम्यङ्मृतमेव शुल्वम् ।।९३ ।।

Therapeutic Properties

Properly prepared *bhasma* of copper does not cause nausea, cracking pain, giddiness and burning sensation. It cures *kuṣṭha* (obstinate skin diseases including leprosy), *gulma* (phantom tumour), diseases of the anus, colic pain, oedema, *udara* (obstinate abdominal diseases including ascites), anemia and *meha* (obstinate urinary diseases including diabetes).

ताम्रं तिक्तं कषायकं समधुरं वीर्योष्णं पाके कटु ।
अर्शःपित्तकफापहं जठरनुत्कुष्ठामाजीर्णान्तकृत् ।।९४।।
ऊर्ध्वाधःपरिशोधनं ज्वरहरं स्थौल्यापहं क्षुत्करम् ।
दुष्टामक्षयशोफपाण्डुशमनं नेत्र्यं तथा लेखनम्[७२] ।।९५।।

।। इति ताम्रोत्पत्ति-लक्षण-शोधन-मारणगुणाः ।।

Another Description of Therapeutic Properties of Copper

Copper is bitter, astringent and sweet in taste. It is hot in potency and pungent in *vipāka* (the taste which emerges after digestion). It cures piles, diseases caused by *pitta* and *kapha*, *udara* (obstinate abdominal diseases including ascites), *kuṣṭha* (obstinate skin diseases including leprosy) and *āmājīrṇa* (indigestion). It cleanses the body through both the upward and downward tracts. It cures fever and obesity. It promotes appetite. It cures serious type of *āma doṣa* (diseases caused by the product of improper digestion), consumption, oedema and anemia. It promotes eye-sight and causes scraping of the tissues (***lekhana***).

Thus, ends the description of origin, characteristics, methods of **purification** and calcination and properties of copper.

VAṄGA (TIN)

खुरकं मिश्रकं चैव द्विविधं वंगमुच्यते ।
खुरकं तु गुणैर्युक्तं मिश्रकं हरितं मतम् ।।९६।।

Varieties of Tin

Tin is of two types, viz., *khuraka* and *miśraka*. *Khuraka* type of tin is very useful and *miśraka* type of tin is inferior in quality.

स्वच्छं सुकोमलं स्निग्धं वंगं योज्यं रसायने ।।९७।।

Useful Characteristics

Tin which is clean, soft and unctuous should be used in recipes for rejuvenation therapy.

कठिनं स्फुटनं रूक्षं श्यामिकादलसंयुतम् ।
पञ्चदोषयुतं वंगं नेच्छेत् रसकर्माणि ।।९८।।

Harmful Characteristics

Tin which is hard, having cracks, ununctuous and having black layer should not be used in the processing of mercury. These are the five defects (*doṣa-s*) of tin.

निर्गुण्डीमूलचूर्णेन सार्कदुग्धेन लेपितम् ।
वंगपत्रं तु संशुष्कं द्रावयित्वा विनिक्षिपेत् ।।९९।।
निर्गुण्डीद्रवमध्ये तु ततः पत्रं तु[73] कारयेत् ।
लिप्त्वा लिप्त्वा पुनः शोष्यं सप्तवारं विशुद्धये ।।१००।।
चक्रिकाक्वाथमध्ये वा सप्तवारं निषेचयेत् ।।१०१।।
ज्वरप्रमेहहृत्कम्पगौरवं वह्निमार्दवम् ।
वंगो दोषान्वितः कुर्यादुदरं नेत्रनाशनम् ।।१०२।।

।। इति मोहापालात् ।।

Purification of Tin
According to Mohāpāla

Tin-leaves should be smeared with the paste prepared by triturating the powder of the root of *nirguṇḍī* with the milky latex of *arka*. Then the tin-leaves should be dried, melted and immersed into the juice of *nirguṇḍī*. Again thin leaves of the tin should be prepared by smearing the above mentioned paste, and then they should be immersed again. This process should be repeated for seven times. This immersion can also be done in the decoctionn of *cakrikā* for seven times.

Properties and Adverse Effects

Purified tin cures fever, *prameha* (obstinate urinary disorders including diabetes), palpitation, heaviness of the heart and suppression of the power of digestion. Impure tin causes *udara* (obstinate abdominal diseases including ascites) and impairement of the eye-sight.

अथ चिन्तामणिः

गोणिकापृथके[74] कृत्वा कटुसर्षपजं खलिम् ।
दशटंकप्रमाणं स्यात्पिप्पलक्षारजं रजः ।।१०३।।
अस्योपरि भवेदेतत्कर्कटास्थिरजः पुनः ।

तस्योपरि भवेत्तोरी मृदिता सूक्ष्मवर्जिता ।।१०४।।
तस्योपरि भवेत्साधु 'वंगपत्राणि विस्तरात् ।
तेषां च तोरिकां दद्यादुपरिष्टादनालसः[७५] ।।१०५।।
पुनः कर्कटजं चूर्णं पिपलस्यापि तत्पुनः ।
पुनः खलिर्विधातव्या तदा संवृत्य पट्टकम् ।।१०६।।
मृत्सया[७६] लिप्यते शुष्कं पुनर्गजपुटे पचेत् ।
एकं वारत्रयं कृत्वा वंगोऽसौ म्रियते ध्रुवम् ।।१०७।।
अरण्यस्थानके[७७] कृत्वा वंगपत्रं विशोधयेत् ।
अरण्यदानकेनैवं कुंजराख्यः पुटो भवेत् ।।१०८।।

Preparation of Tin-Bhasma According to Cintāmaṇi

In a thick cow-dung-cake, the oil-cake of mustard should be kept. Over it, the powder of the *kṣāra* (alkali preparation) of *aśvattha* (ten *taṅka-s* in quantity) should be spread. The powder of the shell of *karkaṭa* should be spread over it. Crushed *torī* (?) without any fine powder should be kept over it. On these layers of paste and powder, tin-leaves should be spread. Over these tin-leaves *torī* (?) should be spread again. Over these, layers of the powder of the shell of *karkaṭa* and *kṣāra* of *aśvattha* should be spread. This should be covered with the oil-cake of mustard and tied with a cloth which should be wrapped with mud. This should be dried and cooked in *gaja puṭa* for one or three times by which tin is reduced to *bhasma* form.

Vaṅga (tin) should be purified with cow-dung cakes collected from forest and in the *gaja puṭa* these should be used as fuel.

रसदर्पणात्
तालकं कर्कटास्थीनि शंखशुक्तिवराटिकाः ।
सिन्धुकर्पूरसंयुक्तं मारयेद्वंगपर्वतम् ।।१०९।।

Second Method of Preparing Tin-Bhasma According to Rasadarpaṇa

Haritāla, bones of *karkaṭa*, *śaṅkh*, *śukti* and *varāṭikā* mixed with rock-salt and camphor help in reducing tin into *bhasma* form.

अथ रत्नाकरात्
चिंचाक्षारालुतुल्यांशं केनाप्यम्लेन मर्दयेत् ।
पलाशोत्थद्रवैर्वापि[७८] लोलयित्वांधसम्पुटे ।।११०।।
उद्धृत्य दशमांशेन तालेन सह मर्दयेत् ।
पलाशोत्थद्रवेणापि रुद्ध्वा गजपुटे पचेत् ।
एवं त्रिंशत्पुटैः[७९] पक्वो मृतो भवति रोगहा ।।१११।।

Third Method of Preparing Tin-Bhasma

Tin should be added with equal quantity of the *kṣāra* (alkali preparation) of *ciñcā* and triturated by adding any sour liquid, or by adding the juice or decoction of *palāśa*. This should then be cooked in *andha-samputa*. This, taken out of the *samputa*, should be added with one tenth of *haritāla* and triturated by adding the juice or decoction of *palāśa*. Keeping in *śarāva-samputa*, it should then be cooked in *gaja-puṭa*. This process should be done for thirty times by which tin is reduced to *bhasma* form.

अन्यच्च
वंगपादेन सूतेन वंगपत्राणि लेपयेत् ।
चिंचावृक्षस्य[८०] संगृह्य अन्तस्थल्यथ तद्दलैः ।।११२।।
पिष्ट्वा तत्पिण्डमध्ये तु वंगपत्राणि मिश्रयेत् ।
निरुन्ध्याथ पुटैः पश्चात्पूर्वसंख्या मृतो भवेत् ।।११३।।

Fourth Method of Preparing Tin-Bhasma

Tin-leaves should be smeared with 1/4th in quantity of mercury. The inner bark of *ciñcā* should be made to a paste by triturating with the juice of *ciñcā*-leaves. Tin-leaves should be smeared with this paste. Then keeping sealed in *śarāva samputa*, these tin leaves should be cooked in *puṭa* by which it is reduced to a *bhasma*-form.

वंगः सार्कपयस्तालः शुष्काश्वत्थपुटैस्त्रिभिः[८१] ।
म्रियते भ्राष्ट्रगो ब्रह्मकाष्ठघर्षणयोगतः ।।११४।।

Fifth Method of Preparing Tin-Bhasma

Tin triturated with the milky latex of *arka*, *haratāla* and powder of the dried bark of *aśvattha* should be given three *puṭa-s*. Then keeping over an oven it should be stirred with the stick of *brahma-kāṣṭha*. Thus, tin is reduced to *bhasma* form.

यवासाह्वेन घृष्टं वा तिन्तिडीकरसेन वा।
रजनीचूर्णेन घृष्टं वंगं निर्जीवतां गतम् ॥१९५॥

Sixth Method of Preparing Tin-Bhasma

Tin [melted over a pan] should be added with either the powder of *yavāsā* or the juice of *tintiḍī* or the powder of *haridrā* and stirred which reduces it to *bhasma* form.

पाक्हीनौ नागवंगौ[८३] गुल्मकुष्ठरुजाकरौ ।
प्रमेहपाण्डूदरदौ कफपित्तामकारकौ ॥१९६॥

Adverse Effects of Imperfect Tin-Bhasma

Tin and lead used in imperfect *bhasma* form or without reducing these to *bhasma* form cause *gulma* (phantom tumour), *kuṣṭha* (obstinate skin diseases), pain, *prameha* (obstinate urinary diseases), anemia, *udara* (obstinate abdominal diseases including ascites) and diseases caused by *kapha, pitta,* as well as *āma* (improper digestion and metabolism).

भस्मंगतोत्थितं वंगं पत्रं कृत्वा पुटेत्पुनः ।
अतसी[८४]चूर्णपुटितो वंगः स्याद्भस्म पाण्डुरम् ॥१९७॥

॥ रससिन्धुतः ॥

Seventh Method of Preparing Tin-Bhasma According to Rasasindhu

Bhasma of tin should be retrieved and this should be made to thin leaves. These tin leaves should be mixed with the powder of *atasī* and given *puṭa* again. Thus, the yellowish-brown coloured *bhasma* of tin is prepared.

रसार्णवात्[८५]

वंगं तिक्तोष्णकं रूक्षमीषद्वातप्रकोपणम् ।
मेहश्लेष्मज्वरहरं कृमिघ्नं बलदं परम् ॥१९८॥

Properties of Tin
According to Rasārṇava

Tin is bitter in taste, hot in potency, ununctuous and slightly aggravator of *vāyu*. It cures *meha* (obstinate urinary diseases including diabetes), diseases of *kapha*, fever and parasitic infestation. It is an excellent promoter of strength.

अन्यथाकरे[८६]
वंगं सुशीतं लवणं रसं भवेत्पाण्डुप्रमेहारुचिदाहहन्मतम्[८७] ।
तिक्तं कृमिघ्नं कफजित्समीरजित्सूतेन युक्तं सकलज्वरापहम् ।।११९।।

।। इति वंगलक्षणशोधनमारणगुणाः ।।

Properties of Tin
According to Another Text

Tin is exceedingly cooling and saline in taste. It cures anemia, *prameha* (obstinate urinarydiseases including diabetes), anorexia and burning sensation. It is bitter in taste. It cures parasitic infestation and diseases caused by *kapha* and *vāyu*. In association with mercury, it cures all types of fever.

Thus, ends the description of characteristics, purification, calcination and properties of tin.

NĀGA (LEAD)

रसदर्पणात्
कोमलं निर्मलं नागं रजतेन समन्वितम् ।
वज्रसंज्ञं[८८] रसे योज्यं स्तब्धं रूक्षं च वर्जयेत्[८९] ।।१२०।।

Characteristics of Lead
According to Rasadarpaṇa

Lead is soft and clean. When it is associated with silver, it is called *vajra* (diamond). Such type of lead should be used for processing mercury. Lead which is stiff and ununctuous is not useful.

गौरीफलानि क्षुरको[९०] रजनी तुम्बुरूणि च ।
कुबेराक्षस्य बीजानि मल्लिकयास्तथैव च ।
पलाशस्नुगपामार्गक्षारांस्तु[९१] क्षीरयोगतः ।

सप्तधा प्रतिवापेन शोधयन्ति भुजङ्गम् ।
गौरीफलं आमलकी ।।१२१।।

Purification of Lead

Lead sheets should be made hot and immersed for seven times in milk added with *āmalakī*, *kṣuraka*, *haridrā*, *tumburu*, seeds of *kuberākṣa* and *mallikā* (*kuṭaja*), and *kṣāra-s* (alkali preparations) of *palāśa*, *snuhī* as well as *apāmārga* by which it gets purified.

वंगवच्छोधयेद्वापि[१२] मारणं कथ्यतेऽधुना ।
शिलाया रविदुग्धेन नागपत्राणि लेपयेत् ।
मारयेत्पुटयोगेन निरुत्थं जायते ध्रुवम् ।।१२२।।

Preparation of Lead-Bhasma

Lead can also be purified on the methods prescribed for the purification of tin.

Thin sheets of lead should be smeared with the paste of *manaḥśilā* and milky latex of *arka*, and cooked in *puṭa*. Thus, the unretrievable (*niruttha*) *bhasma* of lead is prepared.

अथ राजहसमतात्
पुन्नाग-प्रतिनागरोगदमनीनीरेण[१३] नागोत्तमः ।
वासाग्नौ परिपाचितोरगमुखे रामान्वितः पन्नगः ।।१२३।।
सिन्दूरप्रतिपूर-पूरकणिका सिन्दूरसाडम्बरः ।
स्यादाशु क्षयरोगमेहजिदयं श्री पद्मरागानुकः[१४] ।।१२४।।

Second Method of Preparing Lead-Bhasma

Lead should be cooked in the juice or decoction of *punnāga*, *pratināga* and *rogadamanī* with the fuel of *vāsaka* stems. Then it should be cooked in *puṭa*. Thus, red coloured *bhasma* like *sindūra* (vermilion) is prepared which instantaneously cures consumption and *meha* (obstinate urinary diseases including diabetes). This *bhasma* looks like the lotus-petals in colour.

अन्यच्च
नागं सुगलितं कृत्वा भिषग्मातादलं ततः[१५] ।
दत्त्वा[१६] दत्त्वा प्रघर्षेत लोहदण्डेन संततम् ।
यावत्सुवर्णवर्णाभं भवेदिति विनिश्चितम् ।।१२५।।

Third Method of Preparing Lead-Bhasma

Lead should be melted in an iron pan. Over it, the powder of *vāsaka*-leaves should be sprinkled in small quantities and constantly rubbed with an iron pestle till the lead is reduced to golden coloured *bhasma* form.

अन्यच्च

तांबूलीरससंपिष्टशिलालेपात्पुनः पुनः ।
द्वात्रिंशद्भिः पुटैर्नागो निरुत्थो याति भस्मताम् ।।१२६।।

Fourth Method of Preparing Lead-Bhasma

Manaḥśilā should be made to a paste by triturating with the juice of betel-leaf. This paste should be applied over the thin sheets of lead given *puṭa* for thirty two times repeatedly by which lead is reduced to irretrievable (*niruttha*) *bhasma* form.

कुमारीपादघातेन सर्पो मृत्युमवाप्नुयात् ।
भूयस्तत्पुटयोगेन सिन्दूराभं ध्रुवं भवेत् ।।१२७।।

Fifth Method of Preparing Lead-Bhasma

Lead is reduced to *bhasma* form by triturating with the juice of *kumārī* and then by cooking in *puṭa* repeatedly. The *bhasma*, thus produced, is red in colour like that of vermilion.

अन्यच्च

भूभुजङ्गमगस्तिं च पिष्ट्वा पत्रं विलेपयेत् ।
तत्र[17] संविद्रुते नागे वासाकुट्टकभस्मना ।।१२८।।
वासाकाष्ठेन संघृष्टे[18] चतुर्यामिनं तत्परः ।
ततश्चैवं[19] शिलाताप्यैर्वासकक्षारसंयुतैः ।।१२९।।
त्रिभिस्तुल्यं मृतं नागं विंशदेक्पुटैः पचेत् ।
कुमारीस्वरसेनापि दद्याद्गजपुटं पुनः ।।१३०।।
दिक्पुटं चिञ्चिडिक्षारैर्देयं वासान्वितैः रसैः ।
नागैः सिन्दूरवर्णाभो म्रियते सर्वकार्यकृत् ।।१३१।।

Sixth Method of Preparing Lead-Bhasma

Earth-worm and *agasti* should be triturated and made to a paste. Thin sheets of lead should be smeared with this paste and cooked by keeping in an iron pan till it melts. To this, the ash of *vāsaka* and *kuṭaka* (?) should be sprinkled in small quantities and rubbed with pestle prepared of the wood of *vāsaka* for four *yāma-s*.

Thereafter, the *bhasma* of *nāga* (one part) should be added with *manaḥśilā* (one part), *tāpya* (one part) and *kṣāra* (alkali preparation) of *vāsaka* (one part) and cooked in *gaja-puṭa* for twenty one times.

Thereafter, this *bhasma* should be triturated with the juice of *kumārī* and given *gaja-puṭa*. Again, this *bhasma* should be added with the *kṣāra* of *ciñcā* and triturated by adding the juice of *vāsaka*. This should again be given ten *puṭa-s*. Thus, red coloured *bhasma* of lead like vermilion is prepared which is useful in all recipes.

शतनागबलं धत्ते वीर्यायुःकान्तिवर्धकम् ।
प्रमेहं पिडिकायुक्तं शोषं कासं जयेद् ध्रुवम् ।।१३२।।

Properties of Lead-Bhasma

By taking the *bhasma* of lead, a person is endowed with great strength like that of one hundred cobra snakes. It promotes semen, longevity and complexion. It cures *prameha* (obstinate urinary diseases including diabetes) associated with diabetic carbuncles, consumption and bronchitis.

अन्यच्च[100]

नागं च नागशततुल्यं बलं[101] करोति ।
व्याधीन्विनाशयति जीवित[102]मातनोति ।।१३३।।
वह्निं प्रदीपयति कामबलं तनोति ।
दुष्टव्रणान्हरति रोहति पूरणेन ।।१३४।।
गुल्मप्रमेहोदरकुष्ठनाशनम् ।
सकाश्र्यपाण्डुज्वररुक्च[103] नाशनम् ।।१३५।।
प्रोत्साहतेजोजपरं विवर्धनम् ।
नागं च नागेव बलं ददाति ।।१३६।।

।। इति नागलक्षणशोधनमारणगुणाः ।।

Another Description of the Properties of Lead-Bhasma

Bhasma of lead (*nāga*) endows a person with great strength like one hundred cobra-snakes (*nāga-s*). It cures diseases and makes the life purposeful. It promotes the power of digestion and sex. It cures purulent ulcers by healing and filling. It cures *gulma* (phantom tumour), *prameha* (obstinate urinary disorders including diabetes), *udara* (obstinate abdominal disorders including ascites), *kuṣṭha* (obstinate skin diseases including leprosy), emaciation, anemia and fever. It is an excellent promoter of enthusiasm, vigour and complexion. It endows a person with strength like that of a cobra.

Thus, ends the characteristics, purification, calcination and properties of lead.

KĀṂSYA (BRONZE)

कृत्रिमं पित्तलं कांस्यं लोहेषु गणयन्ति ते ।
क्वचिदेव मतं ह्येतत्प्रायशो न वरं मतम् ॥१३७॥

Alloys

Pittala (bell-metal) and *kāṃsya* (bronze)—these two artificially prepared alloys, according to some physicians, are included in the group of *loha-s* (metals). Therapeutically, these two are generally not considered as very useful.

सप्तभागेन ताम्रेण द्विभागं कुटिलेन च ।
विद्रुतेन भवेत्कांस्यं तत्सौराष्ट्रजमुत्तमम् ॥१३८॥

Preparation of Bronze

Seven parts of copper and two parts of tin, taken together, are melted to produce bronze. This alloy prepared in Saurāṣṭra is excellent in quality.

तीक्ष्णशब्दं मृदुस्निग्धमीषच्छ्यामं च सुप्रभम् ।
दाहे रक्तं निर्मलं च सप्तधा कांस्यमुत्तमम् ॥१३९॥

Characteristics of Good Bronze

Bronze which produces sharp sound, which is soft, unctuous, blackish blue in colour and with glaze, which when placed over fire becomes red and which is clear is the best. These are the seven good qualities of bronze.

आपीतं दहने ताम्रं खरं रूक्ष्यं घनासहम् ।
मंदनादं गतद्योतिं सप्तधा कांस्यमुत्सृजेत् ।।१४०।।

Bad Qualities of Bronze

Bronze, having seven bad qualities, viz., which is yellowish in colour, which looks like copper when heated, which is rough and ununctuous, which is incapable of tolerating hard impacts, which produces dull sound and which is free from glaze, should not be used.

कांस्यस्य शोधनं चाथ मारणं ताम्रवन्मतम् ।।१४१।।

Purification and Calcination of Bronze

For purification and calcination of bronze, the methods prescribed for copper should be followed.

अशुद्धं यद्भवेत्कांस्यं[१०४] कामहानिकरं परम्[१०५] ।।१४२।।

Adverse Effects of Impure Bronze

Impure bronze exceedingly diminishes sexual power.

शुद्धं दृष्टिकरं वृष्यं कषायोष्णं कफापहम् ।।१४३।।

Properties of Pure Bronze

Pure bronze promotes eye sight. It is aphrodisiac. It is astringent in taste and hot in potency. It alleviates *kapha*.

लघु लेखनकं कांस्यं रसे तिक्तकषायकम् ।
अञ्जनादौ हितं ज्ञेयं चक्षुरोगहरं परम् ।।१४४।।

।। इति[१०६] कांस्यमारणगुणाः ।।

Another Description of the Properties of Bronze

Bronze is light and *lekhana* (which causes scraping of tissues). It is bitter and astringent in taste. It is an excellent remedy for eye diseases and is useful for recipes of collyrium.

Thus, ends the description of calcination and properties of bronze.

PITTALA (BELL-METAL)

रीतिका काकतुण्डी च द्विविधा पित्तली मता ।।१४५।।

संतप्ता कांजिके क्षिप्ता ताम्राभा रीतिका मता।
एवं कृते च या कृष्णा काकतुण्डीनि सा मता ।।१४६।।

Varieties of Bell-Metal

Bell-metal is of two types, viz., *rītikā* and *kākatuṇḍī*. After heating, it should be immersed in *kāñjī* (vinegar). If it becomes coppery in colour, then it is called *rītikā* and if by doing so, it becomes black in colour, then it is called *kākatuṇḍī*.

गुर्वी मृद्वी च पीताभा[107] स्फराङ्गी त्रोटमक्षमा[108] ।
सुस्निग्धा मसृणाङ्गी[109] च रीतिरेतादृशी शुभा[110] ।।१४७।।

Characteristics of Good Bell-Metal

Bell metal, which is heavy, soft, yellowish in colour and *spharāṅgī* (quivering), which does not break when hammered and which is unctuous and smooth, is auspicious.

रीतिकाशोधनं चैव मारणं चापि ताम्रवत् ।।१४८।।

Purification and Calcination of Bell-Metal

Bell-metal should be purified and calcinated according to the methods prescribed for copper.

रसे लवणतिक्ता च लेखनी पाण्डुनाशिनी ।
शोधिनी कृमिदोषघ्नी रीतिका[111] व्रणनाशिनी ।।१४९।।

।। इति रीतिका लक्षणमारणगुणाः[112] ।।

Properties of Bell-Metal

Bell-metal is saline and bitter in taste. It is *lekhana* (which scraps the tissues). It cures *pāṇḍu* (anemia). It cleanses the body by the elimination of *doṣa-s*. It cures parasitic infestation and ulcers.

Thus, ends the description of the characteristics, calcination and properties of bell-metal.

LAUHA (IRON)

देवासुरसमाजेन मथ्यमाने महोदधौ ।
समुत्पन्नं पुरा तस्मिन्नमृतं देवजीवनम् ।।१५०।।

पीयमानं सुरैस्तस्मादुत्थिताः क्षुद्रबिन्दवः ।
ज्ञात्वा भूमिगतान्यत्नात् गोपयामास धूर्जटिः ।।१५१।।
लोहपाषाणरूपेण कृत्वा तान्वसुधातले ।
पापरोगाभिभूता ये मानवास्ते भजन्तु तम्[११३] ।।१५२।।

Mythology Regarding the Origin of Iron

In the days of yore, the gods and demons churned the ocean which produced ambrosia, the life-giver of the gods. While drinking this, drops of ambrosia sprinkled out and fell down on the earth which were kept secretly by Lord Śiva in the form of iron-stone for the benefit of the humanity suffering from sinful diseases.

नागार्जुनात्

जातं[११४] मारणवस्तु गर्तनियमं संस्कारकर्म क्रमात् ।
संधायाभ्रकसंस्कृतं[११५] च बहुधा चूर्णौषधीनां गणान् ।।१५३।।
पाकं भक्षणकालमाननियमं रक्षानुपानस्थितिम्[११६] ।
पथ्यापथ्यगणान्तथैव च गुणान् लोहस्य वक्ष्याम्यहम् ।।१५४।।

According to Nāgārjuna

The following topics relating to iron will be discussed by me (Nāgārjuna) :

(1) Origin of iron;
(2) Drugs to be used for the calcination of iron;
(3) Rule for preparing the pit [on the earth for cooking iron in *puṭa*];
(4) *Saṃskāra* or processing of iron;
(5) Processing iron with the help of mica [?];
(6) Group of drugs to be used in powder form for processing iron;
(7) Method of cooking iron in *puṭa*;
(8) Time of taking iron-*bhasma*;
(9) Rules regarding dosage of iron-*bhasma*;
(10) Storage of iron-*bhasma*;
(11) *Anupāna* (vehicle or post-prandial drink);
(12) Wholesome and unwholesome food; and
(13) Properties of iron-*bhasma*.

[Note: This premise taken from Nāgārjuna's work does not appear to have been followed seriatum in the present text.]

नाधः पञ्चपला त्रयोदशपलादूर्द्धं न लोहं पचेत् ॥१५५॥

Quantity of Iron to be Taken for Processing

For the purpose of processing (purification, calcination, etc.) the unit quantity of iron should not be less than five *pala-s* and not more than thirteen *pala-s*.

तत्रायःपलपञ्चकस्य पचने निर्वापनादिक्रियाम् ।
उद्दिश्यं त्रिफलापलानि शतकैः निःक्वाथयेत्षोडश ।
प्रक्षिप्याष्टगुणं जलं परिमितं पादेन तच्चोद्धरेत् ॥१५६॥

Preparation of Triphalā-Decoction

For the purpose of *Nirvāpana* (making iron hot and immersing it in liquid) etc., five *pala-s* of iron and one hundred *pala-s* of *triphalā* should be boiled by adding sixteen (?) or eight times of water and reduced to one fourth. [After filtering out the powder, the decoction should be used as follows]:

सकलगुणसमेतं पांडिमादाय लोहम् ।
विगतमलमभवत्तस्य वर्गादिकं वा ॥१५७॥
त्रिफलापयसि सम्यग्यंत्रितं वह्नितप्तम् ।
गिरिमलहरणाय प्रक्षिपेत्सप्तकृत्वः ॥१५८॥

Removal of Giri-Mala

To remove *giri-mala* (impurities of iron associated because of its contact with elements in the mountain), *pāṇḍi* type of good quality iron should be heated over fire by holding carefully and immersed in the decoction of *loha-śodhaka-gaṇa* (group of drugs specially useful for purifying iron) or in the decoction of *triphalā* (described above) for seven times.

अथ तंत्रान्तरात् लोहपद्धतितः
"पुरा लोमिलदैत्यानां"[१७] निहतानां सुरैर्युधि ।

उत्पन्नानि शरीरेभ्यो लोहानि विविधानि च" ।।१५९।।
[आयुर्वेदप्रकाश : ३ : २०४]

According to Another Text and
According to Lohapaddhati

In the days of yore, when the demon called Lomila was killed in war by the gods, different types of iron originated from the body of this demon.

तत्र मस्तकजातानि शीतवीर्याणि तानि च ।
स्थूलदीर्घांगयुक्तानि स्निग्धानि सुरभीणि च ।
वारिदस्निग्धगम्भीरस्वराणि[१८] मधुराणि च ।
पित्तव्याधिहराण्याहुरमूनि सकलानि च ।।१६०।।

Iron Originated from the Head of Lomila

The iron originating from the head of the demon Lomila is cooling in potency. It is bulky, large in size, unctuous and sweet smelling. When struck, it produces sweet and deep sound like cloud. It is sweet in taste. All the types of iron belonging to this category alleviate *pitta*.

सुस्वराणि सुवर्णानि विस्रगन्धीनि[१९] यानि च ।
स्थूलकिञ्चिद्घनाङ्गानि वक्षोजानि[२०] कटूनि च ।
निहन्युः कफजान्येव व्याधीन्येतान्यसंशयम् ।।१६१।।

Iron Originating from the Chest of Lomila

The iron originating from the chest of the demon Lomila produces pleasing sound when struck and is good in colour. But it smells like flesh. It is bulky and slightly compact. It is pungent in taste and it undoubtedly cures diseases caused by *kapha*.

'विच्छिन्नपाण्डुराभानि[२१] पूतीनि कटिजानि च ।
रूक्षाणि रूक्षशब्दानि कषायाणि विनिर्दिशेत्' ।।१६२।।

Iron Originating from the Waist of Lomila

The iron originating from the waist of the demon Lomila is broken, yellowish in colour, foul smelling and ununctuous. When struck, it produces harsh sound and it is astringent in taste.

वाजीकरणयोगेषु वातव्याधौ तथैव च।
भिषग्तमसम्प्रदायाल्लोहान्येतानि योजयेत्[122] ।।१६३।।

Therapeutic Utility of Iron

Different types of iron mentioned above are used in recipes of aphrodisiacs and recipes for the diseases caused by *vāyu*.

रससारात्
मुंडः तीक्ष्णं तथा कान्तं भेदास्तेषां त्रयोदश।
मृदु कुंडं च काण्डारं त्रिविधं मुंडमुच्यते ।।१६४।।
खरसारं च होतालं तडावट्टं चिडं तथा ।
कान्तलोहं गजाख्यं च षड्विधं तीक्ष्णमुच्यते ।।१६५।।
कान्तलोहं चतुर्धोक्तं[123] रोमकं भ्रामकं तथा ।
चुंबकं द्रावकं चैव गुणास्तस्योत्तरोत्तराः ।
पञ्चमं च क्वचित्प्रोक्तं कर्षकं च रसार्णवे ।।१६६।।

Varieties of Iron
According to Rasasāra

Iron is generally classified into three categories, viz., (1) *muṇḍa*, (2) *tīkṣṇa*, and (3) *kānta*. These, in total, are of thirteen types as follows:

(1) *Muṇḍa* type of iron is of three types, viz., *mṛdu*, *kuṇḍa* and *kāṇḍāra*.
(2) *Tīkṣṇa* type of iron is of six types, viz., *kharasāra*, *hotālu*, *taḍāvaṭṭa*, *ciḍa*, *kānta-loha* and *gaja*.
(3) *Kānta-lauha* is of four types, viz., *romaka*, *bhrāmaka*, *cumbaka* and *drāvaka*.

These sucessively more and more useful. According to *Rasārṇava*, *kānta-lauha* is of five types and the fifth one is called *karṣaka*.

यद्यदाकरसम्भूतं तत्तद्देशजरोगनुत् ।।१६७।।

The iron collected from a particular mine is useful for the treatment of diseases of the people of that particular locality.

तेन तस्य परीक्षायां पतेन्मह्यां सहेतुकम् ।
तत्र वीरणपुष्पाभैरंगैः सारं परीक्षयेत् ॥१६८॥
तद्द्विधा स्थूललघ्वंगात्भेदाल्लोहविदो[२४] विदुः ।
औद्रं सेहुण्डपत्रांगं छिद्रांगं च कलिंगजम् ।
शुकपिंजरवर्णं च मृतं तद्गुरुसान्द्रकम् ॥१६९॥

Characteristics of Different Types of Iron

For the examination of iron, [its *sattva* or metallic essence] should be extracted which looks like the flower of *vīraṇa* in colour. According to the expert examiners of iron, it is of two types depending upon its grossness or small size. The *audra* type of iron takes the shape of the leaf of *snuhī* and the *kaliṅgaja* type of iron has holes in its corpus. The *bhasma* of the latter type of iron looks red like the parrot's beak and it is heavy as well as compact in nature.

गोरक्षमतात्
वज्रवल्लीति[२५] विख्याता सर्वलोहस्य मातरा ।
स्थूललघ्वंगभेदेन तस्माद्वज्रादिसंभवः ॥१७०॥

Iron-Ore

According to Gorakṣa

The ore of iron is called *vajravallī* and it is the source (mother) of all types or iron. It is of two types, viz., the one having big mass and the other having small mass. From this ore different types of iron, viz., *vajra*, etc., are extracted.

लोहपद्धतिः
'भद्रमेरण्डबीजांगं[२६] वज्रं च दमनाङ्कम् ।
तत्पीतं रुक्मलोहाख्यं सितं च बलवज्रकम्' ॥१७१॥
असितं[२७] कललोहाख्यं रक्तं लोहितवज्रकम् ।
मयूरवज्रकं चान्यदन्यत्तित्तिरवज्रकम् ॥१७२॥
'रोहिणीवज्रकं[२८] चान्यदन्यद्वा शुकवज्रकम्' ।
एवं दशविधं वज्रं गुणवानुत्तरोत्तरम् ॥१७३॥

Varieties of Iron
According to Loha-Paddhati

Vajra type of iron is of ten types as follows :

(1) *Bhadra* which is like the castor-seeds;
(2) *Damanāṅgaka*;
(3) *Rukmaloha* which is yellow in colour;
(4) *Bala-vajraka* which is white in colour;
(5) *Kāla-loha* which is black in colour;
(6) *Lohita-vajraka* which is red in colour;
(7) *Mayūra-vajraka*;
(8) *Tittira-vajraka*;
(9) *Rohiṇī-vajraka*; and
(10) *Śuka-vajraka.*

The suceeding ones are better in effect than the preceding ones.

क्षयकुष्टज्वरहरं वातरक्तामवातनुत् ।
रक्तपितं प्रमेहं च ग्रहण्यर्शोगदं जयेत् ।
जरापलितखालित्यशमनं स्रंसनं मतम् ।।१७४।।

Properties of Iron

Bhasma of iron cures consumption, *kuṣṭha* (obstinate skin diseases including leprosy), fever, *vāta rakta* (gout), *āmavāta* (rheumatism), *rakta pitta* (an ailment characterised by bleeding from different parts of the body), *prameha* (obstinate urinary disorders including diabetes), *grahaṇī* (sprue syndrome) and piles. It prevents ageing process and cures wrinkling of the skin and graying of hair. It is laxative.

यत्र घृष्टतरो नूनं वर्तुलाङ्गानि सर्वतः ।
रेखा स्यात् हेमनिक्षात् पाड्यं तदभिधीयते ।।१७५।।
यत् सितासितभेदेन द्विधा च स महीण्डकम्[१२९] ।
कांतिजं तण्डुलांगं स्यादन्यलोहनिकृन्तनम्[१३०] ।।१७६।।
निरंगं निखनेन्नित्यं[१३१] निर्मलं सजलच्छविः[१३२] ।
कृष्णायसमिति ज्ञेयं सर्वलोहोत्तमोत्तमम् ।।१७७।।
शुद्धतारप्रभं कान्तं तारेणावर्तितं मिलेत् ।
अहोरात्रस्थितो निंबकल्कस्तु मधुरायते ।।१७८।।

कृष्णाः स्युः श्वेतचरणाः आघृष्टो हिंगुगन्धवान् ।
क्वाथ्यमानं पयो नैव अधश्च परिसर्पति ।।१७९।।

Characteristics of Different Types of Iron

Pāḍya type of iron if rubbed over a touch-stone (whetstone), leaves marks (lines) which are round all through.

Mahiṇḍaka type of iron is of two types, viz., white and black.

Kāntija type of iron is like a rice in shape and it cuts other types of iron.

Kṛṣṇāyasa, which is the best, does not break into pieces while used in the form of a shovel for digging. It remains clean and always appear as if washed with water.

Kānta type of iron which looks like pure silver is generally mixed with the latter. If the paste of *nimba* is kept in it for one day and night then the taste of the paste is changed to sweet. If rubbed, it leaves black lines with white spots and produces smell like asafoetida. [There appears to be some error in this line. Generally, asafoetida gets rid of its acid smell when kept in *kānta*-vessel and this is one of its tests]. If milk is boiled in a vessel of *kānta* type of iron, then the milk does not overflow the vessel when excessive heat is applied.

न सूतेन विना कान्तं न कान्तेन विना रसः ।
कान्तसूतसमायुक्तः प्रयोगो देहधारकः ।।१८०।।

Supplementary Effects of Mercury and Iron

Mercury does not become effective without its mixture with *kānta*-iron and the latter does not produce its effects without being added with mercury. The combination of mercury and *kānta*-iron helps in the sustenance of the body.

लोहं साराह्वयं हन्याद्ग्रहणीं अतिसारकम् ।
औण्ड्रः सर्वांगिनं वातं शूलं च परिणामजम् ।।१८१।।
छर्द्यतीसारपित्तोत्थं ग्रहणीं च विनाशयेत् ।
वन्ध्यायाः गर्भदं बल्यं क्षयहृद्धातुवर्धनम् ।।१८२।।
रसायनेषु सर्वेषु शस्यते च कलिंगजकम् ।।१८३।।
शोषशोथज्वरहरं[१३] तडावट्टं रसायनम् ।

ज्वरं छर्दिं रक्तपित्तं क्षयं भद्राह्वयं जयेत् ।।१८४।।
कान्तलोहगुणाः प्रोक्ताः[१३४] ।।१८५।।

Properties of Different Types of Iron

Sāra type of iron cures *grahaṇī* (sprue syndrome) and diarrhoea.

Auṇḍra type of iron cures *vāyu* diseases affecting the whole body, *pariṇāma śūla* (a type of colic pain), vomiting, *paittika* type of diarrhoea and *grahaṇī* (sprue syndrome).

Kaliṅgaja-iron helps in the conception of sterile women. It promotes strength. It cures consumption and nourishes tissue elements. It is useful in the recipes of rejuvenation therapy.

Taḍāvaṭṭa type of iron cures consumption, oedema and fever. It rejuvenates the body.

Bhadra type of iron cures fever, vomiting, *rakta pitta* (an ailment characterised by bleeding from different parts of the body) and consumption .

Thus, the properties of different types of *kānta*-iron are described.

शोषार्शःश्वासकासांश्च प्रमेहान्विषमज्वरान् ।
गुल्मांश्च पाण्डुरोगांश्च पांडिलोहं नियच्छति ।।१८६।।
कान्तिजं जयति प्लीहमम्लपित्तं शिरोरुजम् ।
गुल्मोदराश्मरीशूलमामवातं भगन्दरम् ।
श्लीपद-कामलाशोफकुष्ठक्षयहरं परम् ।।१८७।।
शक्तिं पुष्टिं बलं स्थैर्यं दत्ते जनयते सुतान् ।
सर्वान्विजयते रोगान्कान्तलोहं न संशयः ।।१८८।।

Another Description of Iron-Properties

Pāṇḍi type of iron cures consumption, piles, asthma, bronchitis, *prameha* (obstinate urinary disorders including diabetes), *viṣama-jvara* (irregular fever), *gulma* (phantom tumour) and anemia.

Kāntija-iron cures splenic disorders, *amla pitta* (hyper acidity), headache, *gulma* (phantom tumour), *udara* (obstinate abdominal diseases iucluding ascites), renal calculi, colic pain, *āma vāta* (rheumatism), anal fistula, filariasis, jaundice, oedema, *kuṣṭha* (obstinate skin diseases including leprosy) and consumption.

Kānta type of iron promotes energy, nourishment, strength and sturdity. It helps a person to procreate progeny. It undoubtedly cures all diseases.

यल्लोहं यद्गुणं दृष्टं तत्किट्टमपि तद्गुणम् ।।१८९।।

Rust of Different Types of Iron

Rust (*kiṭṭa*) of different types of iron produces same therapeutic effects as described in respect of the concerned types of iron.

किट्टाद्दशगुणं मुण्डं मुण्डात्सारं चतुर्गुणम् ।
सारादौंड्रं द्विगुणितं कलिंगं च ततोऽष्टधा ।।१९०।।
तस्माद्भद्रं शतगुणं भद्राद्वज्रं सहस्रधा ।
वज्रात्षष्टिगुणं पाण्ड्यं कान्तिजं शतधा ततः ।
सर्वलोहोत्तमं यस्मात्तस्मात्कोटिगुणं[३५] मतम् ।।१९१।।

Relative Merits of Different Types of Iron

Muṇḍa type of iron is ten times more effective than the iron-rust. *Sāra* type of iron is four times more effective than the *muṇḍa* type of iron. *Auṇḍra* type of iron is twice more effective than the *sāra* type of iron. *Kāliṅga* type of iron is eight times more effective than the *auṇḍra* type of iron. *Bhadra* type of iron is one hundred times more effective than the *kaliṅga* type of iron. *Vajra* type of iron is one thousand times more effective than *bhadra* type of iron. *Pāṇḍya* type of iron is sixty times more effective than the *bhadra* type of iron. *Kāntija* type of iron is one hundred times more effective than the *pāṇḍya* type of iron. It is the best among all the types of iron and it has innumerable (lit. one crore) properties.

जालन्धरे[३६]

कान्तं लक्षगुणं प्रोक्तं शालग्रामसमुद्भवम्[३७] ।
स्फटिकोत्थं कोटिगुणं विद्युत्संभूतं दुर्लभम् ।।१९२।।
रसे[३८] रसायने[३९] योज्यं रोगघ्नं च रसायनम् ।
लिंगाकारांगसहितं जयदं समरे परम् ।
पुत्रदं राजरोगघ्नं महारोगौघनाशनम् ।।१९३।।

Properties of Different Types of Iron According to Jālandhara

Kānta-iron extracted from *śālagrāma* has one lakh properties. The one obtained from crystal stone (*sphaṭika*) has one crore properties. The iron obtained from meteor (lit. lightening) is rarely found. These types of iron should be used in *rasa* (recipes containing mercury) and *rasāyana* (rejuvenating recipes). They cure diseases and rejuvenate the body.

The iron of the shape of a *liṅga* (phallus) endows a person with victory in the war. It helps a person to procreate a male child. It cures tuberculosis and other serious diseases.

रससिन्धुः

यान्रोगान्घ्नन्ति लोहानि शुद्धानि सुमृतानि च ।
तानेव कुर्वतेऽशुद्धान्यमृतानि गुरूणि च ।।१९४।।

Adverse Effects of Impure Iron According to Rasasindhu

Purified and calcinated iron cures certain diseases as described before. These very diseases are caused if iron is used without purification and calcination. In addition, such impure iron is heavy for digestion.

रत्नाकरात्

अशुद्धं तु मृतं लोहं आयुर्हारि रुजाकरम् ।
कुष्टांगमर्दहृत्पीडां दद्यात्तस्मात्सुशोधयेत् ।।१९५।।

Adverse Effects of Impure Iron According to Ratnākara

If iron is calcinated without purification and taken, then it may cause even death. It also causes different types of pain, *kuṣṭha* (obstinate skin diseases including leprosy), malaise and cardiac pain. Therefore, iron should be properly purified before calcination and used.

रसदर्पणात्

गुरुता दृढतोत्क्लेदी कश्मली दाहकारकः ।
अश्मदोषः सुदुर्गन्धो सप्तदोषायसस्य च ।।१९६।।

Defects in Iron
According to Rasadarpaṇa

Heaviness, excessive hardness (unmalleability), *utkledī* (chipping), dirtiness, causing burning sensation when touched, association with the defects of stone and extremely foul smell — these seven are the defects (*doṣa-s*) of iron.

तैले तक्रे गवां मूत्रे कांजिके च कुलत्थके[४०] ।
सप्तधा तापनिर्वापात्सर्वलोहं विशोधयेत् ।।१९७।।

General Method of Purification

Heating and immersing for seven times in each of oil, butter-milk, cow's urine, vinegar and the decoction of *kulattha* purify all types of metal.

माण्डवः
तप्तानि सर्वलोहानि कदलीमूलवारिणि ।
सप्तधा तु निषिक्तानि शुद्धिमायान्ति तत्क्षणात् ।।१९८।।

Second Method of Purification
According to Māṇḍava

All types of metal, when heated and immersed in the juice of the rhizome of *kadalī* for seven times, become purified instantaneously.

रससिन्धुः
शुद्धिमायाति तीक्ष्णं च मुण्डं निर्गुण्डीसेचनात् ।
इतराणि च लोहानि सर्वाण्युलूकविष्ठया[४१] ।।१९९।।
महालोहं तु कक्रिया रेतसा वेतसान्वितम् ।
रेतसा मर्दितं सूर्ये धमितं शुद्धिमृच्छति[४२] ।।२००।।
कान्तं शशकरक्तेन लेपितं सप्तधा पुटात् ।
तडावट्टं लिंगलोहं हिंगुतोयेन सेचितात् ।
सप्तधा शुद्धिमायाति तन्न[४३] कार्या विचारणा ।।२०१।।

Third Method of Purification
According to Rasasindhu

Tīkṣṇa and *muṇḍa* types of iron when heated and sprinkled with the juice of *nirguṇḍī*, get purified. All other types of iron get purified by the stool of *ulūka*.

Mahāloha should be added with *vetasa* and the *retas* (bartholin secretion) of *kākinī* type of woman. After trituration, it should be blown over fire by exposing to the sun by which it gets purified.

Kānta type of iron should be smeared with the blood of rabbit and cooked in *puṭa* for seven times for its purification.

Taḍāvaṭṭa and *liṅga* types of iron should be heated and sprinkled with the solution of *hiṅgu* for seven times as a result of which they get purified.

लोहपद्धतितः

अथाग्नितापतप्तानि[१४४] लोहपत्राणि निक्षिपेत् ।
सप्तधा च वराक्वाथे गिरिदोषप्रशान्तये ।।२०२।।
वरा चतुर्गुणा लोहात्ततो वारि चतुर्गुणम् ।
दत्त्वा निःक्वाथयेत्तावद्यावत्पादः स्थितो भवेत् ।।२०३।।

Fourth Method of Iron-Purification
According to Lohapaddhati

Thin sheets of iron should be heated and immersed in the decoction of *triphalā* for seven times which remove *giri doṣa* (fault accrued because of contacts in the mountain).

Triphalā should be taken four times in quantity of iron. To this, water four times in quantity of *triphalā* should be added and boiled till one fourth of water remains. This decoction should be used for the purification of iron.

रसार्णवात्

न विस्फुलिंगाः न च बुद्बुदाः यदा यदा न चैषां पटलं न शब्दः ।
मूषागतं रत्नसमं[१४५] स्थिरं च तदा विशुद्धं प्रवदन्ति लोहम् ।।२०४।।

Signs of Iron-Purification
According to Rasārṇava

When iron, kept inside the crucible and blown, does not emit dazzling particles or bubbles, when layers (scales) are not produced, when no sound is produced and when it remains stable like a gem, then it is to be determined as purified.

अथास्यैवंविशुद्धस्य मारणे विधिरुच्यते ।
तत्र त्रिगुणितं लोहात्समादाय फलत्रिकम् ।
चतुर्गुणे जले पक्त्वा ग्राह्यं पादावशेषितम् ।।२०५।।

Calcination of Iron

After purification, iron should be taken for calcination with the help of the decoction of *triphalā*. For this purpose, *triphalā*, three times in quantity of iron should be taken and boiled by adding four times of water till one fourth remains.

रसदर्पणात्
रत्नमाला हंसपदी गोजिह्वा त्रिफला तथा ।
गर्त्तालाबू कुमारी च तथा[46] गर्तकलंबुका ।।२०६।।
तिन्दुकस्य फलं चामं तुम्बुरुर्लोहमारकः ।
हिंगुलं च पलान्पञ्च नारीस्तन्येन पेषयेत् ।।२०७।।
तेन लोहस्य पत्राणि लेपयेत्पलपञ्चकम् ।
रुद्ध्वा गजपुटैः पच्यात्कषायैस्त्रैफलैः पुनः ।।२०८।।
तुम्बीजैराररनालैर्वा[47] विंशत्यंशेन हिंगुलम् ।
पिष्ट्वा रुध्वा पचेल्लौहं तथैवं पाचयेत्पुनः ।।२०९।।
चत्वारिंशत्पुटैरेवं कान्तं तीक्ष्णं च मुण्डकम् ।
म्रियते नात्र संदेहो दत्वा दत्वा च हिंगुलम् ।।२१०।।

Method of Iron Calcination According to Rasadarpaṇa

Five *pala-s* of each of *ratnamālā*, *haṁsapadī*, *gojihvā*, *triphalā*, *garttālābū*, *kumārī*, *garta-kalambukā*, unripe fruit of *tinduka*, *tumburu*, *lohamāraka* and *hiṅgula* should be made to a paste by triturating with woman's milk. The thin sheets of iron (five *pala-s*) should be smeared with this paste and cooked in *gaja puṭa*. Then, by adding twenty times of *hiṅgula* it should be triturated with the decoction of *triphalā* or decoction of *tumbī* or *āranāla* (sour vinegar), made to a paste, kept inside *śarāva sampuṭa*, sealed and cooked in *gaja puṭa*. Cooking like this for forty times, each time by adding *hiṅgula*, will cause calcination of *kānta*, *tīkṣṇa* and *muṇḍa* types of iron.

अथ शैवालभक्षः[१४८]

लोहानि च शृगालानि दन्तिनिर्यूहदर्शनात् ।
म्रियन्तेऽत्र विकल्पं च न मीमांस्यः कदाचन ।।२११।।

Second Method of Iron-Calcination According to Śaivālabhakṣa

All metals get calcinated by the association with the decoction of *dantī* and there need not be any doubt about it. This is on the analogy of the death of the jackal by just seeing the *dantī* (elephant).

तद्यथा

सुलोहं रेतितं कृत्वा स्थापयेन्मृन्मये दृढे ।
नवे भिषक्तमः पश्चाद् दन्तीद्रावैः प्रपूरयेत् ।।२१२।।
एवं पुनः पुनस्तावद्यावत्तत्तरते स्वयम् ।
म्रियते तीव्रघर्मेण चूर्णीकृत्य प्रयोजयेत् ।।२१३।।

Good quality of iron should be filed and kept in a new and strong earthen jar which should be filled with the decoction of *dantī* and exposed to strong sun. This decoction should be added repeatedly till the iron-files float over the decoction. Thereafter, these iron-files should be made to a powder by grinding and used.

रसरत्नाकरात्

'तिन्दुफलस्य'[४९] वा मज्जाखंडं लिप्त्वातपे खरे।
धारयेत्कांस्यपात्रे तद्दिनैकेन स्फुटत्यलम् ।
एवं पुनः पुनः कुर्याद्दिनांते तत्प्रपेषयेत् ।।२१४।।

Third Method of Iron-Calcination According to Rasaratnākara

Thin sheets of iron should be smeared with the paste of the fruit-pulp of *tinduka* and kept in a bronze vessel for one day by which it becomes frazile. At the end of the day, it should be pounded. This process should be repeated for several times.

त्रिफलाक्वाथसंयुक्त दिनैकेन मृतिं व्रजेत्' ।।२१५।।

With the decoction of *triphalā*, iron gets calcinated in one day.

दन्तीपत्रद्रवात्तत्स्थं[150] लोहचूर्णं विलेपयेत् ।
दिनैकं धारयेद्धर्मे द्रवं देयं पुनः पुनः ।।२१६।।
रुद्धा रात्रौ पुटेत्पश्चात्तैर्द्रवैश्चैव भावयेत् ।
एवमष्टदिनं कुर्यात्त्रिविधं म्रियते ह्ययः[151] ।।२१७।।

Fourth Method of Iron-Calcination

Filed powder should be smeared with the paste of *dantī*-leaf, dried, soaked in the juice or decoction of *dantī* and exposed to hot sun. As the juice gets dried up, more and more of this juice should be added for one day. At night, this powder should be kept inside *śarāva-sampuṭa*, sealed and cooked in *gaja puṭa*. Then the powder should be soaked in the juice or decoction of *dantī* and cooked again in *gaja puṭa*. Doing like this for eight days three types of iron get reduced into calcined form.

रत्नाकरात्
माक्षिकं च शिलां ह्यम्लैर्हरिद्रा-मरिचानि च।
पिष्ट्वा लेप्यं[152] लोहपत्रं तप्तं तप्तं निषेचयेत् ।।२१८।।
सप्तधा त्रैफले क्वाथे जलेन क्षालयेत्पुनः ।
कुट्टयेल्लोहदंडेन पेषयेत्त्रैफलाह्वये[153] ।।२१९।।
षोडशांशेन लोहस्य दातव्यं माक्षिकं शिला ।
अम्लेन लोडितं रुध्वा[154] गजाख्यैकंपुटे पचेत् ।
निरुत्थं जायते भस्म कान्तं तीक्ष्णं च मुण्डकम् ।।२२०।।

Fifth Method of Preparing Iron-Bhasma According to Ratnākara

Mākṣika, *manaḥ-śilā*, *haridrā* and *marica* should be made to a paste by triturating with any sour juice. Thin sheets of iron should be smeared with this paste, heated and immersed in *triphalā*-decoction for seven times. Then these iron-sheets should be washed, pounded with an iron pestle and triturated by adding sixteen times of *triphalā* decoction. To this, the paste of *mākṣika* and *manaḥ śilā* triturated with sour juice, should be added and keeping sealed in *śarāva-sampuṭa*, it should be cooked in *gaja-puṭa*. Thus, *kānta*, *tīkṣṇa* and *muṇḍa* types of iron are reduced to *niruttha* (unretrievable) *bhasma* form.

अन्यच्च

आलोड्य त्रिफलाक्वाथे मासं धान्योदरे क्षिपेत् ।
बाले वृद्धे प्रयोज्यं च सत्यं वारितरं भवेत् ।।२२१।।

Sixth Method of Preparing Iron-Bhasma

Iron boiled with *triphalā*-decoction should be kept inside a heap of grains for a month and then made to a powder. This calcined form of iron becomes *vāritara* (floating over water) and can be used for children as well as old people.

शैवागमात्

वज्राख्यं रेतितं लोहं[155] पलमात्रं रसं तथा ।
पलमात्रं शोधितं च विमर्द्यैकत्र मिश्रयेत् ।।२२२।।
मिहंदी च कुमारी च देवकंडरिका-बला ।
पुनर्नवा-हंसपादी-रत्नमालारसेन च ।।२२३।।
प्रत्येकं भावनास्तिस्रः प्रदेया मर्दयेत् दृढम् ।
संस्थाप्य चान्धमूषायां दद्यात्करिपुटं ततः ।
स्वांगशीतं प्रगृह्याथ दापयेदमृतोपमम् ।।२२४।।
क्षयं प्रमेहं क्ष्चयथुं शोषं जीर्णज्वरं तथा ।
प्रतिश्यायं महाघोरं हन्यादत्र किमद्भुतम्[156] ।।२२५।।

Seventh Method of Preparing Iron-Bhasma According to Śaivāgama

One *pala* of the purified and filed powder of *vajra lauha* should be added with one *pala* of purified mercury and triturated. This should be impregnated for three times in each of the juice of *mehandī*, *kumārī*, *devakaṇḍarikā*, *balā*, *punarnavā*, *haṃsapādī* and *ratnamālā*, and triturated strongly. The paste should then be kept in *andha-mūṣā* and cooked in *gaja puṭa*. After it becomes cold of its own, the powder should be used in medicine and it is like ambrosia.

It cures serious types of consumption, *prameha* (obstinate urinary diseases including diabetes), sneezing, phthisis, chronic fever and chronic cold.

लोहपद्धतितः[१५७]

अथ मारणकार्यार्थे कथ्यन्ते भेषजानि च ।
तत्र गंडनिका मुख्या क्वचित्सोक्ता[१५८] महौषधिः ।।२२६ ।।
क्वचित्सा शालचिंचेति हरिपिर्णीति सा क्वचित् ।
दिव्यौषधी तु सा क्वापि[१५९] क्वचिद्गर्तकलम्बुका ।।२२७ ।।

Identification of Gaṇḍanikā According to Lohapaddhati

Now, drugs for the calcination of iron will be explained. The chief amongst them is *gaṇḍanikā*. In different places it is known variously as *mahauṣadhi*, *śālaciñcā*, *hariparṇī*, *divyauṣadhi* and *garta-kalambukā*.

अन्यच्च

अमरी[१६०] तत्र चांगेरी कुमारछिन्नसंज्ञके[१६१] ।
विकंकतं तृतीयं च चतुर्थं रक्तमारिषम् ।।२२८ ।।
पंचमं त्वचकं प्रोक्तं षष्ठमुक्तं मनःशिला ।
हिङ्गुलं[१६२] सप्तमं प्रोक्तमष्टमं स्वर्णमाक्षिकम् ।।२२९ ।।
एतानि क्रमशो हन्युः पित्तं कफमसृग्गदम्[१६३] ।
वातं च पाण्डुतां कण्डूं[१६४] अग्निमांद्यं विवर्णताम् ।।२३० ।।
तत्राद्यैः पञ्चभिर्द्रव्यैः सर्वैरेकैकशो द्विशः ।
त्रिंशच्चतुर्भिः सर्वैर्वा बहुसैन्धवसंयुतैः ।।२३१ ।।
अम्लकाञ्जिकसंपिष्टैर्विलिंपेत्पत्रमायसम् ।
चतुःषष्ट्येष्टकाकोष्ठे भूमिन्यस्ता स्थिरीकृताः ।।२३२ ।।
मध्ये गर्तवती कार्या प्रपंचात्पञ्चमिष्टिका ।
इष्टिका कोष्ठकार्द्धेऽस्मिन्[१६५] खदिरांगारपूरिते ।।२३३ ।।
विन्यस्य ध्मापयेद्विज्ञो चिरं भस्त्राद्वयानिलैः ।
ततस्तद् द्रवतां याति स्थितं मध्येष्टकावटे ।।२३४ ।।
लोहांकुशेन त्रिफलाक्वाथे तप्तं विनिक्षिपेत् ।
ततश्च त्रिफलाक्वाथादुद्धृत्य श्लक्ष्णतां नयेत् ।

उलूखलेन श्लक्ष्णेन लोहदंडेन बुद्धिमान् ।।२३५।।

Group of Drugs Useful for Iron-Calcination
Eighth Method of Calcination

The eight drugs useful for the calcination of iron are (1) *amarī*, (2) *cāṅgerī* which is also called *kugara-chinna*, (3) *vikaṅkata*, (4) *rakta-māṅsa*, (5) *tvacaka*, (6) *manaḥ-śilā*, (7) *hiṅgula*, and (8) *svarṇa-mākṣika*. These drugs cure diseases caused by *pitta*, *kapha*, *rakta* and *vāyu*. They also cure anemia, itching, suppression of the power of digestion and discoloration of the skin. One, two, three, four or all of these drugs should be triturated with large quantity of *saindhava* (rock-salt) by adding sour *kānjī* (vinegar) and made to a paste. The thin sheets of iron should be smeared with this paste.

A *koṣṭha* (oven) of sixty four bricks should be prepard by digging the earth and stabilized. Half of this oven should be filled with the charcoal of *khadira*. Five more bricks with holes in their centres should be placed over these charcoal filled in oven in the middle. These holes are to be filled with the iron paste mentioned above. The remaining space over these bricks should be filled with charcoals of *khadira* and blown with the help of two blowers. Thus, the iron in paste form kept in the bricks gets melted. This melted iron should be removed with the help of an iron hook and immersed in the decoction of *triphalā*. Taking out of this decoction, it should be reduced to a fine powder by pounding with a iron-pestle in a smooth mortar.

अन्यच्च
कुनटीहिंगुलमाक्षिकैः[१६७] सर्वै एकैकशो द्विशः ।
जंबीरद्रवसंपिष्टैः[१६८] सैन्धवेन समायुतैः ।
आलिप्तमायसं पत्रं 'त्रिफला[१६९] पिंडमध्यगम् ।।२३६।।
विद्रुतं पूर्ववद्धीमान्' त्रिफलांभसि निक्षिपेत् ।
एवं हि म्रियते लोहं सर्वमेव न संशयः ।।२३७।।

Ninth Method of Iron-Calcination

Kunaṭī, hiṅgula and *mākṣika*—all these drugs or one or two of them should be made to a paste by triturating with the juice of *jambīra* added with rock-salt. Thin sheets of iron should be smeared with this paste and wrapped with the paste of *triphalā*. As mentioned before, this should be melted and then immersed in *triphalā* decoction. In this method, all types of iron are calcined.

अथान्यप्रकारः

सुलोहफलमथवा धमेद्भस्त्राद्वयेन वै ।
कठोरांघ्रिजकल्कं[70] हि दत्वा दत्वा हठाग्निना ।
गलित्वा म्रियते सर्वं सत्यं यामद्वयेन वै ।।२३८।।

Tenth Method of Iron-Calcination

Sheets of iron should be placed over strong fire and blown with the help of two blowers by adding the paste of the root of *kaṭhorā* frequently. Thus, the iron melts and gets calcinated in two *yāma-s.*

अथ अयस्कृतिः

अथ पानीयक्ट्टिादिस्तदधस्त्रिफलाजलात् ।
उद्धृत्य लोहदंडेन लोहं यद्देवि चूर्णयेत् ।।२३९।।
ततोऽसिन्सान्द्रतां नीते क्षालिते सूक्ष्मवाससि ।
स्थालीपाकं यथा कुर्यात्तथापि विधिरुच्यते ।।२४०।।
ताप्यमस्यमिदापिष्टं शृतं कौलत्थवारिणा ।
विचूर्ण्य षोडशांशेन लोहपट्टे विचूर्णयेत् ।।२४१।।
ततोऽस्मिन्माक्षिकेन्मानं हिंगुयुक् त्रिफलाजले ।
लोहपात्रे स्थितं शोष्यमल्पमल्पं सुखाग्निना ।
लोहमेवं निरुत्थं स्यादमृतादधिकं गुणैः ।।२४२।।

Ayaskṛti

[The text appears to be erroneous; hence left untranslated].

अन्यच्च

शुद्धं सूतं द्विधा गंधं खल्वे कृत्वा तु कज्जलीम् ।
द्वयोः समं चूर्णलोहं मर्दयेत्कन्यकाद्रवैः ।।२४३।।
यामद्वयात्समुधृत्य तद्गोलं ताम्रपत्रके ।
आच्छाद्यैरण्डपत्रैश्च यामार्द्धेत्युष्णता भवेत् ।।२४४।।
धान्यराशौ न्यसेत्पश्चात्त्रिदिनान्ते समुद्धरेत् ।

सम्पेष्य गालयेद्वस्त्रे सत्यं वारितरं भवेत् ।
कान्तं मुण्डं तथा तीक्ष्णं निरुत्थं जायते ध्रुवम् ।।२४५।।

Second Method of Ayaskṛti

One part of purified mercury and two parts of purified sulphur should be triturated in a mortar and made to a *kajjalī* (fine black powder like collyrium). To this, three parts of iron powder should be added and triturated by adding the juice of *kumārī* for two *yāma-s*. Thereafter, this paste in a bolus form should be wrapped with thin sheets of copper which should again be wrapped with the leaves of *eraṇḍa* and heated for half-*yāma*. This should then be kept inside a heap of grains for three days. Thereafter, the bolus should be removed and made to a powder by grinding and filtering through a cloth. This powder when sprinkled, floats over the water *(vāritara)*. Thus, *kānta*, *muṇḍa* and *tīkṣṇa* types of iron are reduced to unretrievable *(niruttha)* type of *bhasma*.

कक्षापुटिमतात्
लोहचूर्णं कुकुरुंदुरसेन घर्मे भावनाद्गुरुभाग एकम् [?] कांजिकेन
प्रपिष्य[१७१] भावनासप्तभिःसिन्दूरवर्णं भवति ।।२४६।।

Third Method of Ayaskṛti
According to Kakṣāpuṭi

Powder of iron should be added with the juice of *kukurundu* and impregnated by exposing to the sun. Then this powder should be triturated by adding *kāñjī* (sour vinegar) and impregnated with this *kāñjī* for seven times by which the powder of iron becomes red in colour like vermilion.

अथ राजहंसमतात्
तीक्ष्णादिचूर्णं कलितार्धगन्धं सूतं कुमारीपयसा निघृष्टम् ।
एकीकृतं कांस्यं पुटान्तरस्थं सूर्यातपे तमुपैति मृत्युम् ।।२४७।।

Fourth Method of Ayaskṛti
According to Rājahaṃsa

One part of the powder of *tīkṣṇa* and other types of iron should be added with half part of sulphur and half part of mercury, and triturated by adding the juice of *kumārī*. Taken together, these ingredients should be kept in a bronze vessel and exposed to hot sun by which iron is reduced to *bhasma* form.

अथ रसचिन्तामणिः
शालीचिंचीति शास्त्रेषु लोकेषु छिलहिंडिका ।
गरुडीनी समाख्याता[१७२] पातालस्य महौषधी ।।२४८।।
गर्तालाबुरिति क्वापि प्रसिद्धा भूमिमण्डले ।
तज्जलं[१७३] केवलं नीत्वा हिंगुलेन समं भवेत् ।।२४९।।
तेन लोहस्य जातस्य कान्तस्य च विशेषतः ।
चूर्णं संमिश्रितं कृत्वा शृणु कर्तव्यतामतः[१७४] ।।२५०।।
जायते[१७५] रोटिकाकारं कृत्वा कृत्वा शरावके।
एतैर्बहुपुटैर्भूयाद्रक्तवर्णं[१७६] सुशोभनम्[१७७] ।।२५१।।
माषत्रयमिदं चूर्णं प्रोच्यते लोहमुत्तमम् ।
जरां संजातरूपां तां नाशयेदचिरेण हि ।
श्वासकासादि[१७८]कान्रोगान्प्रमेहान्नाशयेत्परम् ।।२५२।।
सेव्यते शीतकाले[१७९] च वसंते सततं क्वचित् ।
वर्षासु च भवेत्सेव्यं यथा सात्म्यमथापि वा ।।२५३।।
संभावितसमुत्थानं[१८०] नैवाद्याद्विक्रियाभयात् [?]।
सर्वमेतन्मृतं लोहं ध्मातव्यं मित्रपञ्चकैः ।
यद्वैतत्स्यान्निरुत्थानं[१८१] सेव्यं वारितरं हि तत् ।।२५४।।

Preparation of Iron-Bhasma According to Rasacintāmaṇi

The plant known as *śālīciñcī* is called *chilahiṇḍikā*, *garuḍinī* and *pātālasya-mahauṣadhi* in folk-tradition. Sometime, it is also called *gartālābu*.

The juice of this plant should be triturated by adding equal quantity of *hiṅgula*. This paste should be added with *kānta* type of iron in powder form. It should be made to the shape of *roṭikā* (thin and round shape), kept in *śarāva samputa* and cooked with several *puṭa-s*. Thus, the iron is reduced to beautiful and red *bhasma* form which is administered in the dose of three *māṣa-s*.

It instantaneously cures the ageing process which is already manifested. It is an excellent recipe for curing serious type of asthma, bronchitis and *prameha* (obstinate urinary disorders including diabetes). It should be constantly used in winter and spring seasons. In the rainy season, it should be used only occasionally. Alternatively, this should be used keeping in view the *sātmya* (wholesomeness or appropriateness) of the patient.

To avoid the possibility of any adverse effect because of contamination at the source, this *bhasma* of iron should be added with *mitra-pañcaka* and blown over fire. The *bhasma* should thus be ensured to be *niruttha* (irretrievable) and *vāritara* (which, when sprinkled over the surface of water, floats). After these tests, iron-*bhasma* should be administered to a patient.

अन्यच्च

मध्वाज्यं मृतलोहं च सकूप्यमन्धमूषके[८२] ।
रुद्धाध्माते तु संग्राह्यं[१८३] रूप्ये चेत्पूर्वमानकम् ।
तदा लोहं मृतं विद्यादन्यथा[१८४] साधयेत्पुनः ।।२५५।।

Method of Testing

Honey, ghee and iron-*bhasma,* taken together should be kept in a crucible which latter should be kept in an *andha-mūṣā,* sealed and blown by keeping over fire. If it does not revert to its original metallic form, then the iron should be treated as properly calcined. If it does return to its original metallic form, then it should be processed again.

रसरत्नाकरात्

गन्धकंचेत्थितं तुल्यं लोहं खल्वे विमर्दयेत् ।
दिनैकं कन्यकाद्रावैः रुद्धा गजपुटे पचेत् ।
इत्येवं सर्वलोहानां कर्तव्योत्थिनिरुत्थितः[१८५] ।।२५६।।

Preparation of Niruttha Bhasma According to Rasaratnākara

Sulphur and *lauha bhasma* taken in equal quantities should be kept in a mortar and triturated for one day by adding the juice of *kumārī*. Then it should be cooked in *gaja puṭa* as a result of which *niruttha* (irretrievable) *bhasma* of iron is prepared.

नागार्जुनात्

ततो सकृत्त्रैफलेन क्वाथेन पुटयेदयः ।
पुनर्नवारसेनाथ प्रदद्याद्भूयसा[१८६] पुटात् ॥२५७॥
तद्दद्याद्बद्धकोष्ठस्य लोहं स्यादनुलोमनम् ।
दशमूलीक्वाथपुटं त्रिदोषे तु प्रदापयेत् ॥२५८॥
तालमूलीरसपुटाद्दद्यादर्शोनिवृत्तये ।
उक्तैः पुटौषधैरन्यैर्मन्यन्ते भावनाक्रमात् ॥२५९॥

Different Puṭa-s for Different Diseases According to Nāgārjuna

Iron should be triturated by adding *triphalā* decoction and cooked in *puṭa* for once. Then after triturating with the juice or decoction of *punarnavā*, several *puṭa-s* should be given. The iron-*bhasma*, thus prepared, is useful for a person suffering from constipation. It helps in the downward movement of *vāyu*.

For the treatment of diseases caused by the simultaneous aggravation of all the three *doṣa-s*, iron should be impregnated with the decoction of *daśamūla* and then given *puṭa* for calcination.

For the treatment of piles, iron should be impregnated with the juice of *tālamūlī* and given *puṭa* for calcination.

Similarly, iron should be impregnated with appropriate medicines and given *puṭa* for the treatment of other diseases.

अन्ये तु द्वयमिच्छन्ति प्राक्पुटाद् भावनास्ततः ॥२६०॥

According to some other physicians, iron should be given two *bhāvanā-s* (impregnation with juice, etc.) prior to *puṭa pāka*.

घृततुल्यमृतं लोहं कृत्वा पात्रगतं पचेत् ।
फलत्रिकक्कषायेन शनैर्मृद्वग्निना भिषक् ।
जीर्णे घृते समादाय योगवाहे प्रयोजयेत् ॥२६१॥

Further Processing of Iron-Bhasma

Iron-bhasma with equal quantity of ghee and appropriate quantity of the decoction of *triphalā* should be boiled over mild fire till the ghee gets evaporated (digested). Thereafter, this *bhasma* should be collected and used for the purpose of *yogavāha* (which enhances the properties of other drugs added to it).

रसालंकारात्

तीक्ष्णमारणयोगेन कान्तमारणमिष्यते ।
शुद्धिश्च तादृशी ज्ञेया स्वसत्वस्य तथैव च[१८८] ।।२६२।।
लोहशोधनयोगश्च द्रुतियोगस्तथैव[१८९] च ।
अनुभूत्वा शास्त्रदृष्ट्या चोपदेशान्निरूपिता ।।२६३।।
इमे साधारणाः प्रोक्ता यथा शंभुनिरूपिताः[१९०] ।
यस्मिन्यस्मिन्रसे लोहभस्म वक्ष्ये विशेषतः ।।२६४।।
तत्र तद्विनियुञ्जीत तस्य[१९१] साधारणं हि तत् ।
विशेषो यत्र नोक्तः स्यात्तत्र साधारणो मतः ।।२६५।।
विशेषान्मारणं वक्ष्ये सन्निपातादिभेषजे ।
योजनार्थं हि धातूनां रससिद्धिर्भवेद्यथा ।।२६६।।
जंबीरवारिणा पिष्ट्वा रसभस्ममथापि वा ।
पक्वनिंबूरसेनैव स्वर्णपत्राणि लेपयेत् ।।२६७।।
गन्धकत्रिगुणेनैव संपुटं रचयेद् दृढम्[१९२] ।
पुटित्वारण्यजैः छानैर्भस्मीभूतं समाहरेत् ।।२६८।।
पुटेनैकेन भस्म स्यान्नात्र कार्या विचारणा ।
एवं सर्वाणि लोहानि भस्मीकुर्याद्विचक्षणः ।।२६९।।
रसभस्म यदा न स्याद्धेममाक्षिकयोगतः ।
पूर्वोक्तैश्च रसैः पिष्ट्वा लोहपत्राणि लेपयेत्[१९४] ।।२७०।।
ततः परं च[१९५] पुटयेदष्टोत्तरशतं बुधः ।
वज्रीक्षीरेणाष्टवारं शतहृद्या रसेन च ।।२७१।।
वत्सनाभेन च शतमर्कक्षीरैस्तथा पुनः ।
नक्षत्रसंख्यां पुटयेच्छास्त्रवित्सम्प्रदायवित् ।।२७२।।
एवं सिद्धानि लोहानि रसेषु विनियोजयेत् ।

अन्यथा नैव सिद्धिः स्यात्सन्निपातादिभेषजे ।।२७३।।
कफाधिके गदे चापि कुष्ठे च विषमज्वरे ।
कासे क्षये सामवाते यकृत्प्लीहोदरादिषु ।।२७४।।

।।इति सन्निपातादी विशेषप्रकारधातुमारणम्।।

Special Method for Preparing Iron-Bhasma

According to Rasālaṅkāra

For the preparation of the *bhasma* of *kānta* type of iron, the process suggested for *tīkṣṇa* type of iron should be followed. Even for the purification, *sattva pātana* and melting *of kānta,* the same methods as suggested for *tīkṣṇa* should be followed. These methods are based on experience, scriptures and instructions of preceptors. These are the general methods as determined by the Lord Śiva. Now the special methods which are to be generally followed are being described. When special methods are not specifically indicataed, only general methods are to be followed.

For the treatment of diseases caused by *sannipāta* (simultaneous aggravation of all the three *doṣa-s*), the method of preparing *bhasma* of all the metals (including iron) is being described.

Mercury *bhasma* should be triturated by adding the juice of *jambīra* or ripe fruits of *nimbū*. With this paste, gold-leaves should be smeared. By adding three times of sulphur, it should be kept in *śarāva-sampuṭa* and well sealed. This should be cooked in *puṭa* with the cowdung cakes collected from the forest. The *bhasma,* thus prepared, should be collected. It gets reduced to *bhasma* form only by one *puṭa.* The same method should be used for preparing *bhasma* of all other metals.

If mercury *bhasma* is not available, then the *bhasma* of *svarṇa-mākṣika* should be used and made to a paste by triturating with the juice of *jambīra* or ripe fruits of *nimbū*. Thin sheets of iron should be smeared with this paste and given *puṭa* for one hundred eight times. In addition, eight *puṭa-s* should be given by triturating with the milky latex of *snuhī* and juice of *śatāvarī,* one hundred *puṭa-s* should be given by triturating with the decoction of *vatsanābha* and twenty six *puṭa-s* should be given with the milky latex of *arka* according to the scriptures and traditions. The *bhasma* of metals, thus prepared, should be used in recipes. Otherwise, the recipes do not produce the desired effects in the treatment of diseases caused by *sannipāta,* diseases caused by the aggravation of *kapha, kuṣṭha* (obstinate skin diseases including leprosy), *viṣama-jvara* (irregular fever), bronchitis, consumption, rheumatism and abdominal diseases caused by morbidities in the liver and spleen.

रसदर्पणात्

मुनिरसपिष्टं विडंगं मुनिरसलीढं चिरस्थितं घर्मे ।
द्रावयति लोहदोषान् वह्निर्नवनीतपिंडमिव ।।२७५।।
कृमिरिपु-तुंबुरुचूर्णं लीढं स्वरसेन वंगसेनस्य ।
विनिहन्त्यचिरान्नियतं लोहाजीर्णोद्भवं शूलम् ।।२७६।।
पुनर्नवाहतं कांस्यं त्रिफलालोहचूर्णकम् ।
गन्धकेन हतं ताम्रं भवेद् देहस्य रंजकम् ।।२७७।।

Removal of Impurities
According to Rasadarpaṇa

Iron and other metals should be smeared with the paste of *viḍaṅga* and juice of *agasti*. After impregnating with the juice of *agastya*, it should be exposed to the sun rays for a long time. This melts away the impurities of metals as fire melts a bolus of butter.

If the *bhasma* of the metal is not digested and there is colic pain, then patient should be given the linctus prepared of the powder of *viḍaṅga* and *tumburu* by triturating with the juice of *vaṅgasena*.

Bronze calcinated with *punarnavā*, iron calcinated with *triphalā*, and copper calcinated with the help of sulphur, cause *rañjana* (coloration) of the body.

YAŚADA (ZINC)

अथ रससिन्धुः

खर्परं लोणिकातोये क्वथितं प्रहरावधि ।
अथवा चणकक्षारैर्वाजिमूत्रेण शुद्ध्यति ।।२७८।।

Purification of Zinc
According to Rasasindhu

Zinc, boiled with the juice of *loṇikā* or in the solution of the the *kṣāra* (alkali preparation) of *caṇaka* or in the urine of horse, for one *prahara* gets purified.

रसचूडामणे खर्परमारणगुणाः

वंगवन्मारणं प्रोक्तं ताम्रवद्वा भिषक्तमैः ।
नेत्र्यं प्रमेहशमनं ज्वरघ्नं खर्परं मतम् ।।२७९।।
यशद इति लोके।।२८०।।

Calcination and Properties of Zinc According to Rasacūḍāmaṇi

Zinc should be calcinated on the line suggested for the calcination of tin or copper. It promotes eye-sight, cures *prameha* (obstinate urinary disorders including diabetes) and fever.

In folk language, *kharpara* is called *yaśada.*

तालेन वंगं दरदेन तीक्ष्णं नागेन[१६] रुक्मं शिलया च नागम् ।
गन्धाश्मना चैव निहन्ति शुल्वं तारं च[१७] ताप्येन भिषक्
निहन्यात्।।२८१।।

Calcination of Different Metals

Tin should be calcinated with *haratāla* (orpiment). *Tikṣna* type of iron should be calcinated with cinnabar. Gold should be calcinated with lead. Lead should be calcinated with *manahśilā* (realgar). Copper is calcinated by sulphur. Silver should be calcinated by the help of *tāpya* (copper pyrite).

अथ रसचिन्तामणिः

प्रज्वाल्य च खुरं धीमान् समं वाराहजमलम् ।
मूषिकां लेपयेदन्तःस्फुटितं वस्तु यद्भवेत् ।
निक्षिप्याथ[१८] धमेत्सत्यं मृदुतां याति तत्क्षणात्।।२८२।।

।। इति स्फुटितधातु-मृदुकरणम् ।।

Making a Fragile Metal Malleable According to Rasacintāmaṇi

The hoof of pig should be reduced to ash by burning. To this, the stool of the pig should be added and made to a paste. The inside wall of a crucible (*mūṣā*) should be smeared with this paste. If the frazile metal is kept inside this crucible and blown over fire, then it immediately becomes soft (malleable).

मृतानि लोहानि रसीभवन्ति निघ्नन्ति युक्तानि[99] रसेन रोगान् ।
अभ्यासयोगात् पलितादिनाशं कुर्वन्ति रुक्जन्मजराविनाशम् ।।२८३ ।।

General Effects of Metallic Bhasma-s

Calcinated metals become endowed with the property of penitrability (*rasī bhavanti*) and when such *bhasma-s* are added to recipes, they cure diseases. When used habitually (regularly), they cure wrinkling of the skin and such other ailments of old age. They cure different types of pain and prevent the process of ageing.

आयुष्यं बलमारोग्यं वज्रे स्वर्णे रसे स्थितम् ।
अमृतत्रयमेतद्धि[100] दोषत्रयगदापहम् ।।२८४ ।।

।इत्यमृतत्रयम् ।।

Three Nectars

Promotion of longevity, strength and positive health is caused by diamond, gold and mercury. These three taken together are called *amṛta traya* (three nectars) and they cure diseases caused by all the three *doṣa-s*.

रससिन्धुः
इति कथिततया यो मारयेदष्टलोहम् ।
प्रकृतिपुरुषभेदं देशकालं विदित्वा ।।२८५ ।।
उपचरति रुजार्तं धर्ममूर्तिर्यथाशु[101] ।
स भवति नृपगेहे देववत्पूजनीयः ।।२८६ ।।

Importance of Physician According to Rasasindhu

A physician, who prepares the *bhasma-s* of eight types of metal according to the methods described above and administers them to patients keeping in view the individual characteristics (*prakṛti*=constitution), location and seasons, cures the patient instantaneously like the incarnate of Virtue (*dharma*). He is revered in the house of Kings like God.

आमवातहरणे च शोभनः पाण्डु-मेह-गदनाशने गजः।
दुष्टकुष्टपलितार्शनाशकः श्वासयोपमृति[202] रुग्ज्वरापहः ॥२८७॥

Properties of Iron-Bhasma

The iron-*bhasma*, like an elephant, cures rheumatism, anemia, *meha* (obstinate urinary disorders including diabetes), serious types of *kuṣṭha* (obstinate skin diseases including leprosy), graying of hair, piles, asthma, premature death, different types of pain and fever.

लोहं विशुद्धं कृमिजित्सुशीतलम्।
सुस्वादु तिक्तं नयनामयाञ्जयेत्।
सोष्णं [?] कषायं कफपाण्डुपित्तजित्।
दुष्टप्रमेहारुचिनुत्सुलेखनम् ॥२८८॥

Another Description of Properties of Iron-Bhasma

Bhasma of purified iron cures *kṛmi* (parasitic infestation). It is cooling in potency and sweet as well as bitter in taste. It cures eye-diseases. It has slightly heating effect and is astringent in taste. It cures anemia, diseases caused by *kapha* and *pitta*, serious types of *prameha* (obstinate urinary disorders including diabetes) and anorexia. It causes *lekhana* (scraping of tissues.)

लोहं जन्तुविकारपाण्डुपवनक्षीणत्वपित्तामयान्।
स्थौल्यार्शोग्रहणीज्वरार्तिकफनुच्छोथप्रमेहप्रणुत् ॥२८९॥
गुल्मप्लीहगरापहं बलकरं कान्ताजनानन्दकम्।
सौख्यानन्दि[203] रसायनं स्मृतिकरं कांस्यादिकं[204] लोहवत् ॥२९०॥

Third Description of Properties of Iron-Bhasma

Bhasma of iron cures parasitic infestations, anemia, diseases caused by *vāyu*, emaciation, diseases caused by *pitta*, obesity, piles, sprue syndrome, fever, diseases caused by *kapha*, oedema, *prameha* (obstinate urinary diseases including diabetes), *gulma* (phantom tumour), splenic disorders and poisoning. It promotes strength, virility, happiness and cheerfulness. It rejuvenates the body and promotes memory. *Bhasma-s* of bronze, etc., also produce similar effects.

MAṆḌŪRA (RUST OF IRON)

रसराजलक्ष्मीतः

विभीतांगारे सुध्मातं[205] पुराणं त्रिफलाजले।
अक्षु[?]द्रोण्यां सुसंसिक्तं मण्डूरं शुद्धिमाप्नुयात् ॥२९१॥

Purification of Maṇḍūra
According to Rasarājalakṣmī

Old *maṇḍūra* should be heated by blowing over the red hot charcoal of *bibhītaka* and immersed in the decoction of *triphalā* kept in a wide mouth container. Thus, *maṇḍūra* gets purified.

अथ ग्रंथांतरात्

शतोत्थमुत्तमं किट्टं मध्यं चाशीतिवार्षिकम्[206] ।
अधमं षष्टिवर्षीयं ततो हीनं विषोपमम् ॥२९२॥

Selection of Maṇḍūra
According to Another Text

Maṇḍūra (iron-rust) which is one hundred years old is the best. The *maṇḍūra* which is eighty years old is of moderate quality and the one which is sixty years old is of inferior quality. The *maṇḍūra* which is below sixty years old is like poison.

गुरुं च धूमवर्णं च ग्राह्यं सर्वत्र निश्चितम् ॥२९३॥

Characteristic of Good Quality Maṇḍūra

Maṇḍūra (iron-rust) which is heavy and having the colour of smoke is always useful.

अक्षांगारे धमेत् किट्टं सेचयेदक्षपात्रतः ।
गोमूत्रे त्रिफलाक्वाथे 'सप्तवारं[207] पुनः पुनः ।
मण्डूरोयं समाख्यातः शुद्धः कज्जलसन्निभः ॥२९४॥

Second Method of Maṇḍūra-Purification

Maṇḍūra (iron-rust) should be made hot by keeping over the red hot charcoal of *bibhītaka* and then blowing. Then cow's urine and decoction of *triphalā*, kept in a vessel made of *bibhītaka* wood should be sprinkled over it for seven times. Thus *maṇḍūra* becomes pure and it looks black like collyrium.

रसरत्नाकरात्
गोमूत्रे त्रिफला क्वाथ्या' ततूक्वाथे सेचयेच्छनैः ।
लोहकिट्टं सुसंतप्तं यावच्छीर्यति तत्स्वयम् ।
तच्छीर्णं ग्राहयेद्यत्नाच्छुद्धं योगे प्रयोजयेत् ॥२९५॥

Third Method of Maṇḍūra-Purification According to Rasaratnākara

Decoction of *triphalā* should be prepared by boiling with cow's urine. *Maṇḍūra* (iron-rust) should be heated and sprinkled with this decoction frequently till it becomes fragile and is reduced to small pieces of its own. This purified *maṇḍūra* should be reduced to powder form and used in recipes.

इति श्रीमहाराजाधिराजश्रीटोडरमल्लविरचिते टोडरानन्दे आयुर्वेदसौख्ये लोहोपलोहशोधन-मारण-गुणागुण-सन्निपातादौ- विशेषधातुमारण-मलहरण[१०८]-स्फुटितधातुमृदुकरणं नाम दशमो हर्षः ॥

Thus, ends the tenth chapter of *Āyurveda-saukhya* in *Ṭoḍarānanda* composed by the great king Ṭoḍaramalla which deals with purification, calcination, good and adverse effects of *loha-s* (primary metals) and *upaloha-s* (subsidiary metals),their special processings for treatment of diseases caused by *sannipāta* (simultaneous aggravation of all the three *doṣa-s*), removal of their residual poisoning effects and softening the fragile metals.

NOTES AND REFERENCES

(1) This is the beginning of the tenth chapter of *Āyurveda-saukhy* of *Ṭoḍarānanda* and the invocation reads as follows :

ब्रह्मादिमृग्याखिलपद्धतिर्यो गोपाङ्गनानेत्रसरोजमग्नः ।
दधातु धर्मं ससुखं नरेन्द्रं (द्रे) सद्धर्म तुष्टो भुविगोपिनाथः ।

२. वंगः इति द्वितीयपुस्तके पाठः ।

३. देहसिध्यै इति पंचमपुस्तके पाठः।

४. मुण्डकीट्टकम् इति पंचमपुस्तके पाठः।

५. भूतसूतले इति पंचमपुस्तके पाठः।

६. वराल्लभ्यं इति प्रथमचतुर्थपंचमपुस्तकेषु पाठः।

७. स्वर्णताम्रारं इति द्वितीयपुस्तके पाठः।

८. वर्णं इति प्रथमपंचमपुस्तकयोः पाठः।

९. रसेन्द्रभूतसंभूतं इति पंचमपुस्तके पाठः।

१०. खानि इति प्रथमपंचमपुस्तकयोः पाठः।

११. पटुं इति प्रथमपंचमपुस्तकयोः पाठः।

१२. मृत्तिका इति पंचमपुस्तके पाठः।

१३. लेपं इति पंचमपुस्तके पाठः।

१४. भाविताः इति चतुर्थपुस्तके पाठः।

१५. खल्वे कुर्याच्च इति प्रथमपंचमपुस्तकयोः पाठः।

१६. उर्ध्वाधो इति द्वितीयचतुर्थपुस्तकयोः पाठः।

१७. 'सर्वतुल्यं ....शुद्धमाक्षिकं' पाठोऽयं चतुर्थपुस्तके नोपलभ्यते।

१८. त्रिंशद्विवोत्पन्नैर्देयं इति पंचमपुस्तके पाठः।

१९. गन्धं देयं इति प्रथमपंचमपुस्तकयोः पाठः।

२०. 'रसस्य भस्मनाथ रसेनालेप्यरैदली' पाठोऽयं चतुर्थपुस्तके अधिकमुपलभ्यते।

२१. संमर्द्यकांचनद्रवैर्द्विवं कृत्वा गुथगोलिकदतम्।
भाण्डस्त्यतले दत्वा भस्मना पूरयेत् दृढम्।
अग्निम ज्वालेयद्राढंद्युनिशस्वांगशीतलम्।
उधृत्य सावशेषं चेत्पुनः देयं पुटद्वयम्।
अनेन विधिना स्वर्णनितुल्यं जायते मृतम्'।
पाठोऽयं चतुर्थपुस्तके अधिकमुपलभ्यते।

२२. भवेनेह इति द्वितीयपुस्तके पाठः।

२३. सिन्दूरहान्यों इति चतुर्थपुस्तके पाठः।
२४. तन् मलेस्यातो इति पंचमपुस्तके पाठः।
२५. नागहानये इति चतुर्थपुस्तके पाठः।
२६. विनिर्थताः इति पंचमपुस्तके पाठः।
२७. विधां इति पंचमपुस्तके पाठः।
२८. ततोपरि इति प्रथमपंचमपुस्तकयोः पाठः।
२९. आस्थाद्यपरमात्रेण इति चतुर्थपंचमपुस्तकयोः पाठः।
३०. पुटेष्टवेवणमथो इति प्रथमपंचमपुस्तकयोः पाठः।
३१. एकo इति द्वितीयपुस्तके पाठः।
३२. मायेन इति चतुर्थपुस्तके पाठः।
३३. वा इति पंचमपुस्तके पाठः।
३४. oकेशरी इति प्रथमपंचमपुस्तकयोः पाठः।
३५. oकेशरी इति पंचमपुस्तके पाठः।
३६. 'आयुर्वृद्धिं ..... तनोति' पाठोऽयं प्रथमपंचमपुस्तकयोः नोपलभ्यते।
३७. भूतावेशप्राशान्तिं इति चतुर्थपुस्तके पाठः।
३८. सुवर्णमारणं इति प्रथमपुस्तके पाठः।
३९. 'रसदर्पणात् .....सर्वरोगनुत्' पाठोऽयं चतुर्थपुस्तके नोपलभ्यते।
४०. ध्वनासहं इति चतुर्थपुस्तके पाठः।
४१. शुद्धिमृक्षति इति पंचमपुस्तके पाठः।
४२. पिशाचां इति प्रथमपंचमपुस्तकयोः पाठः।
४३. गन्धं इति पंचमपुस्तके पाठः।
४४. पुटियोगेन खर्परं इति पंचमपुस्तके पाठः।
४५. चन्द्रायुधं इति प्रथमपंचमपुस्तकयोः पाठः।
४६. स्वांगशीतं इति प्रथमपंचमपुस्तकयोः पाठः।
४७. कुम्यकं इति प्रथमपंचमपुस्तकयोः पाठः।
४८. शुल्वं इति प्रथमचतुर्थपंचमपुस्तकेषु पाठः।
४९. केद्मारं इति द्वितीयपुस्तके पाठः।

५०. त्रिगुणं हि इति प्रथमपंचमपुस्तकयोः पाठः।
५१. सर्वलक्षणसंयुतं इति प्रथमपंचमपुस्तकयोः पाठः।
५२. रक्तं पत्रामलं इति प्रथमपंचमपुस्तकयोः पाठः।
५३. 'ताम्रं ......श्वेतं' पाठोऽयं प्रथमपंचमपुस्तकयोः नोपलभ्यते ।
५४. निमज्जयेत् इति प्रथमपुस्तके पाठः।
५५. शुल्वं कोष्ठकुष्ठादिकारकम् इति प्रथमचतुर्थपंचमपुस्तकेषु पाठः।
५६. परसमध्ये इति प्रथमपुस्तके पाठः।
५७. मुखेति शेषः दर्शने इति प्रथमपंचमपुस्तकयोः पाठः।
५८. कमचीयंत्रं इति प्रथमपुस्तके पाठः।
५९. तदोनाय इति चतुर्थपुस्तके पाठः।
६०. सेव्यै ताममृतोपमम् इति प्रथमपंचमपुस्तकयोः पाठः।
६१. प्रकाशितम् इति प्रथमपंचमपुस्तकयोः पाठः।
६२. गंधांशां मिश्रीकृतं द्वैगुण्येन ततो मुखं सुपिहितं कृत्वा इति प्रथमपुस्तके अधिको पाठः।
६३. ०वह्निनाथ पुटितं इति प्रथमपुस्तके पाठः।
६४. जयेदाश्च इति प्रथमपुस्तके पाठः।
६५. रक्तवर्णं ताम्रं इति प्रथमपुस्तके पाठः।
६६. ०ज्वरमदापहम् इति द्वितीयपुस्तके पाठः।
६७. हंडिकी इति प्रथमपुस्तके पाठः।
६८. 'उदकाराचूर्णं ....द्रवति' पाठोऽयं प्रथमपुस्तकेअधिकमुपलभ्यते।
६९. सप्ततत् इति प्रथमचतुर्थपंचमपुस्तकेषु पाठः।
७०. 'च........कुरुते' पाठोऽयं प्रथमपुस्तके अधिकमुपलभ्यते।
७१. कलिकं इति पंचमपुस्तके पाठः।
७२. लेखणी इति पंचमपुस्तके पाठः।
७३. च इति प्रथमपंचमपुस्तकयोः पाठः।
७४. टङ्के इति द्वितीयपुस्तके पाठः।
७५. ०रिष्टादनालक्षुः इति चतुर्थपुस्तकेपाठः।

७६. मृण्मया इति पंचमपुस्तके पाठः।
७७. अरण्यदानके इति द्वितीयपुस्तके पाठः।
७८. पलाशोस्थद्रवैर्वाथ लोलिप्तत्वाधसम्पुटे इति पंचमपुस्तकेपाठः।
७९. विंशत्पुटैः इति चतुर्थपुस्तके पाठः।
८०. छिंवावृक्षस्य इति चतुर्थपुस्तके पाठः।
८१. शुष्कास्वस्थपुटैः त्रिभिः इति पंचमपुस्तके पाठः।
८२. तिनीडकरसैः इति पंचमपुस्तके पाठः।
८३. ०वंगयोः इति पंचमपुस्तके पाठः।
८४. अतीसी इति पंचमपुस्तके पाठः।
८५. अथ रसदर्पणात् इति प्रथमपंचमपुस्तकयोः पाठः।
८६. पाठोऽयं पंचमपुस्तके अधिकमुपलभ्यते।
८७. ०हृन्मतम् इति चतुर्थपंचमपुस्तकयोः पाठः।
८८. क विध्वसंज्ञं इति चतुर्थपुस्तके पाठः।
ख. बध्र इति इति प्रथमपंचमपुस्तकयोः पाठः।
९०. क्षुरकी इति पंचमपुस्तके पाठः।
९१. ०मुष्कपामार्ग० इति चतुर्थपंचमपुस्तकयोः पाठः।
९२. वंगवत्साधेयं इति चतुर्थपुस्तके पाठः।
९३. नीरस्य इति द्वितीयपुस्तके पाठः।
९४. क ०रागातुष्टाः इति प्रथमपंचमपुस्तकयोः पाठः।
ख नुं रागाः इति चतुर्थपुस्तके पाठः।
९५. तथा इति पंचमपुस्तके पाठः।
९६. दत्वा इति प्रथमचतुर्थपंचमपुस्तकेषु पाठः।
९७. तत् इति पंचमपुस्तके पाठः।
९८. संपृष्टे इति चतुर्थपंचमपुस्तकयोः पाठः।
९९. तावश्चैवं इति चतुर्थपुस्तके पाठः।
१००. नागं च इति चतुर्थपुस्तके पाठः।
१०१. बल्यं इति चतुर्थपुस्तके पाठः।

१०२. जीवति इति पंचमपुस्तके पाठः।
१०३. ०रक्तघातनः इति प्रथमपंचमपुस्तकयोः पाठः।
१०४. यद्भवेन् कांस्यं इति प्रथमचतुर्थपंचमपुस्तकेषु पाठः।
१०५. मतम् इति प्रथमचतुर्थपंचमपुस्तकेषु पाठः।
१०६. पाठोऽयं द्वितीयपुस्तके नोपलभ्यते।
१०७. स्फाराङ्गा इति चतुर्थपुस्तके पाठः।
१०८. त्रोद्गमक्षमात् इति चतुर्थपुस्तके पाठः।
१०९. मसृष्टांगी. इति चतुर्थपुस्तके पाठः।
११०. सुता इति पंचमपुस्तके पाठः।
१११. रीरिका इति प्रथमपंचमपुस्तकयोः पाठः।
११२. रीरिका इति प्रथमपंचमपुस्तकयोः पाठः।
११३. तान् इति प्रथमपंचमपुस्तकयोः पाठः।
११४. ज्ञातं इति चतुर्थपुस्तके पाठः।
११५. क० ङ्गारायभ्र इति प्रथमपुस्तके पाठः।
ख० गदारायभ्र इति पंचमपुस्तके पाठः।
११६. संस्कारकर्मक्रमानं पारापभ्रकसंस्कृतं च बहुधा चूर्णौषधाणां गणं पाठोऽयं चतुर्थपुस्तके अधिकमुपलभ्यते।
११७. लोभिसैत्यानां इति चतुर्थपंचमपुस्तकयोः पाठः।
११८. स्निस्वगम्भीर० इति प्रथमपंचमपुस्तकयोः पाठः।
११९. विश्वगन्धीनि इति प्रथमपंचमपुस्तकयोः पाठः।
१२०. चक्ष्णो प्रथमपंचमपुस्तकयोः पाठः।
१२१ 'विच्छिन्न० .... विनिर्दिशेत्' पाठोऽयं प्रथमपंचमपुस्तकयोः नोपलभ्यते।
१२२. "लक्षणं लोहयोगानां विज्ञाय च गुणानपि।
यथाविधिक्रियारंभं ततस्तानभिदध्महे।
अमृतसंजीवन्याख्यापातं जलतन्त्रे यथा।
कफपित्तानिलप्राया देहा यत्र महीतले।

पतिताः दानवास्तत्रप्रदेशाश्चापि तादृशाः ।
गिरिसाराम्नतोजाना उत्तमाधममध्यमाः ।
कमक्षेत्रं शिरः प्रोक्तं हृदयं पित्तमण्डलम् ।
वायोर्नाभेरधः क्षेत्रमिति देहविदो जयुः ।
वक्षोजः व्याधिनाशार्थं कीटजः वाजिकर्मसु ।
शिरोजःदेहसिध्यर्थमित्येवं त्रिविधो मतः ।
देहदोषवशादेते उत्तमाधममध्यमाः ।
तेषामेव प्रपंचोयं रूपशब्दादिभेदतः ।
घनास्तथांगसंयुक्तास्तंत्रीनादविधायिनः ।
कांस्यघंटा महानादकारिणोहित चापरो ।
नीलेंदीवरपुन्नागनागवंगकांधिनः ।
पद्मकेतकोपाली चंदनादिसुगंधिनः ।
कज्जलाभः शिरोजास्ते रसायनविधौ मतः ।
कृशांगा धूमवर्णाश्च कोकिलध्वनिकारिणः ।
वीर्यमार्ज्जारहंसादिमांशालध्वनिशालिनः ।
शरधूमसुरामत्स्यलशुनादिविगंधिनः ।
वक्षोनावह्निजननाः सर्वे ते व्याधिनाशनाः ।
छिन्नाणुः पाण्डुराः क्षुद्राः कायदोषयुताश्च ये ।
सर्पन्ककरककादि रूक्षुशब्दैककारिणः ।
उग्रगंधाः सुधाराश्च नानासंकीर्णगंधिनः ।
वाजिकर्मसु ते शस्ताः कीटजाः शुक्रवर्द्धनाः ।
कटुतिक्तकषायादिरसास्ते तु यथामतम् ।
शिशिरस्तु खरस्पर्शा शालिनश्चापि संस्थिताः ।
इति तावदसंकीर्णवर्णाद्यखिललक्षणम् ।
असंकीर्ण फलावाप्तिकरणं हि भिषग्वहाः ।
संकीर्णलक्षणस्यापि संकीर्णफलमिष्यते ।
शंकरस्तस्य विज्ञेयं सकीर्न्नाकरणम् ।

यथा यथैषां वैमल्यं घनस्थूलां गतामपि ।
तथा तथैषां भाद्रव्यं रसायनगुणैषिणाम् ।
निरंगास्तत्र ये लोहापाति मात्रेण पूजिताः ।
कांतिजः पांडिजश्वै कांतिगुणाः ।
कांतिजश्च चतुर्ज्जातिकं विपांडीद्वतारका ।
उद्भश्चदाक्षिणात्यश्च पारसीयश्च सिंधुजः ।
लोहराजाद्रमे प्रोक्ताः सर्वकर्मकरा मताः ।
कांचिकालायशस्तारकस्तथा ।
राजराजाद्रने प्रोक्ता सर्वकर्मकरा मताः ।
निर्मलमेघसंकाशाः सांगसद्गिरिसंभवाः ।
सर्वैत्ते प्रवराः प्रोक्तास्तत्र द्व्याधिप्रशांतये ।
उत्तमाः सर्वे कमार्थाः मध्यमास्तु द्विकर्मकाः ।
अधमास्त्वेककार्यणा इत्येवं त्रिविधा मताः ।
जीवनाथस्त्वाहः
कांवियंडिस्तथाकांतः कलिंगवज्ररादयः ।
इत्येते जातयस्तेषां गुणान्वक्ष्याम्यतः परम् ।
कांचि पांडिकलिंगानामेष वज्ररको मतः ।
वज्रराघसमुद्दिष्टं कांतमेव गुणोत्तरम् ।
कुष्ठामयेषु सर्वेषु ज्वरेषु विविधेषु च ।
पांडि पांड्वामये शस्तं प्रमेहे च यथौ क्षयः ।।
कांचि गुल्मोदरे ख्यातः शूले च परिणामजे ।
भगन्दराश्मरीरोगे यकृत्प्लीह्निकलिंगजम् ।
रक्तपित्ते ग्रहण्यां च रक्तस्रावे सशूलके।
अनुक्तेष्वपि रोगेषु ताम्रवज्जरको हितः ।
अन्ये च मध्यमगुणाः नाना आकरसंभवाः ।
तेषां हीनत एवगाः कालकुग्वालकादयः ।
सर्वलोहवरस्तेषां कालदोषबलाबलः ।

रसायनविधायुक्तः कांतः कांतिबलप्रदः।

अमोघोक्तं यथा

कांचिर्वजजरक पांडिः कलिंगश्चापि कांतजः।

। इति लोहविशेषाः" ।।

प्रमादपूर्णपाठोऽयं चतुर्थपुस्तके अधिकमुपलभ्यते।

१२३. चतुर्च्छोक्तं इति पंचमपुस्तके पाठः।

१२४. लघ्वंगान् इति पंचमपुस्तके पाठः।

१२५. गजवेलीति विख्याता इति चतुर्थपंचमपुस्तकयोः पाठः।

१२६. 'भद्रमेरण्डबीजांगं ....बलवज्रकम्' पाठोऽयं प्रथमपंचमपुस्तकयोः नोपलभ्यते।

१२७. अमितं इति प्रथमपंचमपुस्तकयोः पाठः।

१२८. रोहिणी... शुक्लजक्रम्' पाठोऽयं प्रथमपंचमपुस्तकयोः अधिकमुपलभ्यते।

१२९. महीण्डकम् इति पंचमपुस्तके पाठः।

१३०. निकृत्तकम् इति प्रथमचतुर्थपंचमपुस्तकेषु पाठः।

१३१. विखन्नित्यं इति प्रथमपंचमपुस्तकयोः पाठः।

१३२. सजलच्छवि इति पंचमपुस्तके पाठः।

१३३. ०शोफ० इति चतुर्थपंचमपुस्तकयोः पाठः।

१३४. पाठोऽयं द्वितीयपुस्तके अधिकमुपलभ्यते।

१३५. यस्मात्ततं कोटिगुणं इति प्रथमपुस्तके पाठः।

१३६. जलन्धरे ईति पंचमपुस्तके पाठः।

१३७. शालमाम० इति प्रथमपंचमपुस्तकयोः पाठः।

१३८. 'जालंधरो' पाठोऽयं चतुर्थपुस्तके अधिकमुपलभ्यते।

१३९. रसायनयोज्यं इति पंचमपुस्तके पाठः।

१४०. कुल्लत्थिके इति पंचमपुस्तके पाठः।

१४१. सर्वाण्यूलूक० इति प्रथमपुस्तके पाठः।

१४२. शुद्धिमिच्छति इति चतुर्थपंचमपुस्तकयोः पाठः।

१४३. क तान्नकार्या इति प्रथमपुस्तके पाठः।
ख. नात्र कार्या इति चतुर्थपुस्तके पाठः।
१४४. तम्रानि इति चतुर्थपुस्तके पाठः।
१४५. भूसमं इति पंचमपुस्तके पाठः।
१४६. क तथागर्तलंबुक इति पंचमपुस्तके पाठः।
ख. तथागर्तकलंबुकाति इति चतुर्थपुस्तके पाठः।
१४७. जंबीरै० इति प्रथमपंचमपुस्तकयोः पाठः।
१४८. शैवालभक्ष इति द्वितीयपुस्तके पाठः।
१४९. 'तिन्द०........... व्रजेत्' पाठोऽयं चतुर्थपुस्तके अधिकमुपलभ्यते।
१५०. द्रावत्तत्स्थं इति द्वितीयपुस्तके पाठः।
१५१. कान्तं तीक्ष्णं च मुंडुं च इति प्रथमपुस्तके अधिको पाठः।
१५२. लिप्यं इति द्वितीयपुस्तके पाठः।
१५३. जले इति प्रथमपंचमपुस्तकेषु पाठः।
१५४. रद्धा इति द्वितीयपुस्तके पाठः।
१५५. कृत्वा इति प्रथमपंचमपुस्तकयोः पाठः।
१५६. ०किमद्रुतो इति चतुर्थपुस्तके पाठः।
१५७. इति लोह पद्धतितः इति पंचमपुस्तके पाठः।
१५८. क्वचिग्दते कलंबुक इति चतुर्थपुस्तके पाठः।
१५९. कापि इति पंचमपुस्तके पाठः।
१६०. पाठोऽयं चतुर्थपुस्तके अधिकमुपलभ्यते।
१६१. संज्ञिके इति प्रथमपुस्तके पाठः।
१६२. इङ्गुलं इति प्रथमद्वितीयचतुर्थपुस्तकेषु पाठः।
१६३. कफ्रसमगदम् इति पंचमपुस्तके पाठः।
१६४. कंहू मांद्यं वह्नि विवर्णताम् इति प्रथमपंचमपुस्तकयोः पाठः।
१६५. कोष्ठिका० इति चतुर्थपुस्तके पाठः।
१६६. उलूषलेन इति चतुर्थपंचमपुस्तकयोः पाठः।
१६७. कुटीहिंगु इति प्रथमपुस्तके पाठः।

१६८. ०द्रवनिःपिष्टैः इति प्रथमचतुर्थपंचमपुस्तकेषु पाठः।

१६९. 'त्रिफला ..... ०मान्' पाठोऽयं द्वितीयपुस्तके नोपलभ्यते।

१७०. कठोरांह्रिज इति प्रथमचतुर्थपंचमपुस्तकेषु पाठः।

१७१. "प्रपिष्य भावना चौदह गजपुटं। वासारसेन" पाठोऽयं द्वितीयपंचमपुस्तकयोः अधिकमुपलभ्यते।

१७२. गरुडीति परा ख्याता इति प्रथमपंचमपुस्तकयोः पाठः।

१७३. वज्रकं इति द्वितीयचतुर्थपुस्तकयोः पाठः।

१७४. मताः इति पंचमपुस्तके पाठः।

१७५. युज्यते इति चतुर्थपंचमपुस्तकयोः पाठः।

१७६. ०पुटर्भूयाद्रक्तवर्णं इति पंचमपुस्तके पाठः।

१७७. सुशोधनम् इति प्रथमपंचमपुस्तकयोः पाठः।

१७८. ०कासान् सशोषाश्च प्रमेहाना० इति चतुर्थपुस्तके पाठः।

१७९. वै इति प्रथमपंचमपुस्तकयोः पाठः।

१८०. संछादितः इति द्वितीयचतुर्थपुस्तकयोः पाठः।

१८१. यद्येवं स्यान्निरुत्थानं इति प्रथमपंचमपुस्तयोः पाठः।

१८२. सकुप्यं वान्धमूषिके इति प्रथमपंचमपुस्तकयोः पाठः।

१८३. संग्राह्य रौप्ये चेत्पूर्वमानकम् इति प्रथमपंचमपुस्तकयोः पाठः।

१८४. विंद्यादन्यथा इति प्रथमचतुर्थपुस्तकयोः पाठः।

१८५. कर्त्तव्योत्थे इति प्रथमचतुर्थपंचमपुस्तकेषु पाठः।

१८६. प्रदद्याद् भूयसा इति चतुर्थपंचमपुस्तकयोः पाठः।

१८७. तद्दानाद् बद्धकोष्ठस्य इति प्रथमपंचमपुस्तकयोः पाठः।

१८८. हि इति प्रथमचतुर्थपंचमपुस्तकेषु पाठः।

१८९. क. मृतियोगास्तथैव हि इति प्रथमपंचमपुस्तकयोः पाठः।
ख. प्रतियोगाश्चप्रतियोगा हि इति चतुर्थपुस्तके पाठः।

१९०. यथातकनिरूपिताः इति द्वितीयपुस्तके पाठः।

१९१. भस्म इतिं प्रथमचतुर्थपंचमपुस्तकेषु पाठः।

१९२. रचयेत्तं दृढम् इति चतुर्थपुस्तके पाठः।

१९३. स्थानैर्भ० इति प्रथमपंचमपुस्तकयोः पाठः।

१९४. मारयेत् इति प्रथमचतुर्थपंचमपुस्तकेषु पाठः।

१९५. वक्ष्यमानक्रमे नैव। अर्कक्षीरेण' पाठोऽयं प्रथमचतुर्थपंचमपुस्तकेषु अधिकमुपलभ्यते।

१९६. नागं च इति प्रथमचतुर्थपंचमपुस्तकेषु पाठः।

१९७. च माक्षिक वरेण हन्यात् इति प्रथमचतुर्थपंचमपुस्तकेषु पाठः।

१९८. निक्षिप्यो प्रथमे सत्यं इति प्रथमपुस्तके पाठः।

१९९. रूक्षाणि इति पंचमपुस्तके पाठः।

२००. मेतद् हि इति पंचमपुस्तके पाठः।

२०१. धर्ममूर्तिर्यशोर्थी इति प्रथमपुस्तके पाठः।

२०२. सज्वरापहः इति पंचमपुस्तके पाठः।

२०३. सौख्यानविरसायनं इति प्रथमपुस्तके पाठः।

२०४. कांसादिकं इति प्रथमपुस्तके पाठः।

२०५. सुधानस्रं इति चतुर्थपुस्तके पाठः।

२०६. वासीत इति प्रथमचतुर्थपंचमपुस्तकेषु पाठः।

२०७. 'सप्तवारं .... क्वाथ्या' पाठोऽयं द्वितीयपुस्तके नोपलभ्यते।

२०८. जसदमारण इति प्रथमचतुर्थपुस्तकयोः पाठः।

CHAPTER-IV

PROCESSING OF SUBSIDIARY METALS, GEMS, ETC.

MĀKṢIKA (COPPER PYRITE)

माक्षिकं[1] तुत्थकाभ्रौ च नीलांजनशिलालकाः ।
रसकश्चेति विज्ञेया[2] एते सप्तोपधातवः ।
विमला चाष्टमं[3] चात्र केचिद्रसविदो[4] विदुः ॥१॥

Subsidiary Metals

Mākṣika (copper pyrite), *tuttha* (Copper sulphate), *abhraka* (Mica), *nīlāñjana* (Antimony), *manaḥ-śilā* (Realgar), *haratāla* (Orpiment) and *rasaka* (Zinc ore) - these are the seven *upadhātu-s* (subsidiary metals). According to some scholars, *vimalā* (Iron pyrite) is the eighth *upadhātu*.

रसार्णवात्[5]
"कृष्णस्तु भारतं कृत्वा[6] योगनिद्रामुपागतः ।
तस्य पादतलं[7] विद्धं व्याधेन मृगशङ्कया[8] ॥२॥

ये तत्र पतिता भूमौ क्षताद्रुधिरबिन्दवः ।
ते[8] निम्बफलसंस्थाना जाता वै माक्षिकोपलाः ।।३।।

Mythology About Origin of Mākṣika According to Rasārṇava

After the completion of his role in the *Mahābhārata* war, Lord Kṛṣṇa went into *yoganidrā* (deep sleep by yogic practice) and a hunter, mistaking him as a deer pierced the sole of his foot by an arrow. Because of the injury, blood drops fell down from this wound on the ground and looking like the fruits of *nimba*, these drops gave rise to the stones of *mākṣika*.

माक्षिको द्विविधस्तत्र पीतः[9] कृष्णो विभागतः" ।।४।।
[रसार्णव : सप्तम पटलः २-५]

चतुर्द्धाकारसंस्थानं विज्ञेयं क्षेत्रभेदतः ।
कदंबगोलकाकारं शुक्तिकापुटसन्निभम् ।
तथाङ्गुलीयकाकारं भस्मकर्तरिकासमम् ।।५।।

Varieties of Mākṣika

Mākṣika is of two types, viz., yellow variety and black variety.

On the basis of its shape and location, it is of four types as follows :

(1) Round like *kadamba*;

(2) Like shells of *śuktikā*;

(3) Like fingers (elongated and round); and

(4) Like flakes of ash.

तार्क्ष्यमाक्षिकविमलाः सुपीतश्च सुलोहितः ।
सुवर्णमाक्षिकं तेषु प्रवरं सप्तवर्णकम् ।।६।।
तद्वद्रजतवर्णं च, हीनाः शुक्तिपुटादयः ।
गुणतश्च सुवर्णान्तः[10] प्रवरः परिकीर्तितः ।।७।।

Characteristics of Mākṣika

Tārkṣya (topaz), *mākṣika* (copper pyrite) and *vimalā* (iron pyrite) are exceedingly yellow and red in colour. *Suvarṇa mākṣika* which has seven colours is the best amongst them. The *mākṣika* having white colour like silver has similar properties. *Mākṣika* which is like the shell of *śukti* is inferior in quality. *Mākṣika* of golden colour is excellent in quality.

सिद्धरत्नाकरात्
मन्दाग्निं बलहानिं च व्रणविष्टम्भनेत्ररुक् ।
वरं छर्दिः प्रकुरुते अशुद्धश्चाशु माक्षिकः ।।८।।

Adverse Effects of Impure Mākṣika According to Siddharatnākara

Use of unpurified *mākṣika* instantaneously causes suppression of the power of digestion, loss of strength, ulcers, constipation, eye diseases and excess of vomiting.

सुश्रुतात्
विपाके मधुरं क्षारं[1] हेमवद्हेममाक्षिकः ।
रजताभं रजतवत् पाकेऽम्लं कोष्णमुच्यते ।।९।।

Properties of Mākṣika According to Suśruta

Svarṇa mākṣika (copper pyrite) is sweet in *vipāka* (the taste which emerges after digestion) and alkaline in taste. It is similar to gold in properties.

Raupya mākṣika (iron pyrite) is like silver in properties. It is sour in *vipāka* and slightly hot in potency.

ग्रन्थान्तरात्
शोधयेत्त्रिफलाक्षीरैर्माक्षिकं वह्नितापितम् ।
गिरिदोषप्रशान्त्यर्थं पुटं देयं ततः परम् ।।१०।।

Method of Mākṣika-Purification According to Another Text

Triphalā should be boiled with milk and in this milk heated *mākṣika* should be immersed for the removal of *giri-doṣa* (contamination with foreign elements in the mountain). Thereafter, it should be cooked in *puṭa*.

माक्षिकस्य त्रयो भागाः भागैकं सैन्धवस्य च ।
मातुलुंगोद्भवैर्वाथ जंबीरोत्थैर्द्रवैः पचेत् ॥११॥
चालयेल्लोहजे पात्रे यावत्पात्रं सुलोहितम् ।
भवेत्तत्र तु संशुद्धं स्वर्णमाक्षिकसंज्ञकम्[१२] ॥१२॥

Second Method of Mākṣika-Purification

Three parts of *mākṣika* and one part of *saindhava* (rock-salt) should be triturated by adding the juice of *mātuluṅga* or *jambīra*. This should be kept in an iron pan, heated and stirred till the iron pan becomes red. Thus, *svarṇa mākṣika* is purified.

अगस्तिपत्रनिर्यासैः शिग्रुमूलं सुलेपितम् ।
तन्मध्ये तापितं ताप्यं क्षिपेद् दोषप्रशान्तये ॥१३॥

Third Method of Mākṣika-Purification

Root of *śigru* should be made to a paste by triturating with the juice of the leaves of *agasti*. Inside this paste, heated *mākṣika* should be immersed for purification.

कक्षापुटिः
मन्दानलत्वं बलहानिमुग्रां विष्टंभतां नेत्रगदांश्च कुष्ठान् ।
करोति मालां व्रणपूर्विकां च माक्षीकधातुः सहसा ह्यपक्वः[१३] ॥१४॥

Adverse Effects of Impure-Mākṣika According to Kakṣāpuṭi

Unpurified (lit. uncooked) *mākṣika* instantaneously causes suppression of the power of digestion, excessive loss of strength, constipation, eye diseases, *kuṣṭha* (obstinate skin diseases including leprosy) and cervical adenitis with ulcers.

पाषाणभेदपिण्डस्थं ताप्यं तण्डुलवत्कृतम् ।
वस्त्रबद्धं कुबेराक्षीक्वाथे निःक्वाथयेद्[१४] (पातयेद्) भृशम् ।
एवं विलीते ताप्यस्य क्विांशो शुद्धिरिष्यते ॥१५॥

Fourth Method of Mākṣika-Purification

Mākṣika should be crushed into small pieces like grains of rice and kept inside a bolus prepared of the paste of *pāṣāṇabheda*. This bolus should then be tied in a piece of cloth and cooked with the decoction of *kuberākṣī* till such time as the pieces of *mākṣika* get dissolved. Thus, *mākṣika* becomes purified and free from wastes (*kiṭṭa-s*).

अन्यच्च

तैले तक्रे गवां मूत्रे आरनाले कुलत्थके[५] ।

शोधयेत्त्रिफलाक्षारैर्माक्षिकं वह्नितापितम् ॥१६॥

Fifth Method of Mākṣika-Purification

Mākṣika heated over fire should be immersed in oil, butter-milk, cow's urine, *āranāla* (sour vinegar), decoction of *kulattha* and solution of the *kṣāra* (alkali preparation) of *triphalā* for purification.

ततः परं पुटं देयं कुमारीरसमर्दितम् ।

कृत्वा सुचक्रिकां शुष्कां कुक्कुटाख्ये पुटे पचेत् ।

सप्तविंशतिसंख्याभिस्ततः स्यादमृतोपमम् ॥१७॥

Calcination of Mākṣika

Thereafter, *mākṣika* should be triturated with the juice of *kumārī* and *cakrikā-s* (round and flat pills) should be made out of this paste. These *cakrikā-s* should be dried and cooked in *Kukkuṭa-puṭa* for twenty seven times. Thus, the *bhasma* of *mākṣika* is prepared which works like ambrosia.

राजहंसमतात्

पाषाणभेदभण्डीरं पिष्ट्वा तत्पिण्डमध्यतः ।

ताप्यं तण्डुलवत्कृत्वा न्यसेद् वस्त्रेण वेष्टयेत् ॥१८॥

कुलत्थक्वाथमध्येन दोलायन्त्रे प्रपाचयेत् ।

यामत्रयं भवेच्छुद्धं लोहमारणकर्मसु ।

उक्तस्थाने प्रयोक्तव्यं भवेद्गुणकरं परम् ॥१९॥

Sixth Method of Mākṣika-Purification According to Rājahaṃsa

Mākṣika should be crushed and reduced to small pieces of the size of rice-grains. The powder should then be kept in the middle of a bolus prepared of the paste of *pāṣāṇabheda* and *bhaṇḍīra*. The bolus should then be wrapped in a piece of cloth and cooked in *dolā-yantra* along with the decoction of *kulattha* for three *yāma-s*. This purified *mākṣika* which is exceedingly useful, should be used for the calcination of metals.

रसार्णवात्

"किमत्र चित्रं कदलीरसेन, सुपाचितं सूरणकन्दसम्पुटे ।
वातारितैलेन पुटेन ताप्यं, पुटेन दग्धं वरशुद्धिमेति[१६]" ॥२०॥
[रसार्णव : सप्तपटल : १२]

Seventh Method of Mākṣka-Purification
According to Rasārṇava

Mākṣika should be triturated by adding the juice of *kadalī*. Thereafter, by triturating with castor oil, it should be kept inside a *sūraṇa*, sealed and cooked in *pūṭa* by which it gets excellently purified.

कर्कोटी मेषशृंगी[१७] च द्रवैर्जंबीरजैर्दिनम् ।
पाचयेदातपे तीव्रे विमला शुध्यति ध्रुवम् ॥२१॥
कांस्यमाक्षिकपर्यायां विमलां केचिदूचिरे ॥२२॥

Purification of Vimalā Type of Mākṣika

Vimalā should be triturated with the paste of *karkoṭī* and *meṣaśṛṅgī* by adding the juice of *jambīra*, and kept exposed to hot sun. Thus, it gets purified.

Some physicians consider *kāṃsya mākṣika* and *vimalā* as synonymous.

रसार्णवात्

स्यान्माक्षिकस्तिक्तसुदीपकः[१८] कटुर्दुर्नामकुष्ठामयभूतनाशनः ।
पाण्डुप्रमेहक्षयनाशनो लघुः सत्वं मृतं तस्य सुवर्णवद्गुणैः ॥२३॥

Properties of Mākṣika

Mākṣika is bitter and pungent in taste, excellent stimulant of digestion and light (*laghu*). It cures piles, *kuṣṭha* (obstinate skin diseases including leprosy), *bhūta* (parasitic infestation), anemia, *prameha* (obstinate urinary disorders including diabetes) and consumption. The *bhasma* of its *sattva* (metallic essence) is like gold in properties.

गरज्वरामकफगदग्रहणीश्वासकासनुत् ।
तेजोजःकान्तिजननो माक्षिको लेखनः परः ।।२४।।

Another Description of Mākṣika-Properties

Mākṣika cures poisoning, fever, diseases caused by *kapha* and *āma* (product of improper digestion and metabolism), *grahaṇī* (sprue syndrome), asthma and bronchitis. It promotes lustre, vitality and complexion. It is exceedingly *lekhana* (scraping of tissues).

ताप्यं मध्वाज्यसंपक्वं मत्स्यस्नेहाद्यगोंबुयुक् ।
सछागपयसा धात्रीं दत्त्वा कंकुष्ठटंकणम् ।।२५।।
वटकीकृत्य संशोष्य प्रध्मातं[९] कोष्ठकाग्निना ।
सत्वं मुंचति रक्ताभं लघु द्रवि च रागवत् ।।२६।।

Extraction of Mākṣika-Sattva

Mākṣika should be cooked with honey and ghee by adding the fish-fat and cow's urine. Then it should be triturated by adding goat's milk, *āmalakī*, *kaṅkuṣṭha* and *ṭaṅkaṇa*. This paste should be made to round and flat tablets, dried and blown with a blower by keeping in a *koṣṭhī* (under ground oven). Thus, the *sattva* (metallic essence) of *mākṣika* comes out which is reddish in colour and light. This *sattva* when melted continues to possess the red colour.

अन्यच्च
क्षौद्रगन्धर्वतैलेन[१०] गोमूत्रेण घृतेन च ।
कदलीकन्दनीरेण भावितं माक्षिकं मुहुः ।
मूषायां मुञ्चति ध्मातं सत्वं शुल्वसमं मृदु ।।२७।।

Second Method of Extracting Mākṣika-Sattva

Mākṣika should be frequently impregnated with honey, castor oil, cow's urine, ghee and the juice of the rhizome of *kadalī*, and cooked in a crucible (*mūṣā*) by blowing as a result of which *sattva* (metallic essence) of the colour of copper comes out. It is soft to touch.

अन्यच्च

कांजिके बहुशः स्विन्नं ताप्यचूर्णं कुलत्थके ।
पाच्यं मधुघृताभ्यां तद्वज्रीपयसि टंकणैः ॥२८॥
गृहधूमघृतक्षौद्रसंयुक्तं पुनरेव च ।
धामितं मूकमूषायां सत्वं शुल्वसमं भवेत् ॥२९॥
शोधनं मारणं चाग्रे सत्वानां लिख्यते ध्रुवम् ॥३०॥

Third Method of Extracting Mākṣika-Sattva

Mākṣika, in powder form, should be frequently steamed (boiled) with *kāñjī* (sour vinegar) and the decoction of *kulattha*. Then it should be added with honey, ghee, milky latex of *snuhī* and *ṭaṅkaṇa* and triturated. Again it should be triturated by adding house-soot, ghee and honey. Thereafter, it should be kept in *mūka mūṣā* and blown over fire as a result of which the *sattva* (metallic essence) comes out which is like copper in colour.

The purification and calcination of this *mākṣika-sattva* will be described later.

प्रलेपाख्यज्वरहरं राजरोगनिकृन्तनम् ।
प्रमेहार्शोगरश्वासकासमेदोनिषूदनम् ॥३१॥
रक्तं पीतं सितं नीलं श्वेतं शुक्रोपमं तथा ।
कुणपं मज्जसदृशं सांगमर्दकटिग्रहम् ।
नाशयेत्प्रदरं चैव सत्वं माक्षिकजं[1] ध्रुवम् ॥३२॥

॥ इति माक्षिकशोधन-मारण-सत्वपातन-गुणाः ॥

Properties of Mākṣika-Sattva

The *sattva* (metallic essence) of *mākṣika* undoubtedly cures *pralepa-jvara* (hectic fever), tuberculosis, *prameha* (obstinate urinary disorders including diabetes), piles, poisoning, asthma, bronchitis, adiposity and *pradara* (menorrhagia) which is red, yellow, white, blue, exceedingly white, which is like semen, which smells like a dead-body, which is like bone-marrow and which is associated with malaise and stiffness of the lumber region.

Thus, ends the descriprion of the purification, calcination, *sattva*-extraction and properties of *mākṣika*.

VIMALA (A TYPE OF CHALCO-PYRITE)

रसदर्पणात्

विमलो द्विविधो ज्ञेयः सन्निपातश्च वर्णतः ।
गुरु स्निग्धो घनश्चास्य नाम्ना स्याद्विमलामलौ ।।३३।।

Varieties of Vimala
According to Rasadarpaṇa

Vimala is of two types. It is variegated in colour, heavy, unctuous and compact. These two varieties are called *vimala* and *amala*.

स्निग्धश्चोष्णश्च विमलः कटुतिक्तरसो भवेत् ।
पाके कषायमधुरो दोषहृद्योगवाहिकः[२२] ।।३४।।

Properties of Vimala

Vimala is unctuous, hot in potency, pungent and bitter in taste, and astringent and sweet in *vipāka* (taste that emerges after digestion). It alleviates all *doṣa-s* and it is *yogavāhin* (which enhances the properties of other drugs added to it).

जंबीरस्य रसे स्विन्नो मेषीशृङ्गीरसेन वा ।
आयाति शुद्धिममलो धातवश्च तथाऽपरे ।।३५।।

Purification of Amala

Amala and other metals get purified by boiling with the juice of *jambīra* or *meṣaśṛṅgī*.

कर्कोटीमेषशृङ्ग्युत्थैर्द्रवैर्जम्बीरजैर्दिनम् ।
भावयेदातपे तीव्रे विमलः शुद्धिमृच्छति ।।३६।।

Purification of Vimala

Vimala gets purified by impregnating with the juices of *karkoṭī*, *meṣaśṛṅgī* and *jambīra* and exposing to sun for one day.

अथवा विमलः शुद्धो न जातो येन पाचितः ।।३७।।

[The meaning of this line is not clear; hence left untranslated.]

मारणं ताप्यवज्ज्ञेयं रसतत्त्वविशारदैः ।।३८।।

Calcination of Vimala

Vimala should be calcinated on the lines suggested for *mākṣika*.

ज्वरगलगंडक्षयनुत्प्रमेहरोगं जयेच्छीघ्रम् ।।३९।।

Properties of Vimala

Purified and calcinated *vimala* instantaneously cures fever, goiter, consumption and *prameha* (obstinate urinary diseases including diabetes).

"विमलं शिग्रुतोयेन कांक्षीकासीसटंकणैः ।
वज्रकन्दसमायुक्तं भावितं कदलीरसैः ।।४०।।
मोक्षकक्षारसंयुक्तं धमितं[23] मूकमूषया ।
सत्वं तारार्कसंकाशं प्रयच्छति न संशयः" ।।४१।।

[रसरत्नसमुच्चय : २ : १६-१७]

Extraction of Vimala-Sattva

Vimala should be impregnated with the juice of *śigru* by adding *kāṅkṣī* (alum), *kāsīsa* (iron sulphate), *ṭaṅkaṇa* (borax), *vajra kanda* and juice of *kadalī*. Then by adding the *kṣāra* (alkali preparation) of *mokṣaka*, it should be kept inside *mūka-mūṣā* and blown over fire by which its *sattva* like silver comes out.

विषोन्मादज्वरहरं [24]गलगंडप्रमेहनुत् ।
रसायनं परं नेत्र्यं सत्वं विमलसंभवम् ।।४२।।

।।इति विमलशोधनसत्वपातनगुणाः[25] ।।

Properties of Vimala-Sattva

Vimala-sattva cures poisoning, insanity, fever, goiter and *prameha* (obstinate urinary disorders including diabetes). It causes rejuvenation of the body and is useful for eyes.

Thus, ends the description of purification, *sattva pātana* and properties of *vimala.*

SASYAKA (A VARIETY OF COPPER SULPHATE)

कालकूटं विषं पीत्वा गरुडः सोढुमक्षमः ।
स्वयं निपातितं चंचोः सस्यकोऽभूत्सकालिकः ।।४३।।

Mythology About Origin of Sasyaka

Garuḍa (celestial bird) having taken *kālakūṭa* type of poison became incapable of tolerating it. Thus, this poison came out of its beaks and being polluted [because of its contact with the earth] became *sasyaka*.

एकधा सस्यकस्तुत्थः शिखिकण्ठसमाकृतिः ।।४४।।

A Variety

A type of *sasyaka* is called *tuttha* and in colour it is like the neck of peacock.

शशशोणितमध्ये तत् दिनमेकं निधापयेत् ।
अथवा शुद्धिमाप्नोति रक्तवर्णेन भावितः ।।४५।।

Purification of Sasyaka

Keeping *sasyaka* for one day inside the rabbit's blood or impregnating it with the decoction of drugs belonging to *rakta varga* (a group of drugs having red colour) purifies it.

"तस्य चूर्णं महेशनिपादसौभाग्यसंयुतम् ।
करंजतैलमध्यस्थं दिनमेकं निधापयेत् ।।४६।।
अन्तस्थमंधमूषायां प्रधमेत्कोकिलात्रयम् ।
इन्द्रगोपेन संकाशं सत्वं पतति शोधनम्" ।।४७।।
[रसरत्नसमुच्चय : २ : १२६-१२७]

Extraction of Sasyaka-Sattva

The powder of *sasyaka* should be added with *lākṣā* (lac) and triturated along with the oil of *karañja* for one day. Then it should be kept in *andha-mūṣā* over the fire of three pieces of charcoal and blown with the help of a blower by which its *sattva* like *indra-gopa* (red in colour) comes out.

'सत्त्वो[२६] मयूरतुत्थस्य वह्निकृद्वलिनाशनः ।
रसायने तु योज्यः स्याद् वयस्तम्भकरो भवेत् ।।४८।।
।। इति सस्यकशोधन'सत्वपातनगुणाः ।।

Properties of Sasyaka-Sattva

The *sattva* (metallic essence) of *sasyaka* (*mayūra tuttha*) promotes the power of digestion and cures wrinkling of the skin. It should be added to recipes for rejuvenation therapy. It arrests the process of ageing.

Thus, ends the description of the purification, *sattva-pātana* (extraction of metallic essence) and properties of *sasyaka*.

AÑJANA (DRUGS USED FOR COLLYRIUM)

रसदर्पणात्
सौवीरमंजनं प्रोक्तं रसांजनमतः परम् ।
स्रोतोञ्जनं तदन्यच्च पुष्पाञ्जनमतः परम् ।
नीलांजनं तथा प्रोक्तं स्वरूपमिह कथ्यते[२७] ।।४९।।

Varieties of Añjana
According to Rasadarpaṇa

Añjana is of five types, viz.,

(1) *Sauvīra-añjana* (Stybnite)
(2) *Rasāñjana* (Solid extract of *Berberis aristata*)
(3) *Srotoñjana* (Galena or Lead sulphite)
(4) *Puṣpāñjana* (Zinc oxide)
(5) *Nīlāñjana* (Antimony)

Their specific characteristics will be described hereafter.

सौवीरमंजनं धूम्रं रक्तपित्तहरं हिमम् ।
विषनेत्रामयहरं व्रणशोधनरोपणम् ।।५०।।

Sauvīra Añjana (Stybnite)

Sauvīrāñjana is smoky in colour. It cures *rakta-pitta* (an ailment characterised by bleeding from different parts of the body). It is cooling in potency. It cures poisoning and eye diseases. It cleanses and heals ulcers.

पीतचन्दननिर्यासं रसाञ्जनमितीरितम् ।
तत्क्वाथजं वा भवति[28] पीताभं वक्त्ररोगनुत् ।
श्वासहिक्काहरं वर्ण्यं वातपितास्रनाशनम् ॥५१॥

Rasāñjana (Solid Extract of Berberis Aristata)

Rasāñjana is the exudate of *pīta-candana* (*dāru haridrā* = *Berberis aristata*). Alternatively, this is prepared of its decoction. It is yellow in colour and it cures mouth-diseases. It cures asthma and hiccup. It promotes complexion. It cures diseases caused by *vāyu*, *pitta* and vitiated blood.

नेत्र्यं हिध्माविषछर्दिकफपित्तास्रकोपनुत् ॥५२॥
स्रोतोञ्जनं नदीभवमिति ॥५३॥

Srotoñjana (Galena)

Srotoñjana (galena) is available in rivers. It promotes eye sight. It cures hiccup, poisoning, vomiting and diseases caused by *kapha*, *pitta* and vitiated blood.

पुष्पाञ्जनं सितं स्निग्धं हिमं नेत्रामयापहम् ॥५४॥

Puṣpāñjana (Zinc Oxide)

Puṣpāñjana is white in colour, unctuous and cooling. It cures eye diseases.

नीलाञ्जनं परं नेत्र्यं छर्दिहिक्कानिवारणम् ।
रसायनं सुवर्णघ्नं लोहमार्दवकारकम् ॥५५॥

Nīlāñjana (Antimony)

Nīlāñjana is exceedingly useful for eyes. It cures vomiting and hiccup. It causes rejuvenation and helps in the calcination of gold. It produces malleability in iron.

अञ्जनान्याशु शुद्ध्यन्ति भृङ्गराजनिजद्रवैः ।।५६।।

Purification of Añjana-s in General

All types of *añjana* get purified by the juice of *bhṛṅgarāja*.

रसरत्नाकरात्

नीलाञ्जनं चूर्णयित्वा जंबीरद्रवभावितम् ।
दिनैकमातपे शुद्धं भवेत्कार्येषु योजयेत् ।।५७।।
एवं गैरिककासीसटंकणानि वराटिकाः ।
शंखाटकीटं[29] कंकुष्ठं शुद्धिमायाति निश्चितम्[30] ।।५८।।

Purification of Nīlāñjana
According to Rasaratnākara

Nīlāñjana should be made to a powder, impregnated with the juice of *jambīra* and dried in sun for one day by which it gets purified and can be used in recipes. By this method *gairika*, *kāsīsa*, *ṭaṅkaṇa*, *varāṭikā*, *śaṅkha* and *kaṅkuṣṭha* get purified.

मनोह्वासत्त्ववत्सत्त्वं अञ्जनानां समाहरेत् ।।५९।।

।इत्यञ्जनलक्षणशोधनसत्वपातनगुणाः।।

Extraction of Añjana-Sattva

The *sattva* (metallic essence) of *añjana* is to be extracted in the lines suggested for *manaḥśilā* (realgar).

Thus, ends the description of characteristic features, purification, extraction of *sattva* and properties of *añjana*.

शोधनं मारणं सम्यगभ्रस्य कथितं पुरा ।
तथा सत्त्वनिपातं यद्रीतिरग्रे प्रलिख्यते ।।६०।।

Abhraka-Sattva

Purification and calcination of mica are already described. The method of extracting *sattva* from mica will be described afterwards. [This verse does not appear to be relevant with reference to the context.]

ŚILĀJATU (MINERAL PITCH)

अथ शैवालभक्षमतात्

महार्णवाम्भोमृतमन्थनोत्थः स्वेदो गिरेर्योऽवतरत्ततः प्राक् ।
समंदरस्यामृतमंथनाभिः सोमेन संपर्कमियाय दिव्यम् ।।६१।।
ब्रह्माणमिन्द्रं प्रतिपूज्य सम्यक् हिताय पुंसां प्रददौ च तेभ्यः।
सोमोऽमृतं कल्पगुणं तु भूमौ शिलाजतु स्यादिति निर्विचिन्त्य।
हितं प्रजानां सुखदं निदाघे नगात्स्रवेद्भास्करतापनाच्च ।।६२।।

Mythology About Origin of Śilājatu According to Śaivālabhakṣa

In the days of yore, when the ocean was being churned with the mountain called Mandara, then the sweat of this mountain came in contact with the *soma* (nectar). This substance with innumerable properties, called *śilājatu* (mineral pitch) on the earth, should be useful to creatures, was the desire of the gods. Because of the heat of the sun in summer, it exudes from the mountains.

प्रभावतश्चोत्कटभारभावान्संसृज्यते येन च धातुना तत् ।
तदात्मकंतं प्रवदन्ति तज्ज्ञास्तस्मात्परीक्षेत्तदनन्तवीर्यम् ।।६३।।

Characteristics of Śilājatu

It is very heavy in weight because of its association with different types of metals in the stones. On the basis of the presence of these metals, mineral pitch is named variously with the prefix of these metals to the term *śilājatu*.

सुवर्णरूप्य-त्रपुसीसताम्रलोहसत्वतश्च मनःशिलातः ।
समुद्भवं चास्य वदन्ति वैद्याः सर्वोत्तमं विन्ध्यनगोद्भवं च ।।६४।।

Varieties of Śilājatu

Śilājatu is of different types as follows :

(1) *Suvarṇa* (gold) *śilājatu*;
(2) *Raupya* (silver) *śilājatu*;
(3) *Vaṅga* (tin) *śilājatu*;
(4) *Sīsa* (lead) *śilājatu*;

(5) *Tāmra* (copper) *śilājatu*;
(6) *Lauha* (iron) *śilājatu*, and
(7) *Manaḥaśilā* (realgar) *śilājatu*.

Śilājatu which comes out from the Vindhya mountains, according to physicians, is the best.

मधुरं च सतिक्तं च जपापुष्पनिभं च यत् ।
स्निग्धं घनं गैरिकाभं सुशीतं काञ्चनात्सुतम् ।।६५।।
पाके मिष्टं त्रिदोषघ्नमोजोदं शोषनाशनम् ।
वातव्याध्यश्मरीकुष्टमेहोदरभगन्दरान् ।
अर्शांसि नाशयेच्छीघ्रं ग्रहालक्ष्मीविनाशनम् ।।६६।।

Suvarṇa Śilājatu

Suvarṇa (gold) type of *śilājatu* which exudes from stones containing gold is sweet and bitter in taste, like the flower of *japā*, unctuous, compact, like red-ochre in colour, exceedingly cooling and sweet in *vipāka* (the taste which emerges after digestion). It alleviates all the three *doṣa-s*, promotes *ojas* (vitality) and instantaneously cures consumption, diseases caused by *vāyu*, stones in urinary tract, *kuṣṭha* (obstinate skin diseases including leprosy), *meha* (obstinate urinary disorders including diabetes), *udara* (obstinate abdominal diseases including ascites), anal fistula and piles. It annihilates the effects of evil planets anś inauspiciousness.

रौप्यकराादिन्दुमृणालवर्णां सक्षारकट्वम्लरसं विदाहि ।
प्रमेहजीर्णज्वरपाण्डुशोषप्लीहाढ्यवातं शमयेद्धि सद्यः ।।६७।।

Raupya Śilājatu

Raupya (silver) type of *śilājatu* which exudes from the stones containing silver, is white in colour like that of moon or lotus-stalk, alkaline, pungent and sour in taste and *vidāhi* (which causes burning sensation). It instantaneously cures *prameha* (obstinate urinary diseases including diabetes), chronic fever, anemia, consumption, splenic disorders and gout.

मयूरकण्ठोपमचाषपक्षवर्णं सतिक्तकटु चापि ताम्रम् ।
तिक्तं[?]ह्यनुष्णं[3]' खलु लेखनं च मेहाम्लपित्तज्वरशोषहारि ।।६८।।

Tāmra Śilājatu

Tāmra (copper) type of *śilājatu* is like the throat of pea-cock or the feather of *cāṣa* in colour and bitter as well as pungent in taste. It is not hot in potency. It is *lekhana* (which causes scraping of tissues). It cures *meha* (obstinate urinary disorders including diabetes), gastritis, fever and consumption.

किञ्चित्सतिक्तं कटुसान्द्रमृत्स्नं त्रपुप्रसूतं त्रपुवर्णगन्धम् ।
शोथप्रमेहज्वरशोषहारि शीताम्लपित्तं विनिहन्ति सद्यः ॥६९॥

Vaṅga Śilājatu

Vaṅga (tin) type of *śilājatu* has the colour and smell of tin. It is bitter and pungent in taste, dense and in powder form. It instantaneously cures oedema, *prameha* (obstinate urinary disorders including diabetes), fever, consumption, *śīta pitta* (urticaria) and *amla pitta* (hyper acidity).

सीसात्सतिक्तं मृदु चोष्णवीर्यं वर्णादतः स्यात्कुसुमेन तुल्यम् ।
रसेन तत्स्यात्कटुकप्रधानं वर्णौजतेजः प्रबलं ददाति ॥७०॥

Nāga Śilājatu

Nāga (lead) type of *śilājatu* exudates from the stone containing lead. It is bitter, soft, hot in potency and like menstrual blood in colour (*kusuma* = lit. flower). It is dominated by pungent taste. It promotes complexion, vital essence and lustre exceedingly.

गोमूत्रगन्धिः कृष्णं गुग्गुलाभं विशर्करं मृत्स्नम् ।
सिद्धमनम्लकषायं कृष्णायसं शिलाजतुः प्रवरम् ॥७१॥

Lauha Śilājatu

Lauha (black iron) type of *śilājatu* smells like cow's urine, black in colour, like *guggulu* in colour and consistency, free from sand particles and in powder form. It is neither sour nor astringent in taste. This is excellent therapeutically.

क्षिप्तमग्नौ न दह्यते लिंगाकारमथापि वा ।
जले जटिलतां याति श्रेष्ठं तल्लोहसंभवम् ॥७२॥

Test of Śilājatu

When placed over a burning charcoal, *śilājatu* does not get burnt but remains in the shape of *śiva-liṅga* (cylindrical). When placed in water it gives a matted appearance. These are the characteristic features of *loha* type of *śilājatu* which is the best.

शिलाजतुतुल्यवर्णि[३२] च गन्धेनापि तथैव यत् ।
सुतरां शोधने तेषां गुणं लभ्येत नान्यथा ।।७३।।

Need For Purification

Different types of *śilājatu* are similar in colour and smell of the metals the stone of which it exudes from. Therefore, *śilājatu* should be purified. Otherwise, it will not produce the desired effects.

कुष्ठार्शोवातरक्तं च रक्तगुल्मं च नाशयेत् ।।७४।।

Properties of Śilājatu

Śilājatu cures *kuṣṭha* (obstinate skin diseases including leprosy), piles, gout and *rakta-gulma* (a type of tumour caused by the vitiation of blood).

लक्षणं वर्णभेदं च सर्वेषां शृणु साम्प्रतम् ।
अग्नितोयेन यद्वर्णं तद्वर्णेन परीक्षयेत् ।।७५।।

Characteristic Colours of Śilājatu

The characteristic colours of different types of *śilājatu* are examined by placing it on fire or in water.

सर्वं सुतिक्तं विशदं विकाशि रूक्षं गवां मूत्रविगन्धि मृत्स्नम् ।
वीर्येण चोष्णं कफवातहृत्तत् पित्तस्य विस्रंसि कषायभावात् ।।७६।।
ओजस्करं चेन्द्रियवर्धनं च स्वस्थस्य रोगापहरं परं तत् ।
पांड्वामयार्शोगुदगुल्ममेहशोषेषु नेष्यन्ति तदुष्णवीर्यम् ।।७७।।
कुष्ठे विषे शोषिषु [?] कामलायां विशेषतः पर्वतराज-जातम् ।
विन्ध्याद्रिजं लोहभवं वदन्ति गुणप्रदं वह्निकरं सुतीक्ष्णम् ।।७८।।

Properties of Śilājatu in General

All types of *Śilājatu* are bitter, non-slimy, *vikāśi* (expansive), ununctuous, having the smell of cow's urine, fragile and hot in potency. It alleviates *kapha* and *vāyu*. Because of the astringent taste, it helps in the elimination of *pitta*. It promotes *ojas* (vital essence) and the power of senses. It prevents diseases of a healthy person. It is hot in potency; therefore not useful in anemia, piles, anal fistula, *gulma* (phantom tumour), *meha* (obstinate urinary disorders including diabetes), consumption, *kuṣṭha* (obstinate skin diseases including leprosy), poisoning and jaundice.

The *śilājatu* collected from the Vindhyas is of iron type. It is very useful. It promotes the power of digestion and it is sharp (*tīkṣṇa*) in property.

मधुरं कटुपाके च कदुष्णममृतोपमम्[३३] ।
मेहोन्मादाश्मरीशोफकुष्टापस्मारशर्कराः ।
हन्याच्छिलाजतु क्षिप्रं पुष्टिकृच्च रसायनम् ।।७९।।
सर्वरोगहरं योगवाहिनमुष्णशीतलम् [?] ।
क्षयरोगोदरार्शांसि हन्ति बस्तिरुजं ध्रुवम् ।।८०।।

Another Description of Śilājatu-Properties

Śilājatu is sweet in taste and pungent in *vipāka* (the taste that arises after digestion). It is slightly hot in potency. It is like ambrosia. It instantaneously cures *meha* (obstinate urinary diseases including diabetes), insanity, stone in urinary tract, oedema, *kuṣṭha* (obstinate skin diseases including leprosy), epilepsy and *śarkarā* (presence of sand in the urine). It promotes nourishment and it rejuvenates the body. It cures all diseases. It is *yogavāhin* (which enhances the property of other drugs added to it). It is neither very hot nor very cold. It cures phthisis, *udara* (obstinate abdominal diseases including ascites), piles and pain in the urinary bladder.

'शैलं[३४] तु चूर्णयित्वाथ धान्याम्लोपविषैर्विषैः ।
पिंडं बध्वा तु विधिवत् पातयेच्चपलं यथा' ।।८१।।
सत्वं सीससमं तस्य पतते गुणसागरम् ।
शोषक्षयप्रमेहेषु सूतबन्धेषु योजयेत् ।।८२।।

।।'इति शिलाजतु शोधन-मारण-सत्वपातनगुणाः' ।।

Extraction of Śilājatu-Sattva

Śilājatu is made to a powder kept inside the paste of *dhānyāmla* (sour vinegar), *viṣa-s* (poisons) and *upaviṣa-s* (subsidiary poisons). Making it in a bolus form, it should be blown over fire like *capala* (bismuth). Thus, the *sattva* (mineral essence) of *śilājatu* like lead comes out. It is of several properties. It cures consumption, phthisis and *prameha* (obstinate urinary diseases including diabetes). It is used in *sūta bandha* (making mercury non-volatile).

Thus, ends the description of purification, calcination, extraction of *sattva* and properties of *śilājatu*. [Actually in the texts, the methods of purification and calcination are not described.]

RASAKA (CALAMINE)

रसदर्पणात्
'मृत्पाषाणगुडैस्तुल्यस्त्रिविधो[१६] रसको मतः' ।
पीतस्तु मृत्तिकाकारः श्रेष्ठः स्यात्पत्रपत्तलः ।
गुडाभो मध्यमः स्थूलो पाषाणाभः कनिष्ठकः ।।८३।।

Varieties of Rasaka
According to Rasadarpaṇa

Rasaka (calamine) is of three types depending upon its nature, viz., (1) *mṛt rasaka*, (2) *pāṣāṇa rasaka*, and (3) *guḍa rasaka*.

The *mṛt rasaka* is like mud and yellow. It is the best and it is thin like a leaf.

The *guḍa-rasaka* is of medium quality and it is like jaggery.

The *pāṣāṇa rasaka* is bulky and it is of inferior quality.

पीतः कृष्णस्तथा रक्तः क्वचित् संदृश्यते भुवि ।।८४।।

Another Classification

As *rasaka* of different colours is seen on the earth accordingly it is classified into three types, viz., yellow, black and red.

कटुकालाबुनिर्यासे आलोड्य रसकं पचेत् ।
शुद्धं दोषविनिर्मुक्तं पीतवर्णं प्रजायते ।।८५।।

Purification of Rasaka

Rasaka boiled with the juice of the bitter variety of *alābu* becomes free from impurities and yellow in colour.

खर्परः परिसंतप्तः सप्तवारं निमज्जितः । ।
निम्बूबीजरसस्यान्तर्निर्मलत्वं प्रजायते ॥८६॥

Second Method of Rasaka-Purification

Kharpara (*rasaka*), after heating, should be immersed in the juice of *nimbū*-seeds by which it becomes purified.

खरातपे धारयेद्वा तच्चूर्णरसमज्जितम् ।
नरमूत्रेऽश्वमूत्रे वा तक्रे वा काञ्जिकेऽथवा ।
संताप्य मर्ज्जितः सम्यक् खर्परः परिशुध्यति ॥८७॥

Third Method of Rasaka-Purification

Powder of *rasaka* soaked in the juice of *nimbū*-seeds or in human-urine or in horse urine or in butter-milk or in *kāñjī* (vinegar) should be kept exposed to hot sun. It should then be heated and washed by which it gets purified.

अस्थिरोऽग्निगतोऽत्यर्थः दह्यते क्षणमात्रतः ।
तस्य स्थैर्यकरं द्रव्यं नान्यदस्तीति भूतले ॥८८॥
यद्वा किञ्चुलुजं सत्वं तद्रसैर्वापि मर्दितम् ।
स्थैर्यं भजेत्स रसको नान्यैः कोटिशतैरपि ॥८९॥

To Bring About Stability of Rasaka

Rasaka when placed over fire becomes very unstable and gets burnt instantaneously. The *sattva* (alkali preparation) or the juice of *kiñculu* is the only substance in this earth which can bring about the stability of *rasaka*.

त्रिदोषजित्पित्तकफातिसारक्षयज्वरघ्नो रसकोऽतिरूक्षः ।
नेत्रामयानां प्रकरोति नाशं स्याद्रंजकः कमलानाशनश्च ॥९०॥

Properties of Rasaka

Rasaka alleviates all the three *doṣa-s* and cures diarrhoea caused by *pitta* and *kapha*, phthisis and fever. It is exceedingly ununctuous.

It destroys eye diseases and imparts colour. It cures jaundice.

लाक्षागुडासुरी-पथ्या-हरिद्रासर्जटंकणैः ।
सम्यक् संचूर्णितः पक्वो गोदुग्धेन घृतेन च ।।९१।।
वृन्ताकमूषिकामध्ये निरुध्याद् गुटिकाकृतिः ।
ध्मात्वा ध्मात्वा समाकृष्येद्दालयित्वा शिलातले ।।९२।।
सत्वं नागाकृतिं ग्राह्यं गोभट्टस्य [?] मनोहरम् ।
शलाकां कारयेत्तस्य नेत्राञ्जनविधौ ध्रुवम् ।
त्रिदोषघ्नं तु तत्सत्वं नेत्रामयहरं परम् ।।९३।।

Extraction of Rasaka-Sattva

Powder of *rasaka* should be triturated with *lākṣā*, *guḍa*, *āsurī*, *pathyā*, *haridrā*, *sarja* and *ṭaṅkaṇa*, and cooked with cow's milk or ghee. Then it should be kept in *vṛntāka mūṣā* in the form of a pill. Over fire, this crucible should be repeatedly blown and poured over a stone surface. Thus, the beautiful *sattva* (mineral essence) like lead is collected. Rod for applying collyrium should be prepared out of this *sattva*. It alleviates all the three *doṣa-s* and is an excellent remedy for eye-diseases.

अथ रसचिन्तामणितः

कन्यकादलमादाय तद्दलं कारयेद्द्विधा ।
एकस्मिंस्तद्दले कृत्वा खर्परं माषवत्कृतम् ।।९४।।
द्वितीयमपरं दत्त्वोपरिष्टात्कन्यकादलम् ।
द्वितीयमपरं चास्ते तद् द्विधा कृतमस्ति[३७] तत् ।।९५।।
निरुध्यते दलं तस्याः खरमूत्रस्य मध्यगम् ।
क्रियते स्वेद्यते तावद्यावन्मूत्रक्षयो भवेत् ।।९६।।
एवं दिनत्रयं स्वेदः क्रियते तद्दलस्य च ।
त्रिवारं क्रियतेऽप्येवं तद्दले खर्परस्य च ।
अक्लेशं जायते नूनं अग्निस्थायि च खर्परः ।।९७।।
यदि वह्नौ विनिक्षिप्तः खर्परो धूमवान्भवेत् ।
तदा पुनर्दले देयः खर्परो दृढतां व्रजेत् ।।९८।।

क्षारिकालवणे पश्चात्खर्परः पाच्यते पुनः ।
दिनद्वयं भवेदेवं पाकः खर्परस्य च ।।९९।।
पुनरग्नौ परीक्षेत खर्परो दृढमुत्तमः ।
यदि धूमोद्गमो भूयात्खर्परः पाच्यते तदा ।।१००।।
पुनरादीयते तत्र भूनागतनुजद्रवः ।
भावयेत्पुटयेत्पश्चाद्भावनाभिश्च[२८] खर्परः ।।१०१।।

।। इति खर्परशोधनसत्त्वपातनस्थिरीकरणगुणाः ।।

To Make Rasaka Heat Resistant
According to Rasacinatāmaṇi

A leaf of *kumārī* should be cut side wise into two pieces. On one such piece, *rasaka* made into small pieces of the size of *māṣa*, should be kept and covered with the other piece. Over this, two more pieces of *kumārī*-leaf should be placed and tied together. This should be kept in a jar and filled with the urine of ass. It should then be boiled for three days till the urine evaporates. This process should be repeated for two times more. Thus, *kharpara* (*rasaka*) easily becomes heat-resistant.

If smoke comes out when this processed *kharpara* is placed on fire, then the above mentioned process should be repeated by which it becomes fire-resistant and strong.

Kharpara (*rasaka*) should be added with *kṣārikā lavaṇa* and cooked for two days. It becomes strong and fire-resistant. It should be tested over fire again. If smoke comes out of it, it should be cooked with the juice of earth-worm. Then it should be further impregnated and cooked in *puṭa*.

Thus, ends the description of purification, *sattva*-extraction, stabilization and properties of *kharpara* (*rasaka*).

BHŪNĀGA (EARTH-WORM)

शरन्मासससमुद्भूता भूनागाः गुडमिश्रिताः ।
क्षौद्रटंकणसंयुक्ताः कदलीकन्दमर्दिताः ।।१०२।।
सूरणेन समोपेता विशोष्य गुटिकाः कृताः ।
धाम्यमाना भृशं वह्निमध्ये सत्वं प्रगृह्यते ।।१०३।।
कदलीकन्दजलेनेति ।।१०४।।

Extraction of Bhūnāga-Sattva

Earth-worm should be collected in autumn and triturated by adding *guḍa*, honey and *ṭaṅkaṇa* along with the juice of the rhizome of *kadalī*. By triturating with *sūraṇa* and after drying, it should be made to a pill. This pill should be blown over fire and its *sattva* (mineral essence) is thus collected.

अन्यच्च[39]

शरत्कालभवा ग्राह्या भूनागां तु सुमृत्तिकम् ।
धौतजले तथा ग्राह्या यथाधस्तात्सुतिष्ठति ॥१०५॥
तां नागमृत्तिकां नीत्वा दत्वा[40] माहिषं पञ्चकम् ।
समं मधुगुडं दत्वा ध्मायेत् सत्त्वमुद्धरेत् ॥१०६॥
मुद्रिकां रचयेत्तेन तज्जलं पानमात्रतः ।
विषं सर्पविषं चैव नाशयेच्च किमद्भुतम् ॥१०७॥

Another Method of Bhūnāga-Sattva Extraction

Earth-worm should be collected in the autumn season, mixed with unpolluted earth, and then it should be kept in a jar filled with water so that they settle down at the bottom. To this, the dung, urine, milk, curd and ghee of buffalo should be added along with equal quantities of honey and jaggery. By keeping over fire, the jar should be blown with a blower by which *sattva* (metallic essence) of earth-worm comes out. Wearing a ring made out of this *sattva* or drinking water soaked in this ring cures poisons and snake bite.

एवं मयूरपित्तेन पक्षेनापि भवेद्रविः ।
समस्तविषनाशार्थं मुद्रां कृत्वा विधारयेत् ॥१०८॥

॥इति प्रसंगात् भूनागसत्त्वपातनगुणाः॥

Extraction of Sattva From Pea-cock Feather

Similarly, copper is present in the bile and feather of pea-cock. Their *sattva* should be extracted. Wearing a ring made out of this *sattva* cures all types of poisoning.

Thus, because of the context, the extraction of *sattva* from earth-worm and its properties are described.

HARATĀLA (ORPIMENT)

रसदर्पणात्

संध्यायां नरसिंहेन हिरण्यकशिपुर्हतः ।
तच्छर्दितमभूत्तालस्तत्कक्षालेखनाश्रिताः ।
'मदा''यतनसंभूता मनोह्वा तेन कीर्तिता' ॥१०९॥

Mythology About Origin of Haratāla

The demon Hiraṇya-Kaśipu was killed by Lord Narasiṃha in the evening. The vomit of the demon became *haratāla* which came out from his axillary fossa. Since the demon was indulging in alcohol, *manaḥśilā* or *manohvā* (which pleases the mind) also came into existence.

गोदन्तकश्च पिण्डश्च[42] तृतीयः घटलाकृतिः[43] ।
तुर्यः कीटाननस्तेषु गुणवान्पाटलाकृतिः ॥११०॥

Varieties of Haratāla

Haratāla (orpiment) is of four types, viz., *godanta*, *piṇḍa*, *ghaṭalākṛti* and *kīṭānana*. Amongst them, *kīṭānana* is the best in properties and it is pink (*pāṭala*) in colour.

रससिन्धुः

तापस्फोटांगसंकोच[44]-कफमारुतमेहकृत् ।
अशुद्धस्तालकः शुद्धो वातरक्तादिदोषहा ॥१११॥

Adverse Effects of Unpurified Haratāla According to Rasasindhu

Haratāla, if used without purification, causes burning sensation, pustular eruptions, contraction of limbs, diseases caused by *kapha* and *vāyu*, and *meha* (obstinate urinary disorders including diabetes). The purified *haratāla* cures gout, etc.

केवलं च खलु पुष्पहृत् स्त्रियः कुष्ठहारि हरितालमुच्यते ।
श्लेष्मरक्तविषयुक्तभूतनुत् स्निग्धमुष्णकटुकंच दीपनम् ॥११२॥

Properties of Purified Haratāla

Haratāla, when used, stops the menstruation of women. It cures *kuṣṭha* (obstinate skin diseases including leprosy), diseases caused by *kapha*, vitiated blood, poisoning and parasitic infestation. It is unctuous, hot in potency, pungent in taste and stimulant of digestion.

तालकं पोटलीं बद्ध्वा समूत्रे काञ्जिके पचेत् ।
दोलायन्त्रेण यामेकं ततः कूष्माण्डजे रसे ।।११३।।
तिलतैले पचेद्यामं यामं च त्रैफले जले ।
दोलायन्त्रे चतुर्याममेवं शुध्यति तालकः ।।११४।।

Purification of Haratāla

Haratāla should be made to a *poṭṭalī* by wrapping with a cloth and cooked in *dolā yantra* with *kāñjī* (vinegar), juice of *kūṣmāṇḍa*, sesame oil and *triphalā* decoction, for one *yāma* in each. Thus, by cooking for four *yāma-s*, *haratāla* becomes purified.

हरितालीति विख्याता त्रिषु लोकेषु विश्रुता ।
शृणु तस्यापरं नाम हंसराज इति श्रुतम् ।
तया संभक्षितस्तालः सुधारूपः प्रजायते ।।११५।।

Second Method of Haratāla-Purification

There is a well known plant called *haritālī* which is also called *haṃsa-rāja*. *Haratāla* cooked with this plant becomes pure like nectar.

रसचिन्तामणिः
[४५]वंदालीतालमादाय निर्मलं खल्वमध्यगम् ।
दिनसप्तकपर्यन्तं कुमारीद्रवमर्दितम् ।।११६।।
काचकूपे विनिक्षिप्य मुखमुद्राटयेत्ततः ।
विरच्य बालुकायन्त्रं वह्निं दद्याच्छनैः[४६] शनैः ।।११७।।
याति धूमोऽस्य नीलाभः पीतवर्णस्तु सर्वथा ।
मुखमार्गे ततः प्राज्ञो न्यसेल्लोहशलाकिकाम् ।।११८।।
तस्य तालस्य मध्ये[४७] हि या भ्राम्यते क्षणं क्षणम् ।
आकृष्टानीयते सार्द्रा सा शलाका विलोक्यते ।।११९।।

नीलं पीतं यदा किञ्चित्स्वेदरूपं जलं भवेत् ।
दिनैकं परमं स्वेदं दद्यद्वापि दिनद्वयम् ॥१२०॥
जलरूपं यदा स्वेदो दृश्यते तालकस्य वै ।
शीतलं क्रियते तत्र स्वांगशीतं यदा भवेत् ॥१२१॥
खर्जूरखोटिकाकारं तालसत्वं महोज्ज्वलम् ।
गुरुरूपं दृढं प्राप्य करस्पर्शे च सौख्यदम् ॥१२२॥
टंकमात्रं विचूर्ण्याथ प्रदद्यात्कुष्ठिने परम् ।
क्षुद्बोधो जायतेऽत्यर्थं अत्यर्थं सुभगं वपुः ॥१२३॥
अत्यर्थं पच्यते भक्तमत्यर्थं सुखमाप्नुयात् ।
अरुणौदुंबरं कुष्टमृष्यजिह्वं कपालिकम् ॥१२४॥
काकणं पुण्डरीकं च दद्रुकुष्ठं सुदुस्तरम् ।
तथा चर्मदलं हन्याद्विसर्पं चापि कर्कशम् ॥१२५॥
सिध्मं विचर्चिकां पामां श्वेतकुष्टं च नाशयेत् ।
गरं दूषीविषं हन्यान्मासमात्रोपसेवनात् ॥१२६॥

Extraction of Haratāla-Sattva & Its Properties According to Rasacintāmaṇi

Vandāli type of *haratāla* should be cleaned, kept in a mortar and triturated for seven days by adding the juice of *kumārī*. It should be kept in a glass bottle and its neck should be kept open. Keeping this bottle in *vālukā yantra*, fire should be applied slowly. When blue or yellow coloured smoke comes out of the neck of the glass bottle, then an iron rod which could move freely inside the bottle should be brought and with this rod, the condition of the *haratāla* at the bottom of the bottle should be tested. By giving strong heat for one or two days the *haratāla* at the bottom of the bottle becomes blue and yellow in liquid form. When, by this rod it is ascertained that the *haratāla* is reduced to watery or sweat form, it should be allowed to be cool of its own.

Then the *sattva* of *haratāla* of the shape of the seed of *kharjūra*, which is dazzling, which is heavy and hard and which is pleasant to touch is collected.

Therapeutic Properties of Haratāla-Sattva

This *haratāla-sattva* should be given in the dose of one *ṭaṅka* in powder form to a patient suffering from *kuṣṭha* (obstinate skin diseases including leprosy). It promotes appetite and makes the body beautiful. The patient can digest food in large quantity and becomes very happy. It cures *aruṇa*, *audumbara*, *ṛsyajihva*, *kapāla*, *kākaṇa*, *puṇḍarīka* and *dadru* types of *kuṣṭha-s* (obstinate skin diseases including leprosy), *carma-dala*, serious type of *visarpa* (erysipelas), *sidhma*, *vicarcikā* (eczema), *pāmā* (scabies), *śvitra* (leucoderma), *gara* type of poison and *dūṣī* type of poison in one month.

अन्यच्च

गोमूत्रे भावयेत्तालं दिनैकं सेरमात्रकम् ।
स्फोटयित्वा प्रमाणेन तण्डुलस्य न चाधिकी[४८] ॥१२७॥
हण्डिकायां निवेश्याथ काञ्जिकं तत्र दीयते ।
वस्त्रेणाच्छाद्य यत्नेन पर्णचूर्णेन लिप्यते ॥१२८॥
तस्योर्द्धं दीयते तालं चूर्णं तालोपरि क्षिपेत् ।
उपरिष्टात्पुनः लिप्त्वा तेन चूर्णेन तालकम् ॥१२९॥
पालिकां तु परिप्राज्ञः पुनर्दत्वा मृदालिप्ताम् ।
रुद्ध्वा याममधो वह्निं कुर्याच्चुल्यां समन्ततः ॥१३०॥
पुनस्तेन प्रकारेण द्विवेलं तालकं तथा ।
कदलीफलदण्डस्य द्रवेण तालकं तथा ॥१३१॥
याममेकं पुनस्तालं शोषयित्वा च तत्तथा ।
पुनर्यामं पुनर्यामेव वेलात्रयं बुधः ॥१३२॥
कुरुते मर्दनं शोषं तण्डुलीयरसेन तम् ।
गडदूर्वारसैस्तद्वत्तथाऽपुष्पफलद्रवैः ॥१३३॥
सर्व[४९] तिक्ता काकमाचीरसैस्तद्वत्प्रमर्दयेत्[५०] ।
सेहुण्डपयसा दद्याद्गुडसौभाग्यप्रीतिका[५१] ॥१३४॥
पादं दत्वा काचकुंभे क्षिपेद्यन्त्रेथ[५२] सैकते ।
यामद्वादशपर्यन्तमग्निं कुर्यादहर्न्निशम् ॥१३५॥
कदलीफलादिकर्मयत्कृतं विद्यते पुरा ।
तथैव च पुनः कुर्यात् षड्यामं वह्निदीपकम् ॥१३६॥

पुनस्तदेव तत्कर्म द्वियामं वह्निदीपनम् ।
एवं तालकसत्त्वं स्यादधस्तिष्ठति निश्चितम् ।।१३७।।
खोटिकाभं[५३] गुरुतरं सोज्ज्वलं तारसन्निभम् ।
वह्निसंयोगतो नैव समुड्डीय प्रयाति तत् ।।१३८।।

।। इति हरितालशोधनसत्त्वपातनगुणाः ।।

Second Method of Preparing Haratāla-Sattva

One *sera* of *haratāla* should be impregnated with cow's urine for one day. Then it should be crushed to make the size of *haratāla* particles not bigger than the size of rice grains.

In a jar, *kāñjika* (vinegar) should be kept and its opening should be carefully wrapped with a piece of cloth. This cloth should be smeared with lime powder. Over it, *haratāla* should be kept which should be covered with lime powder. Over it, an earthen plate should be placed and the joint should be sealed with mud-smeared cloth. Below the jar, fire should be applied for one *yāma* in an oven.

Similarly, *haratāla* should be triturated with the juice of *kadalī* stem and in the above manner cooked for two *yāma-s*. Then this should be cooked for one *yāma*. This process should be repeated twice more. The *haratāla* should then be triturated by adding the juices of *taṇḍulīya*, *gaṇḍa-dūrvā*, *udumbara* (*apuṣpa-phala*), *tiktā* and *kākamācī*. This *haratāla* should be added with *guḍa* and *saubhāgya* (*ṭaṅkaṇa*), one fourth in quantity and triturated with the milky-latex of *snuhī*. Then it should be cooked in *sikatā-yantra* for twelve *yāma-s* continuously.

Then again *haratāla* should be processed with the juice of *kadalī-phala*, etc., for six *yāma-s*. For the third time this process should be repeated and cooked in *sikatā yantra* for two *yāma-s*.

Thus, the *sattva* of *haratāla* remains at the bottom of the bottle. It looks like a piece of chalk. It is heavier and with glaze like silver. When kept ove fire, this *haratāla* does not get evaporated.

Thus, ends the description of purification, extraction of *sattva* and properties of *haratāla*.

MANAḤŚILĀ (REALGAR)

रसदर्पणात्

मदायतनसम्भूता मनोह्वा तेन कीर्तिता ।।१३९।।

Mythology About Origin of Manaḥśilā According to Rasadarpaṇa

[When the demon Hiraṇya Kaśipu was killed by Lord Narasiṃha, then from the vomit of this demon *manaḥśilā* (realgar) took its origin.] Since it was the product from the place of alcohol (stomach), it is called *manohvā* (which pleases the mind).

मनःशिला त्रिधा प्रोक्ता श्यामाङ्गी कणयन्तिका ।
खण्डाख्या चेति तद्रूपं विविच्य परिकथ्यते ।।१४० ।।
श्यामा रक्ता सरागा च मृदाढ्या श्यामिका मता ।
निःशर्करासु तेजाढ्या ताम्राभा कणयन्तिका ।।१४१ ।।
चूर्णीभूतातिरक्ताङ्गी सभारा खंडपूर्विका ।
तत्रोत्तरोत्तरं श्रेष्ठा भूरिसत्त्वा प्रकीर्तिता ।।१४२ ।।

Varieties of Manaḥśilā

Manaḥśilā (realgar) is of three types, viz., *śyāmāṅgī*, *kaṇayantikā* and *khaṇḍa*. Their characteristics are as below :

1. *Śyāmāṅgī* is bluish black and reddish in colour and mixed with mud.
2. *Kaṇayantikā* is free from sand particles, glazzy and coppery in colour.
3. *Khaṇḍa* is available in powder form. It is exceedingly red in colour and heavy.

The succeeding ones are better and contain more and more of *sattva* than the preceding ones.

रससिंधु
वह्निमान्द्यं मूत्रदोषमशुद्धं कुरुते शिला ।
रक्तप्रकोपं शूलं च तस्माच्छुद्धामृतोपमा ।।१४३ ।।

Adverse Effects of Unpurified Manaḥśilā According to Rasasindhu

Unpurified *manaḥśilā* causes suppression of the power of digestion, urinary disorders, vitiation of blood and colic pain. Therefore, purified *manaḥśilā* which is like nectar should be used in medicine.

जयन्तिका''द्रवे दोलायन्त्रे शुध्येन्मनःशिला ।

दिनमेकमजामूत्रे भृंगराजरसेन वा ।
शृङ्गवेर'रसैर्वापि[55] विशुद्ध्यति मनःशिला ।।१४४।।

Purification of Manaḥśilā

Manaḥśilā, cooked in *dolā-yantra* for one day by adding the juice of *jayantī* or goat's urine or juice of *bhṛṅgarāja* or juice of ginger, gets purified.

रसदर्पणात्

कटुस्निग्धा शिला तिक्ता कफघ्नी लेखनी सरा' ।
भूतावेशज्वरं[56] कासं श्वासं नेत्रामयाञ्जयेत् ।।१४५।।

Properties of Purified Manaḥśilā According to Rasadarpaṇa

Manaḥśilā is pungent, unctuous, bitter, alleviator of *kapha*, *lekhanī* (which scrapes the tissues) and laxative. It cures fever caused by the affliction of evil spirits (parasitic infection), bronchitis, asthma and eye-diseases.

तालवच्च शिलासत्त्वं गृह्णीयान्नात्र संशयः ।।१४६।।

।। इति मनःशिलाशोधनमारणसत्वपातनगुणाः ।।

।। इत्युपधातुलक्षणशोधनसत्वपातनगुणाः[57] ।।

Extraction of Mnaḥśilā-Sattva

Sattva of *manaḥśilā* should be extracted on the lines suggested for that of *haratāla*.

Thus, ends the description of purification, calcination and *sattva*-extraction of *manaḥśilā*.

Thus, ends the description of the characteristics, purification, *sattva*-extraction and properties of *upadhātu-s* (subsidiary metals).

रसदर्पणात्

रसकश्च रसं शैलश्चपलामलसस्यकाः ।
माक्षिकं दरदश्चेति भवन्त्यष्टौ महारसाः ।।१४७।।

Mahārasa-s (Important Minerals) According to Rasadarpaṇa

Rasaka (calamine), *rasa* (mercury), *śaila* (mineral pitch), *capalā* (bismuth), *vimala* (iron pyrite), *sasyaka* (copper sulphate), *mākṣika* (copper pyrite) and *darada* (cinnabar)—these are the eight *mahārasa-s*.

रससिन्धुः
वैक्रान्तकमयस्कान्तं विमला दरदः पविः ।
ताप्यधातुश्च रसक इत्यष्टौ स्युर्महारसाः ।।१४८।।

Mahārasa-s (Important Minerals) : Another View According to Rasasindhu

Vaikrānta (tourmaline), *ayaskānta* (magnetic iron ore), *vimalā* (iron pyrite), *darada* (cinnabar), *pavi* (diamond), *tāpya* (copper pyrite) and *rasaka* (calamine)-these are the eight [the number actually is seven] *mahārasa-s*

रसालंकारात्
अभ्रकं तुत्थकं कान्तं राजावर्तमथाञ्जनम् ।
वज्रवैक्रान्तकं चैव टंकणं च रसान्विदुः ।।१४९।।

Rasa-s (Minerals) According to Rasālaṅkāra

Abhraka (mica), *tuttha* (copper sulphate), *kānta* (a type of iron), *rājāvarta* (Lapis lazuli), *añjana* (galena, etc.), *vajra* (diamond), *vaikrānta* (tourmaline) and *ṭaṅkaṇa* (borax)-these are the *rasa-s*.

गन्धकतालकशिला क्षितिखेचरगैरिकाः ।
इत्यादयश्चोपरसाः पूर्वाचार्यैरुदीरिताः ।।१५०।।

Uparasa-s (Subsidiary Minerals)

Gandhaka (sulphur), *tālaka* (orpiment), *śilā* (realgar), *kṣiti-khecara* (?), *gairika* (red ochre), etc. are called *uparasa-s*.

रससिंधुः
गन्धतालशिलातुत्थं[८] भूनागं नीलमञ्जनम् ।
कासीसं टंकणं शंखं कंकुष्ठं च वराटकम् ।
एते ह्युपरसाः प्रोक्ता रसशास्त्रानुवर्तिभिः ।।१५१।।

Another View About Uparasa-s According to Rasasindhu

Gandhaka (sulphur), *haratāla* (orpiment), *manaḥśilā* (realgar), *tuttha* (copper sulphate), *bhūnāga* (earth-worm), *nīlāñjana* (antimony), *kāsīsa* (iron sulphate), *ṭaṅkaṇa* (borax), *śaṅkha* (conch-shell), *kaṅkuṣṭha* and *varāṭaka* (cowry shells)—these are called *uparasa-s* according to the experts of *Rasaśāstra*.

अथ रसरत्नाकरात्
गन्धकं वज्रवैक्रान्तं वज्राभ्रं तालकं शिला ।
खर्परं शिखितुत्थं च विमला हेममाक्षिकम् ।।१५२।।
कासीसं कान्तपाषाणं वराटांजनरावटम् ।
कंकुष्टं शंखभूनागं टंकणं च शिलाजतुः ।
एते उपरसाः योज्याः रसकर्मणि सर्वदा ।।१५३।।

Another View About Uparasa-s According to Rasaratnākara

Gandhaka (sulphur), *vajra* (diamond), *vaikrānta* (tourmaline), *vajrābhra* (mica), *haratāla* (orpiment), *manaḥśilā* (realgar), *kharpara* (calamine), *śikhi-tuttha* (Copper sulphate), *vimalā* (Irone pyrite), *hema-mākṣika* (Copper pyrite), *kāsīsa* (Iron sulphate), *varāṭa* (cowry shell), *añjana* (galena), *rāvaṭa* (?), *kaṅkuṣṭha*, *śaṅkha* (conch-shell), *bhūnāga* (earth-worm), *ṭaṅkaṇa* (borax) and *śilājatu* (mineral pitch)—these are the *uparasa-s* which should be used for processing mercury.

रसेन्द्रमङ्गलात्
गन्धकश्च स्वभावेन सत्त्वरूपी स्वरूपतः ।
तेनात्र तु[११] मयाख्यातो रसेन्द्रस्य समं यतः ।।१५४।।

According to Rasendra-Maṅgala

Gandhaka (sulphur) is like a *sattva*. Therefore, it is described along with mercury.

रसदर्पणात्
कंपिलश्चपलो गौरीपाषाणो नवसारकः ।
कपर्दो वह्निजारश्च गिरिसिन्दूरमेव च ।।१५५।।

बोदारशृङ्गेमान्यष्टौ रसाः साधारणा मताः ।
रससिद्धिकराः प्रोक्ता नागार्जुनपुरःसरैः[६०] ।।१५६।।

Sādhāraṇa-Rasa-s
According to Rasadarpaṇa

Kampila, *capala* (bismuth), *gauri-pāṣāṇa* (arsenic), *navasāra* (Ammonium chloride), *kaparda* (cowry-shell), *vahnijāra* (ambargris), *giri-sindūra* (vermillion) and *bodāra śṛṅga* (litharge)-these are the eight *sādhāraṇa* (general) *rasa-s*. They help in the processing of mercury according to Nāgārjuna, etc.

CAPALA (BISMUTH)

चपलस्फटिकाक्वाथः [?] षड्रसः[६१] स्निग्धको गुरुः ।
त्रिदोषघ्नोतिवृष्यश्च रसबन्धविधायकः ।।१५७।।

Properties of Capala

Capala (bismuth) has six tastes. It is unctuous, heavy, alleviator of all the three *doṣa-s* and aphrodisiac. It helps in the solidification of mercury (*rasa-bandha*).

गौरः पीतोऽरुणः कृष्णः चपलस्तु प्रशस्यते ।
हेमाभश्चैव ताराभो विशेषाद्[६२] रसबन्धकः ।
शेषा मध्यावलक्षाश्च[६३] शीघ्रद्रावास्तु निष्फलाः ।।१५८।।

Varieties of Capala

Capala (bismuth) which is white, yellow, pink or black is useful. The *capala* which is like gold (yellow) or silver (white) is useful in *rasa-bandha* (solidification of mercury). Remaining varieties are of medium quality. *Capala* which melts quickly is useless.

वंगवत् द्रवते वह्नौ चपलस्तेन कीर्तितः ।।१५९।।

When placed over fire, it melts like tin because of which it is called *capala* (which melts easily or which is quivering).

क्षीयते नापि वह्निस्थः सह्यरूपो[६४] महाबलः ।
ईदृशश्चपलो वा स्याद्वादिनां वादकर्मणि ।।१६०।।

Characteristics of Good Capala

Capala (bismuth) which does not get reduced (evaporated) when placed over fire, which remains stable like mountain and which is strong is useful for the rejuvenation of the body and transmutation of base-metals into noble-metals.

अथ चूडामणेश्चपललक्षणम्
वस्त्रेण बद्ध्वा चपलं[65] लंघयेद्यदि सागरम् ।
वस्त्रेण वेष्ट्यते सद्यस्तेन तच्चपलः स्मृतः ।।१६१।।

Characteristics of Capala According to Cūḍāmaṇi

If a person, keeping *capala* tied in his cloth, crosses sea, then it gets adhered to the cloth because of which it is called *capala*. [The implication of this verse is not clear].

त्रिंशत्पलमितं नागं भानुदुग्धेन मर्दितम् ।
विलिप्य पुटयेत्तावद्यावत्कर्षावशेषितम् ।।१६२।।
न तत्पुटसहस्रेण क्षयमायाति सर्वथा ।
चपलोऽयं समुद्दिष्टो वार्तिकैर्नागसंभवः ।
तत्स्पृष्ट हस्तसंस्पृष्टः केवलो बध्यते रसः ।।१६३।।

Thirty *pala-s* of lead should be triturated with the milky latex of *arka*. [The *capala*] should be smeared with this paste and cooked in *puṭa* till one *karṣa* of it remains. This never gets reduced in quantity even after giving one thousand *puṭa-s*. This type of *capala* is called *nāga-sambhava* (originating from lead). When added to mercury and mixed by only hand, then the mercury becomes solidified.

मारयेत्पुटपाकेन चपलं गिरिमस्तके ।
ताम्रवन्मारणं चापि चपलस्य प्रशस्यते ।।१६४।।

Calcination of Capala

Capala (bismuth) should be calcinated by *puṭa pāka* over the top of a hill. For its calcination, the method prescribed for copper-calcination should be followed.

'देहवेधं[६६] लोहवेधं करोति रसबन्धनम् ।।१६५।।
चपलो लेखनः स्निग्धो देहलोहकरो मतः' ।
रसराजसहायः स्यात् तिक्तोष्णो मधुरो मतः ।।१६६।।
गुल्मामशूलशोषेषु प्रमेहेषु ज्वरेषु च ।
प्रदरेषु प्रयोक्तव्यः चपलस्त्वमृतोपमः ।।१६७।।

Properties of Capala

Capala bhasma causes *deha-vedha* (rejuvenation of the body), *loha-vedha* (transmutation of metals) and *rasa bandha* (solidification of mercury).

It works as an associate of mercury. It is *lekhana* (which scrapes the tissues), unctuous, bitter in taste, hot in potency and sweet in *vipāka* (the taste that emerges after digestion). Purified *capala* is like nectar. It cures *gulma* (phantom tumuour), *āma-śūla* (colic pain caused by indigestion of food), consumption, *prameha* (obstinate urinary disorders including diabetes), *jvara* and menorrhagia.

चपला धातवः सर्वे जंबीररसभाविताः ।।१६८।।
कर्कोटीकंचुकीतोयैः शुध्यते नात्र संशयः ।।१६९।।

Purification of Capala

All the different types of *capala* should be impregnated with the juice of *jambīra, karkoṭī* and *kañcukī* by which they get purified.

सत्वमम्बरवद्ग्राह्यं सूतबन्धकरः[६७] परम् ।।१७०।।

।।इति चपललक्षणशोधनमारणसत्वपातनगुणाः ।।

Extraction of Capala-Sattva

Sattva of *capala* should be extracted on the line suggested for the extraction of the *sattva* of mica. It is an excellent ingredient for *rasa-bandhana* (to solidify mercury and to make it heat-resistant).

Thus, ends the description of the characteristics, purification, calcination, extraction of *sattva* and properties of *capala* (bismuth).

VAIKRĀNTA (TOURMALINE)

रसार्णवात्

महिषस्यासुरेन्द्रस्य दुर्गाशूलनिघातजम् ।

रुधिरं यत्र पतितं वैक्रान्तस्तत्र तत्र तु ।
निकृन्तनेन लोहानां वैक्रान्तस्तेन कीर्तितः ।।१७१।।

Mythololgy About Origin of Vaikrānta According to Rasārṇava

When the goddess Durgā killed the demon Mahiṣāsura with her spear, then the the blood of the demon fell down on the earth and in these very places *vaikrānta* took its origin. It is called *vaikrānta* because it splits (*nikṛntana*) other metals.

विन्ध्यस्य दक्षिणे सोऽस्ति नोत्तरे सप्तधा हि सः ।
श्वेतः पीतस्तथा रक्तो नीलः पारावतप्रभः ।
मयूरपिच्छसदृशां[६८] श्रेष्ठो मरकतप्रभः ।।१७२।।

Location and Varieties of Vaikrānta

Vaikrānta is available in the south of the Vindhya range and it is not available in its north. It is of seven types, viz., white, yellow, red, blue, brown like pigeon and green like the pea-cock feather and pink like *marakata* (emerald). Of these, the last variety is the best.

देहसिद्धिकरः कृष्णः पीतः शीतो सितोऽसितः ।
सर्वार्थसिद्धिदो रक्तस्तथा मरकतप्रभः ।
शेषौ द्वौ निष्फलौ ज्ञेयौ वैक्रान्तः प्रतिसप्तधा ।।१७३।।

[There are errors in these lines; hence left untranslated.]

वैक्रान्तग्रहणे पूज्यौ द्वौ विनायकभैरवौ ।
यत्र क्षेत्रे स्थितं चैव[६९] वैक्रान्तं तत्र भैरवम् ।।१७४।।

Offering Prayer

For the processing of *vaikrānta*, the physician should first of all offer prayer to the gods Gaṇeśa and Bhairava. Bhairava stays in the very place where *vaikrānta* is located.

कुलत्थक्वाथकेस्विन्नो[७०] वैक्रान्तः परिशुध्यति ।
अथवा लवणक्षारमूत्राम्लेन तु तैलके ।।१७५।।

Purification of Vaikrānta

Vaikrānta boiled with the decoction of *kulattha* gets purified. Similarly, it gets purified by boiling with salt, alkalies, urines, sour juices and oil.

कुलत्थकोद्रवक्वाथे स्वेदयेत्सप्तवासरान्[७१] ।
वैक्रान्तं दोषरहितं जायते नात्र संशयः ।
दोलायन्त्रेण वा स्वेद्यं छागीमूत्रे दिनत्रयम् ।।१७६।।

Second Method of Vaikrānta Purification

Vaikrānta should be boiled with the decoction of *kulattha* and *kodrava* for seven days by which it becomes free from adverse effects *(doṣa-s)*. Alternatively, *vaikrānta* should be fomented in a *dolā yantra* for three days along with the urine of she-goat by which it gets purified.

हयमूत्रेण सिञ्चेत्तु तप्तं तप्तं द्विसप्तधा ।
ततश्च मेषीदुग्धेन स्नुग्दुग्धेन हि गोलकम् ।।१७७।।
मूकमूषां पुटेत्पश्चात्कुर्यादिवं हि सप्तधा ।
गोनसो भस्मतां याति वज्रस्थाने नियोजयेत् ।।१७८।।

Calcination of Vaikrānta

Purified *vaikrānta* should be heated and sprinkled with the urine of horse for fourteen times. Then it should be triturated by adding sheep-milk and the milky latex of *snuhī* and made to a bolus form. It should be kept in *mūka mūṣā* and cooked for seven times. Thus, *vaikrānta* gets calcinated and can be used in the place of *vajra* (diamond).

अथवा गोनसं शुद्धं कुमारीरसमर्दितम् ।
दद्यात्कुम्भं पुटं सप्त म्रियते नात्र विस्मयः[७२] ।।१७९।।

Second Method of Vaikrānta-Calcination

Purified *vaikrānta* should be triturated with the juice of *kumārī* and cooked in *kumbha-puṭa* for seven times by which it gets calcinated.

स्याद्गोनसः कुष्ठविषक्षयघ्नः सुवज्रदेहकरो ज्वरघ्नः ।
आयुर्बलाग्निसुखरूपदःस्यात्कुर्याच्छरीरंच महत्सुसंहतम्[७३] ।।१८०।।

Properties of Vaikrānta

Vaikrānta cures *kuṣṭha* (obstinate skin diseases including leprosy), poisoning and phthisis. It makes the body like a thunder bolt. It cures fever. It promotes longevity, strength, power of digestion, happiness and complexion. It makes the body large and compact.

विषघ्नो गोनसः प्रोक्तो क्षयकुष्ठज्वरापहः[७४] ।
रसायनेषु सर्वेषु पूर्वं गण्यः प्रतापवान् ।।१८१।।
अशुद्धो विपरीतः स्यात्संशुद्धो योजयेत्ततः ।
वृद्धानां पुष्टिदं हृद्यं दृष्टिकान्तिसुखप्रदम् ।।१८२।।

Second Description of Vaikrānta-Properties

Vaikrānta cures poisoning, phthisis, *kuṣṭha* (obstinate skin diseases including leprosy) and fever. It is very powerful rejuvenating drug.

Unpurified *vaikrānta* has the opposite effects. Therefore, only purified *vaikrānta* should be used for the above mentioned ailments.

It provides nourishment to old people. It is cardiac tonic. It promotes eye sight, complexion and happiness.

"मूर्वापाटलपलाशक्षारगोमूत्रभावितम् ।
वज्रकन्दशिफाकल्कं[७५] लाक्षाटंकणसंयुतम् ।।१८३।।
वैक्रान्तसम्भवं चूर्णं मेषशृङ्गीरसान्वितम् ।
मूकमूषागतं[७६] ध्मातं सत्त्वं मुञ्चति गोनसः" ।।१८४।।
[रसार्णव : षष्ठपटल : १३५]

गोनसः वैक्रान्तः ।।१८५।।

Extraction of Vaikrānta-Sattva

Vaikrānta should be impregnated with the solution of the *kṣāra* (alkali preparation) of *mūrva*, *pāṭala* and *palāśa* and cow's urine. Then it should be triturated with the paste of the root of *vajrakanda* added with *lākṣā* and *ṭaṅkaṇa* and made to a *bhasma* form. This *bhasma* should be triturated with the juice of *meṣa śṛṅgī* and blown over fire by keeping in *mūka-mūṣā*. Thus, the *sattva* (metallic essence) of *vaikrānta* comes out.

वैक्रांतं[७७] वज्रकन्दं च पेषयेद्द्रवारिणा ।

माहिषं नवनीतं च सक्षौद्रं पिण्डितं ततः ।
शोषयित्वा धमेत्सत्त्वमिन्द्रगोपसमं पतेत् ।।१८६।।

Second Method of Extracting Vaikrānta-Sattva

Vaikrānta and *vajrakanda* should be triturated by adding the juice of *vajra* (*snuhī*). Then it should be triturated by adding the butter of buffalo-milk and honey. This should be made to a bolus form and dried. When placed over fire and blown, *sattva* of *vaikrānta* with the colour of *indragopa* (the insect cochineal) comes out of it.

केतकीस्वरसं कांक्षी माणिमन्थं सखेचरम् ।
स्वेदनाज्जायते देवि वैक्रान्तं रक्तसन्निभम्[७८] ।
[रसार्णव : षष्टपटल : १३६-१३७]
को वा चास्य गुणवक्तुं शक्नोति पृथिवीतले ।।१८७।।
।।इति वैक्रान्तलक्षणशोधनमारणसत्वपातनगुणाः।।

Red Coloration of Vaikrānta

Vaikrānta, fomented in *dolā-yantra* by adding the juice of *ketakī*, *kāṅkṣī*, *maṇi-mantha* and *khecara* (mercury) becomes red like blood. It gets endowed with excellent and innumerable properties.

Thus, ends the description of characteristics, purification, calcination, extraction of *sattva* and properties of *vaikrānta*.

SASYAKA (A TYPE OF COPPER SULPHATE)

भवानीमतम्
छेदे रक्तं कषे पीतं दाहे कुङ्कुमसन्निभम् ।
ताडने मार्दवं याति एतत्सस्यकलक्षणम् ।।१८८।।

Characteristic Features of Sasyaka According to Bhavānī

Sasyaka is red in cut surface, yellow when rubbed over touch-stone, pink like saffron when burnt, and malleable when hammered. These are the specific features of *sasyaka*.

सस्यकं ताप्यवच्छोध्यं मारयेत्ताम्रवच्छुभम् ।
ताप्यवत्सत्त्वपातं च मारणं चापि ताप्यवत् ।।१८९।।

Purification, Etc., of Sasyaka

Sasyaka should be purified on the line suggested for *mākṣika*. It should be calcinated according to the method prescribed for either copper or *mākṣika*. Its *sattva* should be extracted on the line suggested for *mākṣika*.

स्यात्सस्यको मारुतजिद्बलाग्निकृद्
भवेत् वयस्तम्भकरो रसायनः ।
बलासकासज्वरपाण्डुगुल्मरुक्
क्षयामछर्दिं जयति प्रभावात् ।।१९०।।

।। इति सस्यकलक्षणशोधनमारणसत्त्वपातनगुणाः ।।

Properties of Sasyaka

Sasyaka alleviates *vāyu*, promotes strength and the power of digestion and arrests the process of aging. It effectively and specifically cures diseases caused by *kapha*, bronchitis, fever, anemia, *gulma* (phantom tumour), pain, phthisis, *āma* (product of improper digestion) and vomiting.

Thus, ends the description of characteristics, purification, calcination, *sattva* extraction and properties of *sasyaka*.

KĀNTA LAUHA (A TYPE OF IRON)

रसार्णवात्
"भ्रामकं चुंबकं चैव कर्षकं द्रावकं तथा ।
रोमकं पञ्चधा प्रोक्तं कान्तलोहं सुरेश्वरि ।।१९१।।
एकद्वित्रिचतुःपञ्चमुखान्येतेषु वा मुखम् ।
पीतं रक्तं तथा कृष्णं त्रिवर्णं[71] स्यात्पृथक् पृथक् ।।१९२।।
क्रमेण देवतास्तत्र ब्रह्माविष्णुमहेश्वराः ।।१९३।।
स्पर्शवेधी भवेत्पीतं कृष्णं श्रेष्ठं रसायने ।
रक्तवर्णं महाभागे रसबन्धे प्रशस्यते ।।१९४।।

Varieties of Kānta-Lauha
According to Rasārṇava

Kānta-lauha is of five types, viz., *bhrāmaka*, *cumbaka*, *karṣaka*, *drāvaka* and *romaka*.

It might have one, two, three, four or five sharp-edges *(mukha?)*.

It might be yellow, red or black in colour and they represent Brahmā, Viṣṇu and Maheśvara respectively.

Yellow variety of *kānta-lauha* when added to processed mercury helps the latter in the transmutation of base metals. Black variety of *kānta-lauha* is very useful in rejuvenation therapy. Red variety of *kānta-lauha* is useful in *rasa-bandha* (making mercury solid and non-volatile).

भ्रामकं तु कनिष्ठं स्याच्चुंबकं मध्यमं प्रिये ।
उत्तमं कर्षकं प्रोक्तं द्रावकं चोत्तमोत्तमम् ।
रोमकं च कनिष्ठं स्याच्छृणु देवि मम प्रिये ।।१९५।।

Relative Merits

Among the different types of *kānta-lauha, bhrāmaka* is inferior in quality; *cumbaka* is medium; and *karṣaka* is excellent. *Drāvaka* type of *kānta-lauha* is the best amongst them. *Romaka* is of inferior quality.

भ्रामयेल्लोहजातं तु तत्कान्तं भ्रामकं प्रिये ।
चुंबयेच्चुंबकं कान्तं कर्षयेत्कर्षकं प्रिये ।
यत्साक्षाद्द्रावयेल्लोहं तत्कान्तं द्रावकं भवेत् ।
तद्रोमकान्तं लोहस्य यथा रोमोद्गमो[८०] भवेत् ।।१९६।।

Characteristics of Different Types of Kānta-Lauha

Bhrāmaka type of *kānta-lauha* causes round movement of other iron products when brought near it.

Cumbaka type of *kānta-lauha* embraces other iron products placed nearby.

Karṣaka type of *kānta-lauha* attracts other iron products.

Drāvaka type of *kānta-lauha* causes melting of other iron products.

Romaka type of *kānta-lauha* causes horripilation.

कनिष्ठं स्यादेकमुखं मध्यमं त्रिमुखं च यत् ।
चतुःपञ्चमुखं श्रेष्ठमुत्तमं सर्वतो मुखम् ।।१९७।।

Second Description of Relative Merits

Kānta-lauha having one sharp-edge (*mukha*) is inferior in quality, the one having three *mukha-s* is medium in quality and the ones having four and five *mukha-s* are of superior quality. The type of *kānta-lauha* having *mukha* (sharp edge) in all sides is the best amongst them.

भ्रामकं चुंबकं चैव व्याधिनाशे प्रशस्यते।
रसे रसायने चैव कर्षकं' द्रावकं हितम्" ।।१९८।।
[रसार्णव : षष्टपटल : ४०-४८]

Specific Properties

Bhrāmaka and *cumbaka* types of *kānta-lauha* are useful in curing diseases. For processing of mercury and for the purpose of rejuvenation, *karṣaka* and *drāvaka* types of *kānta-lauha* are useful.

"मारुतातपविक्षिप्तं वर्जयेत्सुखंदिते! ।।१९९।।

Kānta-Lauha to be Rejected

Kānta-lauha kept exposed to wind and air should not be used.

वह्निस्थितमयस्कान्तं छागरक्तेन भावयेत् ।
छागरक्तप्रलिप्तेन वाससा तत्र वेष्टयेत् ।।२००।।
छागचर्मपरिवेष्ट्य विन्यसेत्पूर्ववत्क्षितौ ।
उद्धृतं सप्तभिर्मासैस्तोयकुम्भे विनिक्षिपेत् ।।२०१।।

Purification of Kānta-Lauha

Kānta-lauha should be heated over fire and impregnated with goat's blood. A piece of cloth soaked in goat's blood should be wrapped over it. It should then be covered with goat's skin, tied and kept in a pit made in the earth for seven months. Thereafter, it should be taken out and kept in a jar filled with water. This, thus, becomes purified.

रक्तपुष्पैः सदा पूज्यं रक्तमाल्यानुलेपयेत् ।
पूजितं मद्यमांसैश्च योज्यं रसरसायने ।।२०२।।

Sacred Rituals

Purified *kānta-lauha* should be offered prayer with red-flowers, garlands prepared of red-flowers, alcohol and meat. Then it should be used for processing mercury and preparation of rejuvenating recipes.

संस्कृतं छागरक्तेन भ्रामकं चुम्बकं भवेत् ।
अनेन क्रमयोगेन द्रावकं च भवेत्प्रिये ।।२०३।।

Bhrāmaka type of *kānta-lauha* impregnated with goat's blood becomes converted into *cumbaka* type and by subsequent such processings, it gets converted into *drāvaka* type.

कान्तलोहं विना सूतो देहे न क्रमते क्वचित् ।
वेधयेद् व्यापयेत्सिद्धं[८२] तैलविन्दुरिवाम्भसि" ।।२०४।।
[रसार्णव : षष्ठपटल : ५०-५६]

Mercury without *kānta-lauha* does not permeate through the body. When processed with *kānta-lauha*, mercury permeates throughout the body quickly as a drop of oil spreads over the surface of water.

[८३]मतोन्मत्तगजः सूतः कान्तमंकुशमुच्यते ।
क्षेत्रं ज्ञात्वा ग्रहीतव्यं तत्प्रयत्नेन भूयसा ।।२०५।।

Power of Controlling Mercury

Mercury is like a rogue elephant and *kānta-lauha* works like an iron hook. It should be carefully collected from suitable locations.

गुडः पुरस्तथा लाक्षा पिण्याकं टंकणं तथा ।
ऊर्णा सर्जरसश्चैव क्षुद्रमीनसमन्वितम् ।।२०६।।
एतत्सर्वं तु संचूर्ण्य छागदुग्धेन पिण्डका ।
कृताध्माता खराङ्गारैः सत्वं मुञ्चति नान्यथा ।।२०७।।
पाषाणमृत्तिकादीनि सर्वलोहानि च पृथक् ।
अन्यानि यानि[८४] साध्यानि भ्रामकादेस्तु का कथा ।।२०८।।

Extraction of Kānta-Sattva

Kānta-lauha should be triturated by adding jaggery, *guggulu*, lac, oil-cake, borax, wool, *sarja-rasa* and small-fish. This powder should be made to a bolus by triturating with goat's milk and blown over strong fire by which the *sattva* of *kānta-lauha* comes out. By this process, *sattva* of *pāṣāṇa-mṛttikā* (red ochre) and all types of iron including *bhrāmaka* type of *kānta-lauha* is extracted.

लोहानां मारणस्थाने मारणं कथितं पुरा ।।२०९।।

।। इति कान्तपाषाणशोधनसत्त्वपातनं च ।।

Calcination of Kānta-Lauha

The calcination of *kānta-lauha* is done on the line already suggested earlier for the calcination of iron.

Thus, ends the description of the purification and *sattva*-extraction of *kānta-lauha*.

VAJRA (DIAMOND)

सुरासुरैर्मथ्यमाने समुदायान्महोदधौ ।
पुरातनामृतं जातं जरामृत्युविनाशनम् ।।२१०।।
पीयमानं सुरैस्तस्मादुत्थिताः क्षुद्रविन्दवः ।
ततो भूमिमनुप्राप्ताः शुक्लवर्णातिभास्वराः[८५] ।
शुष्कास्ते वज्रतां जाताः[८६] नानावर्णा महाबलाः ।।२११।।

Mythology About Origin of Vajra

When the gods and demons churned the ocean, in the days of yore, ambrosia, which annihilates ageing process and death, came out. When the gods were drinking this ambrosia, small drops of it fell down on the earth and coming in contact with the earth, these drops became white and exceedingly dazzling. When these drops got dried up, they gave rise to very strong (hard) diamonds of different colours.

अन्ये चोपरसाः सर्वे ये प्रोक्ता महारसाः ।
वज्रानां[८७] तु वरिष्ठत्वं तेषु प्रोक्तं शिवेन तु ।।२१२।।

Importance of Diamond

Diamond is the best among the different types of *uparasa-s* and *mahārasa-s* as instructed by Lord Śiva.

ब्राह्मणाः क्षत्रिया वैश्या शूद्राश्चैव[८८] चतुर्विधाः ।
स्त्रीपुन्नपुंसकमिति त्रिधैषां लिंगनिर्णयः ।

श्वेता रक्ताश्च पीताश्च कृष्णाश्चैव चतुर्विधाः ।।२९३।।

Varieties of Diamond

Diamond is of four types, viz., *brāhmaṇa*, *kṣatriya*, *vaiśya* and *śūdra*.

It is also of three types on the basis of sex, viz., male, female and neuter.

On the basis of colours, it is also classified into four categories, viz., white, red, yellow and black.

वृताः[८९] फलकसंयुक्तास्तेजोवन्तो बृहत्तमाः[९०] ।
पुरुषास्ते समाख्याता [९१]रेखाबिन्दुविवर्जिताः ।।२९४।।

Male Type of Diamond

Male type of diamond is round with flat surfaces, dazzling, very big in size and free from dots and lines.

रेखाबिन्दुसमायुक्ताः षट्कोणास्ताः स्त्रियः स्मृताः ।
त्रिकोणाः पत्तलाः दीर्घाः कृष्णाश्चापि नपुंसकाः ।।२९५।।

Female and Neuter Types of Diamond

Diamond having dots and lines and having six angles is of female type.

Diamond having three angles, thin, long and black in colour is of neuter type.

सत्ववन्तो बलोपेताः क्रामणे परमं हिताः ।
रसबन्धकराः ख्याताः पुरुषा वज्रसंज्ञकाः ।।२९६।।

Importance of Male-Diamond

Male-diamond is full of *sattva* (essence) and strength (hardness). It is very useful for the *krāmaṇa saṃskāra* of mercury. It causes *rasabandhana* (making mercury solid and fire-resistant).

शरीरकान्तिजनकाः भोगदाः वज्रयोषितः ।।२९७।।

Properties of Female-Diamond

Female-diamond promotes the body complexion and pleasure in life.

अल्पवीर्यास्तथा स्वल्पाः कमकास्ताः [?] प्रकीर्तिताः।
नपुंसकाः सत्वहीनाः कोष्टाल्लोहं क्रमन्ति च।।२१८।।

Properties of Neuter-Diamond

Neuter-diamond is low in potency, very small in size, without any *sattva* (essence), and when heated in an oven it gets mixed up (*kramaṇa*) with metals.

स्त्रियः स्त्रीषु प्रयोक्तव्याः क्लीबे क्लीबं तथैव च।
सर्वेषु सर्वदा योज्याः पुरुषा बलवत्तराः।।२१९।।
रसायने भवेद्विप्रो ह्यणिमादिगुणप्रदः।
क्षत्रियो मृत्युनाशाय वलीपलितरोगहृत्[१२]।।२२०।।
द्रव्यकारी तथा वैश्यः शरीरदृढतां नयेत्।
व्याधिप्रशमनः शूद्रो वयस्तम्भं करोति च।।२२१।।

Specific Utilities of Different Types of Diamond

Female types of diamond should be used for females and neuter types of for neuters. But male type of diamond is useful for all at all times and it is the strongest (hardest) one.

Brāhmaṇa type of diamond is useful in rejuvenation. It endows a person with eight *siddhis*, viz., *aṇimā*, etc.

Kṣatriya type of diamond prevents death and it cures wrinkling, graying of hair and other diseases.

Vaiśya type of diamond endows a person with wealth and makes for the sturdiness of the body.

Śūdra type of diamond cures diseases and maintains youth.

षट्कोणं लघुतीक्ष्णं च बृहदष्टफलं च यत्।
जले तरति यद्वज्रं तद्वज्रं[१३] रसकर्मणि।।२२२।।

Diamond Useful for Processing Mercury

The diamond having six angles, which is light and sharp, which is big in size, which has eight flat surfaces and which floats over water is suitable for processing mercury.

कृते युगे कलिंगे च कौशले वज्रसंभवः।

हिमालये मतंगे च त्रेतायां वज्रसंभवः ॥२२३॥
पौण्ड्रके च सुराष्ट्रे च द्वापरे पविसंभवः ।
वैरगिरौ च सोपारे क्लौ हीरकसंभवः ॥२२४॥

Availability of Diamond in Different Ages

During the *satya* age, diamond was available in Kaliṅga and Kauśala. During *tretā* age, diamond was available in the Himalayas and Mataṅga. During *dvāpara* age, diamond was available in Pauṇḍraka and Saurāṣṭra. In this *kali* age, it is available in Vairagiri and Sopāra.

वर्णरश्मिसमस्वच्छं[१४] तीक्ष्णधारामलं लघु।
फले शुद्धं च षट्कोणं वज्रं ग्राह्यं रसे शुभे ॥२२५॥

Selection of Suitable Diamond

Diamond, which is of good colour, which emits rays appropriately, which is transparent, which has sharp edges, which is free from dirt, wihch is light, whose flat surfaces are clean and which has six angles is suitable for processing mercury.

उत्तमं तद्धृते हस्ते सर्वोपद्रवनाशनम् ।
तथापमृत्युशमनं सत्सुवर्णेन[१५] संयुतम् ॥२२६॥

Wearing of Diamond-Ring

Wearing of good quality diamond in a gold ring in the hand annihilates all complications including untimely death.

यत्र तिष्ठति तद्रत्नं तत्र श्रीर्नात्र संशयः ।
पुण्यवृद्धिकरं हृद्यं मनैश्वर्यकरं परम् ॥२२७॥
गुर्विणीभिर्न धर्तव्यो बालरक्षाकरो मणिः।
कदाचिद् वज्रसंस्पर्शाद् गर्भस्तम्भः प्रजायते ॥२२८॥

Properties of Diamond

Where ever diamond is placed, it undoubtedly becomes the location of *Śrī* (goddess of wealth). It promotes *puṇya* (virtuousness). It is cardiac tonic. It gives excellent happiness to the mind. It should not be worn by the pregnant woman as a talisman for protecting the foetus (*bāla-*

rakṣākara-maṇi) because at times because of the touch of diamond which is worn, the foetal development gets arrested (*garbha-stambha-kara*):

रुजासमूहं हरते च वज्रं
देहस्य रूपं विदधाति युक्त्या[१६] ।
पुष्टिं च सौख्यं प्रबलं चिरायु-
र्जराबलानां निधनं करोति ।।२२९ ।।

Diamond cures all types of pain, promotes the complexion and nourishment of the body, happiness and longevity. It counteracts the factors responsible for ageing.

अदाह्यं[१७] च अभेद्यं च अमूल्यं स्वप्रकाशता ।
यथैवात्मा तथा वज्रं सेवनीयं प्रयत्नतः ।।२३० ।।

Soul and Diamond

Both the soul and the diamond are not amenable to burning, cutting and valuation. They have their own lights. Therefore, like soul, a person should carefully wear diamond.

पीडां विधत्ते विविधां नराणाम्
वज्रं रुजाः पोषयति हि काये ।
कुष्ठं ज्वरं पाण्डुगदं क्षयं च ।
हृत्पार्श्वपीडां कुरुतेऽतिरौद्री ।।२३१ ।।

Adverse Effects of Unpurified Diamond

Diamond, [when used internally without purification], causes different types of pain, makes the body abode of several diseases including *kuṣṭha* (obstinate skin diseases including leprosy), fever, anemia, pthisis, excessive pain in the cardiac region and side of the chest.

रसार्णवात्
"श्यामा शमी घनरवो वर्षाभून्मत्तकोद्रवः ।
आखुकर्णी मुनिलता: कुलत्थं चाम्लवेतसम् ।।२३२ ।।

मेषशृङ्गीरसं चैषां कन्दस्य सूरणस्य तु ।
शोधयेत्त्रिदिनं वज्रं शुद्धिमेति सुरेश्वरि" ।।२३३।।
[रसार्णव : षष्ठपटल : ७९-८४]

Purification of Diamond According to Rasārṇava

Diamond gets purified in three days with the juices of *śyāmā*, *śamī*, *ghana-rava*, *punarnavā*, *dhustūra*, *kodrava*, *ākhukarṇī*, *agasti*, *kulattha*, *amla-vetasa*, *meṣa-śṛṅgī* and the tuber of *sūraṇa*.

गृहीत्वा तं[८] शुभं वज्रं व्याघ्रीकंद्रोदरे क्षिपेत् ।
लिप्त्वा कंद्रं माहिषेण करीषेणाग्निना पचेत् ।
निशायां च चतुर्यामं वज्रं शुध्यति नान्यथा ।।२३४।।

Second Method of Diamond-Purification

Diamond of good quality should be kept inside *vyāghrī-kanda* and thereafter, the paste of *vyāghrī-kanda* should be smeared around it. Then it should be cooked in the fire of the cake of buffalo-dung at night for four *yāma-s* by which diamond gets purified.

द्रुतिः भक्तं भस्म त्रिविधं वज्रमारणम् ।
उत्तमं द्रुतिरूपं तु मध्यमं चान्नसन्निभम् ।
अधमं भस्मसदृशं वज्रस्य त्रिविधा गतिः ।।२३५।।

Calcination of Diamond

The *māraṇa* (calcination-lit. killing) of diamond is done in three different ways, as follows :

(1) *Druti* (when diamond remains in liquid form);
(2) *Bhakta* (when diamond becomes soft and swollen like boiled rice);
(3) *Bhasma* (when diamond is calcinated and reduced to powder form).

Of these, *druti* is the best; *bhakta* is medium; and *bhasma* is infeior in quality.

रसे रसायने योज्यं द्रुतिरूपं गुणाधिकम् ।
धातुवादे च विदितं भक्तरूपं सुपोषकम् ।।२३६।।

क्षयशोषप्रमेहेषु तथा जीर्णज्वरेषु च ।
कुष्ठेषु भस्मरूपं च वज्रं योज्यं सुरेश्वरि ।।२३७।।

Specific Utilities of Different Types of Diamond

The diamond in *druti* form is excellent in property; hence it is to be used in processing mercury and for the purpose of rejuvenation.

The diamond in *bhakta* form is nourishing and it is useful in *dhātu-vāda* (processing mercury for the transmutation of base metals into noble ones).

The diamond in *bhasma* (calcinated) form is useful in the treatment of phthisis, consumption, *prameha* (obstinate urinary disorders including diabetes) and chronic fever.

अस्थिसंहारमध्यस्थं कृत्वा वज्रं सुरंध्रितम् ।
जलभाण्डे तु तत्स्विन्नं सप्ताहाद्द्रवतां व्रजेत् ।।२३८।।

Preparation of Diamond-Druti

In a piece of *asthi-saṃhāra*, a small hole should be made and steamed over a jar containing water for seven days by which diamond gets liquefied.

क्षारत्रयं रामठं च चणकाम्लाम्लवेतसम् ।
क्षिप्त्वा ज्वालामुखीक्षारं स्थलकुंभीरसेन च ।।२३९।।
एतानि पेषयेद्गाढं स्नुह्यर्कमयसा सदा[99] ।
तत्कल्कगोलकं कृत्वा वस्त्रबद्धं दृढं ततः ।।२४०।।
वज्रमुख्यानि रत्नानि क्षिप्त्वा तस्मिञ्च[100] तं पचेत् ।
दोलायन्त्रेण धान्याम्लैर्दिनरात्रक्रमेण तु ।
वज्रमुख्यानि रत्नानि रसरूपं प्रजायते ।।२४१।।

Second Method of Preparing Diamond-Druti

Three types of *kṣāra* (alkali preparations), *hiṅgu*, *caṇakāmla* and *amla-vetasa* added with the *kṣāra* (alkali preparation) of *jvālāmukhi* should be triturated strongly along with the juice of *sthala-kumbhi* and the milky latex of *snuhi* and *arka*. This paste should be made to a round bolus and tied with a cloth. Inside this bolus, diamond and other gems should be placed and cooked in *dolā-yantra* along with *dhānyāmla* (a type of sour vinegar) for a day and a night when these gems including diamond get liquefied and look like mercury.

कान्तस्य पिष्टिकामध्ये वज्रं देवि विनिक्षिपेत् ।
कार्पासनिंबपत्रं च बदरीपत्रसंयुतम् ।।२४२ ।।
एकत्र पेषयेत्तत्तु कान्तगोलकवेष्टितम् ।
बाह्ये ताम्बूलपत्रेण स्थापयेज्जानुमध्यतः ।
यामद्वयेन तद्वज्रं भवेदन्धसमं ध्रुवम् ।।२४३ ।।

Third Method of Preparing Diamond-Druti

In the paste of *kānta-lauha* diamond should be placed. By adding the leaves of *kārpāsa*, *nimba* and *badarī*, this should be triturated. This paste should be kept inside a ball of *kānta-lauha* which is to be wrapped with betel-leaves and in the fossa at the back of the knee joint *(jānu-madhya?)* for two *yāma-s* by which it gets liquefied (*andha-sama*=lit. like a blind person).

जंबीरफलमध्यस्थं वस्त्रपोटलिकागतम् ।
क्वाथयेत्कोद्रवक्वाथैः क्रमेणानेन तु त्र्यहम्[101] ।
तद्वज्रं 'जायते[102] खोटं[103] हेम्न मिलति तत्क्षणम् ।।२४४ ।।

Fourth Method of Preparing Diamond-Druti

Diamond should be kept inside a fruit of *jambīra* which should be kept in a *poṭṭalī* prepared of cloth. It should be boiled in the decoction of *kodrava* for three days. Thus, diamond becomes *khoṭa* (liquefied) and it immediately gets mixed up with gold.

मातृवाहकजीवस्य मध्ये वज्रं विनिक्षिपेत् ।
दोलास्वेदात्त्र्यहं स्वेद्यं' भवेत्सिक्थसमं[104] ध्रुवम् ।।२४५ ।।

Method of Preparing Diamond-Bhakta

Diamond should be kept inside the animal called *mātṛvāhaka* and cooked in *dolā-yantra* for three days by which it becomes soft like wax.

मत्कुणस्तालकं पिष्ट्वा यावद् भवति गोलकम् ।
तद्गोले निहितं वज्रं तद्गोलं च क्षिपेद् बुधः ॥२४६॥
रुध्वाध्मातं पुनः पेष्यं एवं कुर्याच्च सप्तधा ।
एवं च जायते भस्म वज्रोत्थं नैव संशयः ॥२४७॥

Preparation of Diamond-Bhasma

Haratāla should be made to a paste by triturating with *matkuṇa* and made to a round bolus form. Diamond should be kept inside this bolus. It should be kept in *śarāva-sampuṭa* and sealed. Then it should be placed over fire and blown. This process should be repeated for seven times by which diamond undoubtedly gets reduced to a *bhasma*-form.

मंडूकं कांस्यजे पात्रे निगृह्य स्थापयेत्सुधीः ।
स भीतो मूत्रयेत्तत्र तन्मूत्रे वज्रमारणम् ।
तप्तं तप्तं च निर्वाप्यं शतवारं मृतिं व्रजेत् ॥२४८॥

Second Method of Preparing Diamond-Bhasma

A frog should be kept in a bronze vessel. Because of fear, it will void urine in the vessel. Diamond should be repeatedly heated and immersed in the frog-urine for one hundred times by which it gets reduced to *bhasma* form.

ताप्य[१०५] ताप्य खरे वह्नौ सेहुण्डपयसा क्षिपेत् ।
वेलाचतुर्दश प्राज्ञः पिष्ट्वा वज्रं विचूर्णयेत् ॥२४९॥

Third Method of Preparing Diamond-Bhasma

Diamond should be repeatedly heated over strong fire an immersed in the milky latex of *snuhī* for fourteen times. Then it shoul be triturated and made to a powder form.

रसचिन्तामणिः

इंगुदस्य च तैलेन काचपात्रकृतेन च ।
तप्त्वा निर्वाप्यते हीरं चतुर्धातिमृतिं[१०६] व्रजेत् ॥२५०॥

Fourth Method of Preparing Diamond-Bhasma According to Rasa-cintāmaṇi

Oil of *iṅgudī* should be kept in a glass vessel. Heated diamond should be immersed in it. Doing like this for four times [and triturating thereafter] reduces diamond into *bhasma* form.

अश्वत्थबदरीमिंडीमाक्षिकं कर्क्टास्थि च ।
तुल्यं स्नुहीपयः क्षिप्त्वा[१०७] वज्रं तद्गोलकं भवेत्[१०८] ।
रुद्ध्वा गजपुटे पाच्यं विप्रजातिः मृतिर्भवेत् ।।२५१।।

Preparing Bhasma of Brāhmaṇa Type of Diamond

Aśvattha, *badarī*, *miṇḍī* [?], *mākṣika* and the bone of *karkaṭa* should be taken in equal quantities and triturated by adding the milky latex of *snuhī*. This paste should be made to a bolus. Inside this, diamond should be kept, covered with *śarāva-sampuṭa*, sealed and cooked in *gaja puṭa* by which the *brāhmaṇa* type of diamond gets reduced to *bhasma* form.

करवीरमेषशृंगं दरदं च उदुम्बरम् ।
अर्कदुग्धैः समं पिष्ट्वा विप्रवन्मारयेन्नृपम् ।।२५२।।

Preparing Bhasma of Kṣatriya Type of Diamond

Karavīra, *meṣaśṛṅga*, *hiṅgula* and *udumbara*, taken in equal quantities, should be triturated by adding the milky latex of *arka*. By keeping diamond inside the bolus of this paste, further processing should be continued as suggested for the *brāhmaṇa* type of diamond by which *kṣatriya* type of diamond gets reduced to *bhasma* form.

बला चातिबला गन्धं विडालं कच्छपास्थि च ।
उत्तरावारुणीदुग्धैर्वैश्योऽपि म्रियते ध्रुवम् ।।२५३।।

Preparing Bhasma of Vaiśya Type of Diamond

Balā, *atibalā*, sulphur and bones of cat and tortoise should be triturated by adding the milky latex of *uttarā-vāruṇī*. *Vaiśya* type of diamond should be further processed [like *brāhmaṇa* type of diamond] by which it gets reduced to *bhasma* form.

सूरणं लशुनं शंखं समं पेष्यं मनःशिला ।

चतुष्टयमिदं पिष्टं वटक्षीरेण लेपयेत् ।
एवं कृते तदा सम्यक् सिद्ध्यते शूद्रवज्रकम् ।।२५४।।

Preparing Bhasma of Śūdra Type of Diamond

Sūraṇa, *laśuna*, *śaṅkha* and *manaḥśilā* should be triturated by adding the milky latex of *vaṭa*. *Śūdra* type of diamond should be further processed [like *brāhmaṇa* type of diamond] by which it gets reduced to *bhasma* form.

रत्नाकरात्
स्त्रियस्तेषां म्रियन्ते तु तत्तदौषधयोगतः ।
[109]नपुंसकमृतिस्तेषां चतुर्णामौषधैः सदा[110] ।।२५५।।

Preparing Bhasma of Female & Neuter Diamond According to Ratnākara

By adding the drugs mentioned above and cooking on the line suggested before, female and neuter types of diamond get reduced to *bhasma* form.

रेखाबिन्दुसमायुक्तं भग्नकं ह्येकतोन्नतम् ।
सत्रासं चिपिटं वृत्तं वज्रं काकपदं त्यजेत् ।।२५६।।

।। इति वज्रलक्षण-मारण-गुणागुणम् ।।

Characteristics of Defective Diamond

Diamonds with lines and dots, which are broken, which are more elevated in one side, which look fearful, which have depressions, which are round in shape and which have marks like the foot of crow should not be used.

Thus, ends the description of characteristics, calcination, properties and adverse effects of diamond.

RĀJĀVARTA (LAPIS LAZULI)

राजावर्तो द्विधा प्रोक्तो गुटिकाचूर्णभेदतः ।।२५७।।

Varieties

Rājāvarta is of two types, viz; one in the form of pills and the other in the form of powder.

शिरीषपुष्पार्द्रकरसैः संतप्तश्च निमज्जितः।
सप्तवारं भवेच्छुद्धो राजावर्तो न संशयः ।।२५८।।

Purification of Rājāvarta

Heated *rājāvarta* should be immersed in the juice of the flower of *śirīṣa* and *ārdraka* for seven times by which it gets purified.

क्षयशूलप्रमेहघ्नो राजावर्तो ज्वरापहः ।।२५९।।

Properties of Rājāvarta

Rājāvarta cures phthisis, colic pain, *prameha* (obstinate urinary disorders including diabetes) and fever.

तच्चूर्णं देवदेवेशि महिषीक्षीरसंयुतम् ।
विपचेदायसे पात्रे गोघृतेन विमिश्रितम् ।।२६०।।
तच्चूर्णं तु सुरेशानि कुनटीघृतमिश्रितम् ।
सौभाग्यं पञ्चगव्येन पिण्डीबद्धं तु कारयेत् ।
धमितं रक्तपीताभं सत्त्वं मुञ्चति शोभनम् ।।२६१।।

।। इति राजावर्त्तशोधनसत्त्वपातनगुणाः ।।

Extraction of Rājāvarta-Sattva

Powder of *rājāvarta* should be added with buffalo-milk and cooked in an iron vessel along with cow's ghee. The powder, thus obtained, should be added with realgar, ghee, borax, *pañca-gavya* (five products of cow, viz; milk, ghee, urine, stool and curd) and made to a paste which further should be made to a bolus form and blown by keeping over fire. Thus, its beautiful *sattva* which is reddish yellow in colour comes out.

Thus, ends the description of purification, *sattva*-extraction and properties of lapis-lazuli.

BRAHMA-PIŚĀCIKĀ (A TYPE OF BORAX)

श्वेतटंकणसंकाशा मता ब्रह्मपिशाचिका ।।२६२।।

Brahma piśācikā is like white variety of *ṭaṅkaṇa* (borax).

सुशीता रक्तपित्तघ्नी तृष्णोरःक्षतनाशिनी ।
रसबन्धकरी नेत्र्या धातुवादेषु पूजिता ।।२६३।।

Properties of Brahma-Piśācikā

Brahma-piśācikā is cooling in potency. It cures *rakta-pitta* (a disease characterised by bleeding from different parts of the body), morbid-thirst and phthisis. It causes *rasa-bandhana* (to solidify mercury and to make it non-volatile). It is useful for the eyes. It is also useful in *dhātu-vāda* (to process mercury for the transmutation of base metals into noble ones).

टंकणवल्लभेच्छुद्धिं'' प्रोक्ता ब्रह्मपिशाचिका ।।२६४।।

Purification of Brahma Piśācikā

Brahma-piśācikā may be purified on the lines suggested for the purification of borax.

ṬAṄKAṆA (BORAX)

धूर्जटिः
टंकणस्त्रिविधः प्रोक्तः स्फटिकाभो गुडप्रभः ।
तृतीयः पाण्डुरः प्रोक्तः शृणु तस्य गुणागुणम् ।
पर्यायो पाण्डुरस्यापि नीलकंठेति विश्रुतः ।।२६५।।

Varieties of Ṭaṅkaṇa
According to Dhūrjaṭi

Borax is of three types as follows :

(1) *Sphaṭikābha* (like crystal stone).
(2) *Guḍa-prabha* (like jaggery); and
(3) *Pāṇḍura* (brownish yellow in colour). It is also called *nīla-kaṇṭha*.

प्रोत्तमो नीलकण्ठश्च स्फटिकाख्यश्च मध्यमः ।
गुडाभश्चाधमः प्रोक्तो रसशास्त्रविशारदैः ।।२६६।।

Relative Merits

According to experts in Iatro-Chemistry *(rasa-śāstra)*, *pāṇḍura* or *nīla-kaṇṭha* type of borax is the best; the *sphaṭika* type of borax is of medium quality; and the *guḍābha* (*guḍa-prabha*) type of borax is inferior in property.

टंकणो द्रावणो भेदी विषहारी ज्वरापहः ।
गुल्मामशूलशमनो वातश्लेष्महरः परः ।।२६७।।

Properties of Borax

Borax helps in the melting of metals. It is purgative. It cures poisoning, fever, *gulma* (phantom tumour), *āma* (diseases caused by the product of improper digestion), colic pain and diseases caused by *vāyu* and *kapha*.

जंबीरजरसेनैव अहोरात्रं विभावयेत् ।
टंकणः शुद्धिमायाति नात्र कार्या विचारणात्[112] ।।२६८।।

।। टंकणशुद्धिः ।।

Purification of Borax

Borax should be impregnated with the juice of *jambīra* for one day and night by which it gets purified.

KAMPILLAKA

रसदर्पणात्
इष्टिकाचूर्णसंकाशश्चन्द्रिकावान्प्रभेदतः ।
सौराष्ट्रदेशे जनितः[113] स हि कम्पिल्लको मतः ।।२६९।।

According to Rasadarpaṇa

Kampillaka is like the powder of brick with dazzling particles. It is available in Saurāṣṭra. [This is a controversial drug. From the description given here, it appears to be a mineral available in Saurāṣṭra. Generally, the pollens of the plant *Mellotus phillipinensis* are used as *kampillaka]*.

पित्तज्वराध्मानविबन्धनिघ्नः
श्लेष्मोदरार्तिकृमिगुल्मवैरि ।

व्रणामशूलज्वरशोफहारी
कंपिल्लको नेत्रगदापहश्च[१४] ।।२७०।।

।। कम्पिल्लकगुणाः ।।

Properties of Kampillaka

Kampillaka cures *paittika* type of fever, flatulance, constipation, diseases caused by *kapha*, *udara* (obstinate abdominal diseases including ascites), parasitic infestations, *gulma* (phantom tumour), ulcers, diseasas caused by *āma* (product of improper digestion), colic pain, fever (in general), oedema and eye-diseases.

Thus, ends the description of the properties of *kampillaka.*

GAURĪ-PĀṢĀṆA (ARSENIC)

गौरीपाषाणकः पीतो विकटो हतचूर्णकः ।
रसबन्धकरः स्निग्धो दोषघ्नो वीर्यकारकः ।।२७१।।

।। गौरीपाषाणगुणाः ।।

Properties of Arsenic

Arsenic is yellow and unpleasant to look at. Its *bhasma* causes *rasa bandha* (making mercury solid and nonvolatile). It is unctuous. It alleviates *doṣa-s* and promotes semen.

NAVAṢĀRA (AMONIUM CHLORIDE)

करीरपीलुजैः कोष्टे पच्यते नेष्टकोद्भवः ।
क्षारोऽसौ नवसारः स्याच्चूलिका लवणश्च सः ।।२७२।।

The *kṣāra* (alkali preparation) prepared by burning *karira* and *pīlu* in an oven *(koṣṭha)* is called *navasāra*. It is not the ash of bricks. It is also called *cūlikā-lavaṇa.*

रसेन्द्रजारणं लोहजारणं जठराग्निकृत् ।
प्लीहगुल्मामशोषघ्नं[१५] भुक्तमांसादिजारणम् ।।२७३।।

Properties of Navasāra and Viḍa Type of Salt

Navasāra helps in the *jāraṇa* (digesting other metals) of mercury and of different other metals. It promotes the power of digestion. It cures splenic disorders, *gulma* (phantom tumour), *āma* (diseases caused by the product of improper digestion) and consumption. It helps in the digestion of the ingested meat, etc.

विडाख्यं[११६] च त्रिदोषघ्नं चूलिकालवणं मतः[११७] ।।२७४।।
।। नवसारगुणाः ।।

Viḍa type of salt, which is also called *cūlikā lavaṇa*, alleviates all the three *doṣa-s*.

VARĀṬIKĀ (COWRIE-SHELL)

पीताभां ग्रन्थिला पृष्ठे दीर्घवृत्तवराटिका ।
रसवैद्यैर्विनिर्दिष्टा सा बराबरसंज्ञका ।।२७५।।

Characteristic Features

Cowrie-shells are yellowish in colour and knotty in their back. These are either long or round in shape. According to experts in Iatro-chemistry (*rasa-śāstra*), this type of cowrie-shells are more useful. This *varāṭikā* is also known as *barābara (varāvara).*

सार्धनिष्का मता श्रेष्ठा दन्तैर्द्वादशभिर्युता ।
रसे रसायने योज्या निष्कभारा च मध्यमा ।
पादोननिष्कभारा च कनिष्ठा परिकीर्तिता ।।२७६।।

Relative Merits of Cowrie-Shells

Cowrie-shells which are one and half *niṣka* in weight and which have twelve teeth are of superior quality. Those, which are only one *niṣka* in weight, are of medium quality. Those, which are only 3/4th of a *niṣka* in weight, are of inferior quality.

परिणामादिशूलघ्नी वृष्यातीसारनाशिनी ।
नेत्र्या संग्रहणीं हन्ति कटूष्णा दीपनी मता ।।२७७।।
पाचनी वातकफहा श्रेष्ठा सूतस्य मारणे[११८] ।
तदन्ये पुंसदारा स्युः[११९] गुरवः श्लेष्मपित्तलाः ।।२७८।।

Properties of Cowrie-Shell

Cowrie-shell cures *pariṇāma-śūla* (colic pain which occurs during the digestion of food). It is aphrodisiac. It cures diarrhoea. It promotes eye-sight and cures *saṅgrahaṇī* (sprue syndrome). It is pungent in taste and hot in potency. It stimulates the power of digestion. It is carminative and it alleviates *vāyu* as well as *kapha*. It is an excellent ingredient for the calcination of mercury.

There are other types of cowrie-shells which are either of male or female types. They aggravate *kapha* and *pitta*.

वराटाः कांजिकेस्विन्नाः यामाच्छुद्धिमवाप्नुयात्[२०] ।।२७९ ।।

।। इति वराटगुणाः ।।

Purification of Cowrie-Shell

Cowrie-shells steam-boiled in a *dolā-yantra* with *kāñjī* (sour vinegar) for one *yāma* gets purified.

रसदर्पणात्

शंखशुक्तिवराटाद्यैः योऽसौ संबध्यते रसः ।

क्षारबद्धः परं दीप्तिपुष्टिकृत्स्थौल्यनाशनः ।।२८० ।।

According to Rasa-darpaṇa

Mercury solidified and made non-volatile by the addition of conch-shell, *śukti* (sea-shell), *varāṭikā* (cowrie-shell), etc., and with *kṣāra-s* (alkali preparations) promotes lustre and nourishment and reduces obesity.

AGNIJĀRA (AMBERGRIS)

सामुद्रेणाग्निनक्रस्य जरायुर्वै समुत्थितः ।

संशुष्को भानुतापेन सोऽग्निजार इति स्मृतः ।।२८१ ।।

Characteristics of Agnijāra

The *jarāyu* (placenta) of *agni-nakra* (a type of whale) in the ocean which gets dried up because of exposure to the sun rays is called *agnijāra* (ambergris).

अग्निजारस्त्रिदोषघ्नो धनुर्वातादिवातनुत् ।
वर्धनो रजवीर्यस्य जीवनो जारणस्तथा ।।२८२।।

।। अग्निजारगुणाः ।।

Properties of Agnijāra

Agnijāra alleviates all the three *doṣa-s*, cures *vātika* diseases including *dhanurvāta* (tetanus), promotes the ovulation in ladies and sperm formation in males and longevity. It helps in the *jāraṇa-karma* (digestion of other metals) of mercury.

GIRI-SINDŪRA (RED OXIDE OF MERCURY)

महागिरिषु '१२१'चाल्पीयात्पाषाणान्तःस्थितो रसः ।
शुष्कः शोणः स निर्दिष्टो गिरिसिन्दूरसंज्ञया ।।२८३।।

Characteristics of Giri-Sindūra

In big mountains, mercury in small quantity comes out of cracks in stones which is dry and red in colour. It is called *giri-sindūra*.

त्रिदोषशमनभेदिः रसबन्धन'मग्निदम् ।
देहलोहकरं नेत्र्यं गिरिसिन्दूरमीरितम् ।।२८४।।

।। गिरिसिन्दूरगुणाः ।।

Properties of Giri-Sindūra

Giri-sindūra alleviates all the three *doṣa-s*. It is purgative. It causes *rasa-bandhana* (solidification of mercury and making it non-volatile). It promotes the power of digestion and causes *deha-siddhi* (rejuvenation of the body) and *lauha-siddhi* (transmutation of base metals into noble ones). It promotes eye sight.

VEDĀRA (LEAD OXIDE)

सदलं पीतवर्णं च भवेद्दुर्जरमण्डले ।
अर्बुदस्य गिरेः पार्श्वे जातं[122] वेदारसंज्ञितम् ।।२८५।।

Characteristics of Vedāra

Vedāra (*mṛddāra-śṛṅga*) is obtained from the Mount Abu of

Gujarat [at present, this mountain forms a part of Rajasthan state]. It is available in the form of scales (having layers) and it is yellow in colour

ससत्वं च मरुत्श्लेष्मशमनं पुंगदापहम् ।
'रसबंधकरं'[२३] श्रेष्टं केशरंजनमग्रिमम्' ।।२८६ ।।

।। वेदारगुणाः ।।

Properties of Vedāra

Vedāra contains *sattva* (metallic essence). It alleviates *vāyu* and *kapha* and cures impotency etc., of males. It causes *rasa bandhana* (solidifying mercury and making it non-volatile). It imparts black colour to hair.

AMṚTĀ-ŚṚṄGA (A TYPE OF COPPER-SULPHATE)

शिखिखर्परकलुषं यज्जातं धान्ययोगतः ।
संज्ञाममृतशृङ्गेति प्रसिद्धं श्रीमते श्रुतम् ।।२८७ ।।

The waste of *śikhī* (Copper sulphate) and *kharpara* (calamine) which comes out by their processing with grains is called *amṛtā-śṛṅga*.

मुखरोगप्रशमनं पाण्डुमेहक्षयापहम् ।
रसबन्धनकार्येषु प्रसिद्धं व्रणनाशनम् ।
प्रस्वेदं गात्रदौर्गन्ध्यं[२४] सरोमंतीं च नाशयेत् ।।२८८ ।।
मुदारशंख इति लोके।।२८९ ।।

।। अमृतशृंगगुणाः ।।

Properties of Amṛtā-Śṛṅga

Amṛtā-śṛṅga cures mouth diseases, anemia, *meha* (obstinate urinary diseases including diabetes) and phthisis. It is famous as an ingredient for *rasa bandhana* (solidifying mercury and making it non-volatile). It cures ulcers, exeessive perspiration, foul smell coming out of the body and *romāntikā* (measles).

It is also called *mudāra-śaṅkha* in vernacular.

साधारणरसा[२५] सर्वे मातुलुंगनिजाम्बुना ।

त्रिरात्रं भाविताः शुष्काः भवेयुर्दोषवर्जिताः ।।२९०।।
सत्वमभ्रकवच्चापि पातयेन्नात्र संशयः[१२६] ।।२९१।।
।। इति साधारणरसाः ।।

Sādhāraṇa Rasa

All the ingredients belonging to the category of *sādhāraṇa rasa* should be impregnated with the juice of *mātuluṅga* for three nights and then dried by which they become purified. Their *sattva* (metallic essence) should be extracted on the line suggested for extraction of *sattva* from mica.

Thus, ends the description of *sādhāraṇa rasa-s*.

KAṄKUṢṬHA (RHEUM EMODI?)

हिमवत्पादशिखरे[१२७] कंकुष्ठमुपजायते ।।२९२।।

Source of Kaṅkuṣṭha

Kaṅkuṣṭha is available in the valley and mountain tops of the Himalayas. [From this description, it appears to be a mineral product but generally a plant product is used.]

तत्रैकं तालिकाख्यं हि द्वितीयं रेणुकं मतम्[१२८] ।
पीतप्रभं गुरु स्निग्धं कंकुष्ठं श्रेष्ठमादिकम् ।
श्यामं पीतं लघुतरं तत्तु नेष्टं हि रेणुकम् ।।२९३।।

Varieties of Kaṅkuṣṭha

It is of two types, viz., *tālika* (with layers) and *reṇuka* (in powder form). The former is yellow in colour, heavy and unctuous. It is of superior quality. The latter is bluish yellow and light, and it is of inferior quality.

केचिद्वदन्ति कंकुष्ठं सद्यो जातस्य दन्तिनः ।
वर्चस्तच्छ्यामपीताभं[१२९] रेचनं परिकीर्त्यते ।।२९४।।
अन्ये तु तेजिवाहानां नालं कंकुष्ठसंज्ञितम् ।
वदन्ति श्वेतपीताभं तदतीव विरेचनम् ।
रसे रसायने नेष्टं निःसत्त्वं बहुवैकृतम् ।।२९५।।

Controversy About Identification of Kaṅkuṣṭha

According to some scholars, *kaṅkuṣṭha* is the stool of the freshly delivered calf of the elephant. It is greenish yellow in colour and it causes purgation.

According to some others, *kaṅkuṣṭha* is the umbilical cord of the calf of the horse. It is white and yellow in colour. It is a strong purgative.

These two ingredients should not be used in the processing of mercury and in the preparation of rejuvenating recipes. Because they are free from *sattva* (essence) and give rise to several adverse effects.

कंकुष्टं तिक्तकटुकं वीर्योष्णं चातिरेचनम् ।
व्रणार्तिशूलगुल्मघ्नं प्लीहार्शःकृमिनाशनम् ।
रसशुद्धिकरं ख्यातं सत्त्वरूपं च केवलम् ।।२९६।।

Properties of Kaṅkuṣṭha

Kaṅkuṣṭha is bitter and pungent in taste, hot in potency and a strong purgative. It cures painful ulcers, colic pain, *gulma* (phantom tumour), splenic disorders, piles and parasitic infestation. It helps in the purification of mercury. It is full of *sattva* (essence).

कंकुष्टं शुद्धिमायाति त्रिधा शुंठ्यम्बुभावितम् ।।२९७।।

।। कंकुष्ठगुणाः ।।

Purification of Kaṅkuṣṭha

Kaṅkuṣṭha, impregnated with the decoction of dry-ginger for three times, gets purified.

VIḌA (CATALYTIC AGENT)

रसार्णवात्

मूलकार्द्रकचिंचानां[३०] क्षारैर्गोमूत्रभावितैः ।
गन्धकः शतशो भाव्यो विडोऽयं हेमजारणे ।।२९८।।

According to Rasārṇava

Sulphur should be impregnated for one hundred times with the solution of the *kṣāra* (alkali preparation) of *mūlaka*, *ārdraka* and *ciñcā* and with cow's urine. Thus, a *viḍa* (catalytic agent) is prepared and it is useful for *hema-jāraṇa* (gold-digestion) of mercury.

चूलिका गन्धपाषाणं कान्तस्य च मुखं प्रिये ।
घृष्टैकमेकपर्यासं लोहमारणजारणे ।।२९९।।

Cūlikā (*navasādara* or *viḍa* salt) and *gandha-pāṣāṇa* (sulphur) promote the appetite of *kānta lauha*. These ingredients should be triturated together and used for the calcination of iron and *jāraṇa* (digestion) of iron by mercury.

एकविंशतिपर्यायं देवदालीदलद्रवैः ।
भावितो निचुलक्षारः सर्वसत्त्वानि जारयेत् ।।३००।।
[द्रष्टव्यम् : रसार्णव : नवमपटल : १५-१७]

The *kṣāra* (alkali preparation) of *nicula* should be impregnated with the juice of *devadālī*. With the help of this, mercury becomes capable of digesting (*jāraṇa*) all types of *sattva-s* (metallic essence).

KĀSĪSA (IRON SULPHATE)

"[131]कासीसं त्रिविधं प्रोक्तं[132] सितं श्यामं च पीतकम् ।
पीतं च पुष्पकासीसं[133] न गरीयो भवेन्मृदुः ।।३०१।।

Varieties of Kāsīsa

Kāsīsa is of three types, viz., white, black and yellow. The yellow variety is called *puṣpa-kāsīsa*. It is not heavy and is soft.

तैजिकं कालमेघाभं नीलं स्यान्मुक्तकालिकम् ।
श्यामपीतं[134] भवेच्चापि उत्तमाधममध्यमम् ।।३०२।।

[The meaning of this verse is not clear; hence left untranslated.]

कासीसं[135] शीतलं चैव श्वित्रनेत्रगदापहम् ।
पित्तापस्मारशमनं रसवद्गुणकारकम् ।।३०३।।

Properties of Kāsīsa

Kāsīsa is cold in potency. It cures leucoderma, eye-diseases, diseases caused by *pitta* and epilepsy. It is useful like mercury.

सकृद्भृङ्गाम्बुना स्विन्नं कासीसं[१३६] निर्मलं भवेत् ।
अथवा भावयेद्धर्मे दिनं जंबीरवारिणा ।।३०४।।

।। कासीसशोधनम्[१३७] ।।

Purification of Kāsīsa

Kāsīsa steam-boiled with the juice of *bhṛṅgarāja* becomes purified. Alternatively, impregnating it with the juice of *jambīra* and exposing it to sun for one day makes it purified. Thus, ends the description of the purification of *kāsīsa*.

GAIRIKA (RED-OCHRE)

गैरिकं तु भवेद्रक्तं भग्नं तु कनकप्रभम् ।।३०५।।

Characteristics of Gairika

Gairika is red in colour but when broken, the broken surface looks like gold.

रक्तघ्नं गैरिकं स्निग्धं हिमं रक्तप्रसादनम् ।
कषायमधुरं हृद्यं चक्षुष्यं कफनाशनम् ।।३०६।।

Properties of Gairika

Gairika is hemostatic, unctuous, cooling and promoter of blood. It is astringent and sweet in taste. It is cardiac-tonic and wholesome for the eyes. It alleviates *kapha*.

गैरिकंतु[१३८] गवां दुग्धैर्भावितं शुद्धिमाप्नुयात् ।।३०७।।

।। गैरिकगुणाः ।।

Purification of Gairika

Gairika, impregnated with cow's milk, gets purified.

SAURĀṢṬRĪ (A TYPE OF ALUM)

कृष्णा पीता तथा कांक्षी चूर्णिकंद्वात्मिका खरा ।।३०८।।

Varieties of Saurāṣṭrī

Saurāṣṭrī is of two types, viz., black and yellow. It is available in the form of powder or *kanda* (?). It is rough to touch.

सौराष्ट्री च भवेदुष्णा विषघ्नी कटुका मता ।
कफपित्तार्त्तिशमनी त्वग्दोषव्रणशोधनी ।।३०९।।

Properties of Saurāṣṭrī

Saurāṣṭrī is hot in potency. It cures poisoning. It is pungent in taste. It cures diseases caused by *kapha* and *pitta* and skin diseases. It cleanses ulcers.

तुंबरी[१३९] कांजिकैः स्विन्ना त्रिदिनाच्छुद्धिमृच्छति[१४०] ।।३१०।।

।। सौराष्ट्रिकागुणाः ।।

Purification of Saurāṣṭrī

Saurāṣṭrī boiled in *dolā-yantra* along with *kāñjī* (vinegar) for three days gets purified.

SPHAṬIKĀ (ALUM)

सुसैन्धवसमाना च कषाया स्फटिका मता ।।३११।।

Characteristics of Sphaṭikā

Sphaṭikā is like rock-salt of good quality. It is astringent in taste.

व्रणोरः[१४१]क्षतशूलघ्नी स्फटिकी भूतनाशिनी[१४२] ।।३१२।।

Properties of Sphaṭikā

Sphaṭikā cures ulcers, phthisis and colic-pain. It also cures parasitic infestation (*bhūta*).

सुराष्ट्रिकावच्छोधनं[१४३] कारयेद्रसविंदकः ।।३१३।।

।। फटिकीगुणाः ।।

Purification of Sphaṭikā

Sphaṭikā should be purified on the line suggested for the purification of *saurāṣṭrī*.

GENERAL METHODS OF PURIFICATION, ETC.

अथ रसालंकारात्

सत्वपातनार्थे सामान्यशोधनम्

महारसानां सर्वेषां रसानां[१४४] शुद्धिरुच्यते ।
तथा चोपरसानां च शास्त्रदृष्टेन वर्त्मनी ।।३१४।।
वन्ध्याकंदपीतवेनी[१४५] स्नुह्यर्कावर्तवायसी ।
चारिः पिप्पलिका चैव कदली सपुनर्नवा ।।३१५।।
कोशातकी मेघनादा वज्रकंदश्च लांगली ।
एषां चैव रसैः[१४६] सम्यक् पटुक्षीराम्लसंयुतैः ।।३१६।।
भावितव्याः रसाः सर्वे चोपविंशोपरिक्रमात् ।
महारसाश्च सर्वेऽपि शुध्यन्त्युपरसास्तथा ।
पश्चाद् ध्माता विमुञ्चन्ति सत्वं बहुलमुत्तमम् ।।३१७।।

General Method of Purification
According to Rasālaṅkāra

Before *sattva*-extraction, all the *mahārasa-s*, *rasa-s* and *uparasa-s* are to be purified on the lines suggested in the scriptures as follows :

All the *rasa-s* numbering more than about twenty, all the *mahārasa-s* and *uprasa-s* get purified by boiling with the juice of *vandhyā-kanda*, *pīta-venī*, *snuhī*, *arka*, *āvarta*, *vāyasī*, *cāri*, *pippalikā*, *kadalī*, *punarnavā*, *kośātakī*, *megha-nādā*, *vajrakanda* and *lāṅgalī* along with pungent, alkaline and sour ingredients.

After purification, these *rasa-s*, etc., should be blown over fire to produce large quantity of excellent *sattva-s*.

गुडगुग्गुलुसौभाग्यं लाक्षासर्जरसः पटुः ।
ऊर्णा गुंजा क्षुद्रमीनमस्थीनि शशकस्य च ।।३१८।।
तथा मध्वाज्यपिण्याकं तुल्यं पेष्यमजापयैः ।
सर्वतुल्यं च धान्याभ्रं भूनागमृत्तिकाऽथवा ।।३१९।।
कान्तपाषाणचूर्णं वा कठिनोपरसाश्च ये ।
मेलयेन्माहिषैः पञ्च दृढा सर्वगुटीकृताः ।।३२०।।

कर्षमात्रप्रमाणा च कोष्ठयन्त्रे दृढं धमेत् ।
अंङ्गारैः खदिरोद्भूतैः त्रिवारं धमनाद्ध्रुवम् ।
निर्मलं पतते सत्त्वमसाध्यस्याप्यसंशयम् ।।३२१ ।।

Extraction of Sattva From Rasa-s, Etc.

Guḍa, guggulu, saubhāgya (*ṭaṅkaṇa*), *lākṣā*, *sarja rasa*, salt, wool, *guñjā*, small fish, bones of rabbit, honey, ghee and oil-cake, taken in equal quantities, should be triturated by adding goat's milk. This paste should be added with equal quantity of either *dhānyābhra* or *bhūnāga-mṛttikā* or powder of *kānta-pāṣāṇa* or the *uparasa-s* which are hard. This should be triturated along with *pañca-māhiṣa* (milk, urine, dung, curd and ghee of buffalo) and made to tablet form of one *karṣa* each. In an oven filled with the fire of the charcoal of *khadira*, these tablets should be blown for three times by which the *sattva* (metallic essence) of even obstinate metals, etc., comes out.

शुक्लदीप्तः[१४७] सशब्दश्च यदा वैश्वानरो भवेत् ।
तदा सत्त्वं तु पतितं जानीयान्नान्यथा क्वचित् ।
तथाग्नौ दक्षिणावर्ते सत्वं प्रपतितं वदेत् ।।३२२ ।।

Nature of Flame During Sattva-Extraction

When the flame of the oven becomes white and bright along with noise, then it should be known that the *sattva* of the ingredient has come out and not otherwise.

When *sattva* comes out from the metal, the flame moves clockwise (*dakṣiṇāvarta*).

यदि सत्वं तु कठिनं भवेत्तत्र मृदुक्रिया ।
सत्वं समस्तं संग्राह्यं काचकिट्टं विवर्जयेत् ।।३२३ ।।

Softening of Sattva

If the *sattva* which comes out of the metal is hard, then it should be further processed to make it soft. While collecting the entire amount of *sattva*, one should reject the glass particles [and waste material mixed with it during the process of extraction].

निक्षिप्य वज्रमूषायां वक्रनालेन संधमेत् ।

स्तोकं स्तोकं ददन्नागं समं द्वि-त्रि-चतुर्गुणम् ।
यावत्सकोमलं तावत्तत्सत्वं योजयेद्रसे ।।३२४।।

Extraction of Soft Sattva

The *sattva* should be kept in *vajra-mūṣā* and blown over fire with the help of an instrument called *vakra-nāla*. While blowing, lead in small quantities should be sprinkled over it. The lead may be added in equal, double, three or four times in quantty till the *sattva* becomes soft and this softened *sattva* should be used for softening mercury.

अथवा कठिनं सत्वं वज्रमूषान्तरे स्थितम् ।
[समं] टंकणसौवीरपिष्टं द्रोणपुष्पीरसेन वै ।।३२५।।
खदिराङ्गारके ध्मातं ढालयेद् गोघृतेन वै ।
कोमलं जायते सत्वं नात्र कार्या विचारणा ।।३२६।।

Second Method of Softening Sattva

The hard *sattva* should be kept in *vajra-mūṣā* after mixing with the paste of *ṭaṅkaṇa* and *sauvīra* made by triturating with the juice of *droṇa-puṣpī*. The crucible should be blown by placing it over the fire of *khadira*-charcoal. The melted *sattva*, thus obtained, should be poured into a vessel containing cow's ghee. Thus, the *sattva* becomes soft.

न सत्वं कठिनं सूते देहे वा क्रमते क्वचित् ।
तस्मात्सत्वं च लोहं च मृदु कृत्वा प्रयोजयेत् ।।३२७।।

Need for Softening Sattva

Hard *sattva* never permeates the mercury or the body. Therefore, *sattva-s* and *loha-s* (metals) should be softened before use.

अथ रसार्णवात्

सत्वपातनकाले हि वह्निलक्षणमुच्यते[१४८] ।
आवर्तमाने कनके पीता तारे सितप्रभा ।।३२८।।
शुल्वे नीलनिभा तीक्ष्णे कृष्णवर्णा सुरेश्वरि ।
वंगे ज्वाला कपोताभा नागे मलिनधूसरा ।

शैले तु धूसरा देवि आयसे कपिलप्रभा ।।३२९।।
अयस्कान्ते धूम्रवर्णा शस्यके लोहिता भवेत् ।
वज्रे नानाविधा ज्वाला स्यात्सत्वे[४९] पाण्डुरा प्रभा ।।३३०।।

Characteristics of Flame During Sattva-Extraction According to Rasārṇava

Durig the process of *sattva*-extraction the flame of the fire depicts different types of colour as follows :

(1) gold-*sattva* produces yellow flame.
(2) silver-*sattva* produces white flame.
(3) copper-*sattva* produces bluish flame.
(4) *sattva* of *tīkṣṇa* type of iron produces black flame.
(5) tin-*sattva* produces flame having the colour of *kapota* (pigeon = brown).
(6) lead-*sattva* produces flame which is dirty and gray in colour.
(7) *śilājatu-sattva* produces gray flame.
(8) iron-*sattva* produces flame of *kapila* colour (brownish black).
(9) *ayaskānta-sattva* produces smoky coloured flame.
(10) *śasyaka-sattva* produces red flame.
(11) diamond-*sattva* produces flame of variegated and yellowish colour.

न विस्फुलिंगा न च बुद्बुदा यदा
यदा न चैप्यां पाटलं [?] न शब्दाः ।
मूषागतं रत्नसमं स्थिरं च
तदा विशुद्धं प्रवदन्ति लोहम् ।।३३१।।

Signs of Purified Loha (Metal)

When the *loha* (metal) remains stable like a gem inside a [crucible placed over fire] without sparkling, bubbling and noise, then it is to be known as purified.

शुल्वे दीप्तिः सशब्दः स्यात्तदा वैश्वानरो भवेत् ।
लोहावर्त्तसमं ज्ञेयं सत्त्वं पतति निर्म्मलम् ।।३३२।।

Characteristics of Flame During the Extraction of Copper-Sattva

While extracting *sattva* of copper, the flame becomes bright with noise like the flame of iron. Thereafter, *sattva* comes out of the metal.

KOṢṬHĪ (OVEN)

षोडशाङ्गुलविस्तीर्णं हस्तमात्रायतं शुभम् ।
धातुसत्वनिपातार्थं कोष्ठकं वरवर्णिनी ।।३३३।।

Preparation of Koṣṭhī (Oven)

For the extraction of *sattva*, the *koṣṭhī* (oven) should be sixteen *aṅgula-s* in diameter (*vistīrṇa*) and one cubit in depth (*āyata*).

वंशखादिरमाधूकबदरीदारुसंभवैः ।
परिपूर्णदृढाङ्गारैरधोवातेन[150] कोष्ठकैः ।
भस्रया ज्वालमार्गेण ज्वालयेच्च हुताशनम् ।।३३४।।

Fuel for Oven

For the extraction of *sattva* of metals, in the oven charcoal of the wood of *vaṃśa*, *khadira*, *madhūka* and *badarī* should be used. The pit should be filled with these charcoal. A tubular hole connecting the outside with the bottom of the oven should be made. Blown with a blower, the charcoal should be ignited in the oven.

रससिन्धुः
यस्य द्रव्यस्य यत्सत्वं तद्गुणैस्तच्छताधिकम् ।
द्रुतिः शतगुणास्तस्माद्रसयुक्तात्ततोऽधिकम् ।।३३५।।

Relative Merits of Sattva, Etc.
According to Rasasindhu

The *sattva* of a substance is one hundred times more potent (than the original substance). The *druti* (liquid form) is one hundred times more potent than the *sattva*. If added with mercury, the *druti* of a metal becomes much more potent.

प्रविततमुखभागः संवृत्तान्तः प्रदेशः ।
स्थलविरचितं चान्तर्जालकं कोष्ठकं स्यात् ।।३३६।।

बकगलकसमानं वक्त्रनालं[५१] विधेयम् ।
सशुषिरनलिकान्या मृन्मयी दीर्घवृत्ता ।।३३७।।

Construction of Koṣṭhī (Oven)

The *koṣṭhī* (oven) should have an open mouth and its interior should be well covered. It should be constructed in a dry land. A wire-net should be fixed below it (leaving space over the ground at the bottom). Like the neck of a crane, the instrument called ***vaka-nāla*** (*vaktra-nāla*) should be fitted at the bottom from out side. There should be another tubular opening from its bottom to the exterior. This tube should be made of mud and it should be long and round.

सिद्धाः सिद्ध्यै समाः नित्यं शूरास्त्यागसमन्विताः ।
असिद्धेनोपहास्येत सिध्ये तु अभिवन्दति ।।३३८।।

।। इति वह्निलक्षणम् कोष्ठलक्षणं[५२] च ।।

Attributes of Physician

Physicians who have attained spiritual perfection (*siddha*) or those who have similar attributes and those who are brave and dedicated should venture into these alchemical processes.

If the aim is not achieved then they are rediculed and if the aim is achieved then they are praised.

Thus, ends the description of the characteristics of the flame and *koṣṭha* (oven).

भवानीमतात्

यस्मादोजः प्रवृत्तिश्च शक्तिवृद्धिस्तथा परम् ।
विना सत्त्वान्न लभ्येत तस्मात्सत्त्वं सुमारयेत् ।।३३९।।

Need for Preparing Bhasma of Sattva According to Bhavānī

Without making *bhasma* of *sattva,* its potency is not manifested and its strength (efficacy) is not enhanced. Therefore, all *sattva-s* should be reduced to *bhasma* form before use.

यस्य धातोश्च यत्सत्त्वं रसोपरसयोस्तथा ।
शोधयेत्तं तथैवात्र यथा धात्वादिशोधनम् ।।३४०।।

।। सत्त्वशोधनम् ।।

Purification of Sattva

Sattva should be purified according to the process prescribed for the respective *dhātu-s*, *rasa-s* and *uparasa-s*.

क्रमशो यद्भवेत्सत्त्वं मूषायां प्रणिधापयेत् ।
मित्रपंचकवत् ध्मातमेकीभवति खोटवत् ।।३४१।।

।। इति सत्वैकीकरणम् ।।

Combination of Sattva-s

Particles of different *sattva-s* should be added with *mitra-pañcaka*, kept in a crucible and blown over fire by which they get mixed up in a liquid form (*khoṭa*).

रससिन्धुः
योषारंगेन संताप्यं सत्वं हन्याच्च ताम्रवत् ।
अन्यानि सर्वसत्वानि ताम्रवन्मारयेद्बुधः ।
मारयेत्स्वर्णवद्वापि[१५३] सत्वानि विविधानि च' ।।३४२।।

।। इति समस्तसत्वमारणम् ।।

Calcination of Sattva-s

Sattva mixed with lac should be cooked on the lines suggested for the calcination of copper by which it is reduced to a *bhasma* form. All the different *sattva-s* should be reduced to *bhasma* form by processing according to the methods prescribed for the calcination of copper or gold.

रसदर्पणात्
कान्तं गगनसत्वं च तथा पाण्ड्यं सुरायसम् ।
पौण्ड्रदेशोद्भवं कांस्यं विद्युज्जं मद्ररंगजम् ।।३४३।।
वानाहं लिंगवानाहं [?] कान्तिसारं च चुम्बकम् ।
एतैस्तु[१५४] बध्यते सूतो भूतिदस्तु परः स्मृतः ।।३४४।।

।। इति रसलोहानि ।।

Metals Useful for Processing Mercury According to Rasadarpaṇa

Kānta-lauha, *sattva* of mica, *pāṇḍya* type of iron, iron from thunder-bolt, iron from Pauṇḍra (name of an ancient kingdom), bronze, meteoric stone, produced in the country of Madra, *vānāha* (?), *liṅgavānāha* (?), *kānti-sāra* (*sattva* of *kānta-lauha*?) and *cumbaka* when, mercury is processed with these metals, it gets solidified and nonvolatile. Thus, ends the description of mercury and other metals.

LAVAṆA (SALT)

लवणानि षडाख्यैषां सामुद्रं सैन्धवं विडम् ।
सौवर्चलं गिडं चैव चूलिकालवणं तथा ।।३४५।।

Varieties of Salt

Salt is of six types, viz., *sāmudra*, *saindhava*, *viḍa*, *sauvarcala*, *giḍa* (?) and *cūlikā*.

अथ रसराजलक्ष्मीतः

क्षारो वा लवणो वाथ जलपाषाणमृण्मयः ।
वृक्षोद्भवो यवक्षारो लवणाश्च चतुर्भवाः ।।३४६।।

Alkalies and Salts
According to Rasarāja-Lakṣmī

Kṣāra-s (alkali preparations) and *lavaṇa-s* (salts) are generally associated with water, stone and mud. The alkali preparation, called *yava-kṣāra,* is made out of the ash of the plant called *yava* (barley). Salts originate from four different sources.

सैन्धवं भूमिसंभूतं सैन्धवं जलसंभवम् ।
सैन्धवं तरुसारोत्थं सैन्धवं गिरिशैलजम् ।।३४७।।

Saindhava Salt

Saindhava type of salt is obtained either from ground or from water or from the heart-wood of trees or from the stones in the mountains.

'समुद्रे'[५५] तत्तु सामुद्रं सैन्धवं सिंधुदेशजम्' ।
सिन्धुकोटरसंभूतं सिन्धोर्यातं तु सैन्धवम् ।
सिन्धुराजसरोजातं[५६] सैन्धवं दुर्लभं भुवि ।।३४८।।

The salt collected from the sea (*samudra*) is called *sāmudra*-salt. *Saindhava* type of salt is obtained from Sindhu-*deśa* (Sindha). It is called *saindhava* because it is available in the crevices by the side of the river Sindhu or inside the river Sindhu (Indus). The *saindhava* salt obtained from the pond of the King of Sindhu is rare.

सैन्धवं मेरुसंभूतं धातुवेधकरं[157] परम् ।
क्वचित्स्याज्जीवसंभूतं विषशान्तिकरं परम् ।।३४९।।
सैन्धवं भूमिसंभूतं त्रिदोषघ्नं गरापहम् ।
जलजं दृष्टिदं[158] शीतं विबन्धघ्नं ज्वरापहम् ।।३५०।।
तरुसारसमुद्भूतं धातुवादे हितं मतम् ।
लोहादिमारणे ज्ञेयं शूलगुल्मामनाशनम् ।।३५१।।

Specific Properties of Different Types of Saindhava

Saindhava salt obtained from the hills is useful in *dhātu-vedha* (transmutation of base metals into noble ones).

A variety of *saindhava* is an animal product and it cures poisoning.

Saindhava obtained from the ground alleviates all the three *doṣa-s* and cures pisoning.

Saindhava obtained from water promotes eye-sight. It is cold in potency. It cures constipation and fever.

Saindhava obtained from the heart-wood of trees is useful in *dhātu-vāda* (transmutation of base metals into noble ones). It helps in the calcination of *loha* (metals), etc. It cures colic pain, *gulma* (phantom tumour) and *āma* (ailments caused by the product of improper digestion).

सुगन्धगन्धकोपेतं लवणं गन्धनादनम्[159] ।
रसायनं परं वृष्यं क्षयपाण्डुहरं परम् ।।३५२।।

Smelling Salt

Salt which is mixed with sulphur produces aroma and it helps in the *jāraṇa* (digestion and assimilation) of sulphur by mercury. It is rejuvenating and excellent aphrodisiac. It excellently cures consumption and anemia.

कुण्डे तु कुण्डलाकारं लोणोरकुण्डसम्भवम् ।।३५३।।

।। इति लवणानि ।।

The salt which is obtained from a tank of saline water is round (whirled) in shape.

Thus, ends the description of different types of salt.

क्षौद्रं घृतं गुडं चेदं विज्ञेयं मधुरत्रयम् ।।३५४।।

।। इति मधुरत्रयम् ।।

Madhura-Traya (Three Sweet Ingredients)

Honey, ghee and jaggery, these three ingredients, taken together, are called *madhu-traya* (three sweet ingredients).

मधुघृतगुग्गुलुगुंजाटंकणमेकत्र पंचकं मित्रम् ।
मेलयति सप्तधातूनंगारारग्नौ तु धमनेन ।।३५५।।

।। मित्रपञ्चकम् ।।

Mitra-Pañcaka (Five Friendly Ingredients)

Honey, ghee, *guggulu, guñjā* and boraxthese five ingredients, taken together, are called *mitra-pañcaka* (five friendly ingredients). These ingredients when added to seven types of metals, etc., and blown over fire help in their combination.

आर्द्रकमूलकबीजं चित्रकमेतत्कटुत्रयं ख्यातम् ।
सूतकदोषविनाशं कुर्यादत्यन्ततीव्रत्वात् ।।३५६।।

Kaṭu-Traya (Three Pungent Ingredients)

Ginger, seed of *mūlaka* and *citraka,* taken together, are called *kaṭu-traya* (three pungent ingredients). They help in correcting the *doṣa-s* (faults) of mercury because of their excessive sharpness.

KṢĀRA-S (ALKALI PREPARATIONS)

तिलापामार्गकदलीचित्रकार्द्रकमूलकान् ।
शिग्रुमुष्ककपलाशान्सर्वमेतत्पुटे दहेत् ।।३५७।।
समालोड्य जलैर्वस्त्रैर्बध्वा ग्राह्यमधोजलम् ।
शोषयेत्पाचयेत्सर्वं मृद्भाण्डेन तु तज्जलम् ।
ग्राह्यं क्षारावशेषं तु धूतक्षारमिदं स्मृतम् ।।३५८।।

।। इति धूतक्षारः ।।

Dhūta-Kṣāra (Washed Alkali Preparation)

Tila, apāmārga, kadalī, citraka, ārdraka, mūlaka, śirgru, muṣkaka and *palāśa,* all these should be burnt in *puṭa*, added with water, stirred and tied through a cloth. The water which comes out of the cloth is dried and cooked in an earthen pot. The *kṣāra* (alkali preparation), thus obtained, is called *dhūta-kṣāra*.

वृन्तक्षारपलाशोत्थो मोचजः कदलीभवः ।
निंबापामार्गजौ शिग्रुमूलकार्द्रकवह्निजाः ।।३५९।।

Vṛnta Kṣāra

The *kṣāra-s* (alkali preparations) of *palāśa, moca, kadalī, nimba, apāmārga,* root of *śigru, ārdraka* and *citraka* are called *vṛnta-kṣāra*. [There appears to be some errors in this verse.]

चरकः

क्षारस्तु न रसो द्रव्यमग्निसंस्कारसंस्कृतम् ।
लवणोषणभूयिष्टं क्षरणात्क्षारसंज्ञितम् ।।३६०।।
[द्रष्टव्यम् : चरक : सूत्र २६:९]

Charateristics of Kṣāra
According to Caraka

Kṣāra (alkaline) does not constitute one of the tastes. It is processed by burning plants, etc., with fire. It is dominated by saline and alkaline tastes. Since it is obtained by filtration *(kṣaraṇa)* it is called *kṣāra*.

रसावतारात्

मालतीरससंभूतं स्वर्जिकायावशूकजम् ।
चर्मकारश्च चत्वारो मुख्यक्षाराश्च कीर्तिताः ।।३६१।।

।। इति क्षाराः ।।

Four Important Kṣāra-s
According to Rasāvatāra

Kṣāra obtained from the juice of *mālatī, svarji-kṣāra, yava-kṣāra* and *carmakāra* (?) are the four important *kṣāra-s* (alkali preparations).

Thus, ends the description of *kṣāra-s* (alkali preparations).

VIṬ (STOOL)

पारावतस्य चाषस्य कपोतस्य कलापिनः ।
गृध्रस्य कुक्कुटस्यापि विड्ढिर्दृष्टो हि विड्गणः ।
शोधनः सर्वलोहानां पुटनाल्लेपनात्खलु ।।३६२।।

The stool of *pārāvata, cāṣa, kapota, kalāpī, gṛdhra* and *kukkuṭa* helps in the purification of all metals. These are also used for smearing the metals and for their calcination.

KṢĪRA (MILK AND MILKY-LATEX)

हस्त्यश्ववनिताधेनुर्गर्दभीछागिकाविका ।
उष्ट्रिकोदुम्बिकाश्वत्थभानुन्यग्रोधतिल्वकाः ।।३६३।।
दुग्धिकानिहुडुंगाश्च तथैवोत्तरकर्णिकाः ।
एषां दुग्धैर्विनिर्दिष्टो दुग्धवर्गो रसादिषु ।।३६४।।

।। इति दुग्धवर्गः ।।

Milk of she-elephant, mare, woman, cow, she-ass, she goat, female-sheep and female-camel, and the milky-latex of *udumbara, aśvattha, arka, nyagrodha, tilvaka, dugdhikā, nihuḍuṅgā* and *uttara-karṇikā* constitute *dugdha-varga* (group of milk and milky latex) for use in processing mercury.

Thus, ends the description of *dugdha-varga* (group of milk and milky-latex).

UPAVIṢA-S (SUBSIDIARY POISONS)

स्नुह्यर्कौ करवीरश्च[160] लांगली विषमुष्टिका ।
एतान्युपविषाण्याहुः पंच नागार्जुनादयः ।।३६५।।

।। इत्युपविषाणि ।।

Nāgārjuna, etc., have described five drugs, viz., *snuhī, arka, karavīra, lāṅgalī* and *viṣa-muṣṭi* as *upaviṣa-s* (subsidiary poisons).

TAILA-S (OILS)

कंगुनी तुंबिनी वेनी करंजश्रीफलोद्भवः ।
घोंटावातारिसिद्धार्थसोमराजीविभीतजम् ।।३६६।।
महाकालातसी निंबकुंसुंभं किणिही[161] धरा ।
अंकोलोन्मत्तभल्लातछानपालासविग्रहान् ।
पुत्रंजीवान्नृकेशांश्च तैलं संग्राहयेद्रसे ।।३६७।।

धराधराधरणीदन्तीति ।।३६८।।

[द्रष्टव्यम्ः रसरत्नसमुच्चय : १०:७१-७३]

।। तैलानि ।।

Kanguni, tumbini, veni (?), karañja, śriphala, ghoṇṭā, eraṇḍa, siddhārtha, somarāji, bibhitaka, mahākāla, atasi, nimba, kusumbha, kiṇihi, dharā, aṅkola, unmatta (dhustūra), bhallātaka, chāna (?), palāsa, putrañjivaka and human hair—these are the sources of oil for processing mercury.

VASĀ (FAT)

मर्कटीहरिमार्जारीकच्छपोष्ट्रजलौकजा ।
शिशुमाराजवाराहखरमेषोभ्रगोभवा ।
नमाहिषगजोद्भूता वसा स्याद्रससाधने ।।३६९।।

।। इति वसाः ।।

Markaṭi, hari (lion), *mārjāri, kacchapa, uṣṭra, jalaukas, śiśumāra, aja, vārāha, khara, meṣa, u(ra)bhra*, cow, human beings, buffalo and elephant—these are the sources of *vasā* (fat) for processing mercury.

URINE, SEMEN AND MENSTRUAL BLOOD

मूत्राणि हस्तिकरभमहिषीखरवाजिनाम् ।
गोजावीनां स्त्रियाः पुंसां पुष्पबीजं च योजयेत् ।।३७०।।

[रसरत्नसमुच्चय : १०:७५]

।। इति मूत्रपुष्पबीजानि ।।

Urine of elephant, *karabha,* buffalo, ass, horse, cow, goat and sheep, the semen of their males and menstrual blood of their females are useful for processing mercury.

PAÑCA-GAVYA, ETC.

गोमूत्रविड्दधिक्षीरघृतं स्यात्पञ्चगव्यकम् ।
एवं माहिषगोजानां [?] पशूनामपि सर्वतः ।।३७१।।

।। इति गोमहिष्यजाविपंचकानि ।।

The urine, stool, curd, milk and ghee taken together are called *pañca-gavya* (five products of cow). Similarly, urine, etc., of buffalo are called *pañca-māhiṣa,* those of goat are called *pañcāja* and those of sheep are called *pañcāvi.* The urine, etc., of other animals are also used for processing mercury.

PAÑCĀMLA (FIVE SOUR DRUGS)

कोलदाडिमवृक्षाम्लचुक्रिकानुक्रिका रसाः ।
पञ्चाम्लकं समुदिष्टमम्लवर्गमतः[१६२] शृणु ।।३७२।।

Kola, dāḍima, vṛkṣāmla, cukrikā and *anukrikā (?)*—the juices of these five sour drugs taken together are called *pañcāmla*. Hereafter, the group of sour drugs will be described.

AMLA VARGA (GROUP OF SOUR DRUGS)

अम्लवेतसजंबीरलकुचं बीजपूरकम् ।
चांगेरी चणकाम्लं च तथा शंखवराटिका ।।३७३।।
अम्बाडं करमर्दं च कपित्थकरुणादिकम् ।
चिंचकं चाथ धान्याम्लमम्लवर्गः प्रकीर्तितः ।।३७४।।
चणकाम्लं तु सर्वेषां एक एव प्रशस्यते ।
अम्लवेतसमेकं च सर्वेषामुत्तमोत्तमम् ।।३७५।।

।। अम्लवर्गः ।।

Amla-vetasa, jambīra, lakuca, bīja-pūraka, cāṅgerī, caṇakāmla, śaṅkha, varāṭikā, ambāḍa, karamarda, kapittha, karuṇa, ciñcā and *dhānyāmla*-these are ingredients of *amla-varga* (group of sour-drugs).

Caṇakāmla, amongst these is very useful. *Amla-vetasa* is the best amongst these sour drugs.

RAKTA VARGA (GROUP OF RED DRUGS)

दाडिमं किंशुकं चैव बंधूकं च कुसुंभकम् ।
समंजिष्ठा हरिद्रा च लाक्षारससमन्विता ।।३७६।।

रक्तचन्दनसंयुक्ता रक्तवर्गः प्रकीर्तितः ।
तीक्ष्णादिसम्यक्शुद्ध्यर्थमिष्टो नागार्जुनादिभिः ।।३७७।।

।। रक्तवर्गः ।।

Dāḍima, kiṃśuka, bandhūka, kusumbha, mañjiṣṭhā, haridrā, lākṣā and *rakta-candana,* taken together are called *rakta-varga* (group of red drugs). Nāgārjuna, etc., have advocated the use of these drugs for proper purification of *tīkṣṇa-lauha,* etc.

PĪTA VARGA (GROUP OF YELLOW DRUGS)

किंशुकः कर्णिकारश्च हरिद्राद्वितयं तथा ।
पीतवर्गोऽयमुद्दिष्टः रसराजस्य कर्मणि ।।३७८।।

[रसरत्नसमुच्चय : १०:८९]

।। पीतवर्गः ।।

Kiṃśuka, karṇikāra, haridrā and *dāru-haridrā* constitute *pīta-varga* (group of yellow drugs). These are useful in processing mercury.

ŚVETA VARGA (GROUP OF WHITE DRUGS)

स्नुह्यर्कश्चेङ्गुदी गन्धाकरवीरपुनर्नवा ।
वर्षाभूश्च सिता दूर्वा कंचुकी क्षीरिणी तथा ।।३७९।।
शंखिनी चार्कपुष्पी च चित्रकः शंखपुष्पिका ।
चन्द्रवल्ली च दुर्गन्धा कुटजः क्षुद्रशंखिनी ।।३८०।।
सितपुष्पास्तथौषधयो[६३] जीवन्त्यः क्षीरसंयुताः ।।
शंखशुक्तिवराटाश्च कूर्माश्मशर्करास्तथा ।
रसकार्यार्थं सिद्ध्यर्थं शुक्लवर्गोऽयमुत्तमः ।।३८१।।

।।शुक्लवर्गः ।।

Snuhī, arka, iṅgudī, aśvagandhā, karavīra, punarnavā, varṣābhū, white variety of *dūrvā, kañcukī, kṣīriṇī, śaṅkhinī, arka-puṣpī, citraka śaṅkha puṣpī, candra valli, durgandhā , kuṭaja, kṣudra-śaṅkhinī, sita-puṣpā, jīvantī,* milk, *śaṅkha, śukti, varāṭaka, kūrpāśma* and sugar these drugs belong to *śukla-varga* (group of white drugs). These are useful for processing mercury.

KṚṢṆA-VARGA (GROUP OF BLACK DRUGS)

कदली कारवल्ली च त्रिफला नीलिका नलः ।
पंकः कासीसं बालाम्रं कृष्णवर्गोऽयमीरितः ।।३८२।।
[रसरत्नसमुच्चय : १०:९१]
।। कृष्णवर्गः ।।

Kadalī, kāravallī, triphalā, nīlikā, nala, paṅka (mud), *kāsīsa* and tende fruits of *āmra* constitute *kṛṣṇa-varga* (group of black drugs).

PAÑCA-DRĀVAṆA (FIVE DRUGS FOR MELTING METALS)

गुडटंकणमध्वाज्यगुंजाद्रावणपञ्चकम् ।।३८३।।
।। पञ्चद्रावणम् ।।

Guḍa, ṭaṅkaṇa, madhu, ghṛta and *guñjā*—these five drugs taken together are called *pañca-drāvaṇa* (five drugs which help metals to melt quickly).

ŚODHANA-TRAYA (THREE PURIFICATORS)

काचटंकणसौवीरं शोधनं त्रितयं परम् ।।३८४।।
।। शोधनत्रयम् ।।

Kāca (a type of salt), *ṭaṅkaṇa* (borax) and *sauvīra* (vinegar)-these are the three excellent drugs for purification of metals, etc.

DRĀVAKA-S (MELTERS)

सूर्यावर्तश्च कदली वन्ध्याकोशातकी तथा ।
वज्रकन्दोदकरसा काकमाची च शिग्रुकः ।

देवदाली च देवेशि! द्रावकाः परिकीर्तिताः[१६४] ।।३८५।।

।। एते द्रावकाः ।।

Sūryāvarta, kadalī, vandhyā-kośātakī, vajra-kanda, udaka-rasā, kāka mācī, śigru, and *devadālī*— these are called *drāvaka-s* (when added to metals, etc., and heated, melting takes place at lower temperature).

KRĀMAKA (HELPERS IN PERMEATING DRUGS)

काचमाची घनरवः[१६५] कासमर्दः कृताञ्जलिः ।
वाराहकर्णी पेयरी हंसपादी शतावरी ।।३८६।।
ताम्बूली नागिनी ब्राह्मी हंसपादी [?] च लक्ष्मणा।
अर्जुनीक्षारनाली[१६६] च कारवेल्लोकपत्रिका ।
व्याघ्री च भीरुपत्री च क्रामिका सुखन्दिते।।३८७।।

।। एते क्रामकाः ।।

Kākamācī, ghana-rava, kāsa-marda, kṛtāñjali, vārāha-karṇī, peyarī, haṃsa-pādī, śatāvarī, tāmbūlī, nāginī, brāhmī, lakṣmaṇā, arjunī, kṣāra-nālī, kāra-vella, oka-patrikā, vyāghrī and *bhīru-patrī* - these help mercury to assimilate other metals and get permeated with them.

EIGHT ROOTS

भूपाटली च गोमारी सिंहवल्ली च सूकरी ।
हेमकर्णी पोटली च नागदेवी च भृंगराट् ।
इत्यष्टमूलिकाः प्रोक्ताः पञ्चरत्नं शृणु प्रिये ।।३८८।।

।। इत्यष्टमूलिकाः ।।

Bhū-pāṭalī, gomārī, siṃha-vallī, sūkarī, hema-karṇī, poṭalī, nāga-devī and *bhṛṅgarāṭ*-the roots of these plants taken together are called *aṣṭa-mūlikā* (eight-roots). Hereafter, five gems will be described.

PAÑCA-RATNA (FIVE GEMS)

मंत्रसिंहासना देवि तथा कंकालखेचरी ।

इन्दिरा च क्षमापाला पंचमं तु निशाचरी ।
पञ्चरत्नमिदं प्रोक्तं रसबन्धनजारणे ।।३८९।।

।। इति पञ्चरत्नम् ।।

Mantra-siṃhāsanā, Kaṅkāla-khecarī, Indirā, Kṣamā-pālā and *Niśācarī*—these taken together are called *pañca-ratna* (five gems) which are used for the *bandhana* (solidification and making thermostable) and *jāraṇa* (stimulating digestive power) of mercury.

MĀRAKA-VARGA(DRUGS FOR CALCINATION)

चाण्डाली राक्षसी व्याघ्री खंगारी[१६७] गजकर्णिका ।
शरपुंखाग्निदमनी लाङ्गली स्थलपद्मिनी ।।३९०।।
रक्तस्नुही रक्तदन्ती[१६८] रुदन्ती हनुमन्तिका ।
त्रिविधाश्चित्रकश्चैव उच्चटा श्वेतगुंजिका ।।३९१।।
काकतुण्डी कलिका च अजभारीन्द्रवारुणी।
ताम्बूली सूर्यभक्ता च बाकुची कृष्णजीरकम् ।।३९२।।
कंगुणी कृष्णकनकं श्वेतार्क चापि पीलुकम् ।
यवः चिंचा च कर्कोटी दन्तिनी कारवेल्लिका ।।३९३।।
गोजिह्वा काकजंघा च सितमंकोलमेव च ।
एकैकमौषधीबीजैर्मारयेद्रसभैरवम् ।।३९४।।

।। इति मारकवर्गः[१६९] ।।

Cāṇḍālī, rākṣasī, vyāghrī, khaṅgārī, gaja-karṇī, śara-puṅkhā, agni-damanī, lāṅgalī, sthala-padminī, rakta-snuhī, rakta-dantī, rudantī, hanumantikā, three varieties of *citraka, uccaṭā, śveta-guñjā, kāka-tuṇḍī, kalikā, ajabhārī, indra-vāruṇī, tāmbūlī, sūrya-bhaktā, bākucī, kṛṣṇa-jīraka, kaṅguṇī, kṛṣṇa-kanaka, śveta-arka, pīlu, yava, ciñcā, karkoṭī, dantinī, kāravellikā, gojihvā, kāka-jaṅghā* and white variety of *aṅkola*-in the *bīja* (essence) of each of these drugs mercury should be calcinated.

APUNARJANMAKĀ VARGA

रंभा चक्रा स्नुहीक्षीरं कंचुकी च विदारिका ।

गोरम्भा चैव मत्स्याक्षी सहसोमा बला निशा ।।३९५।।
सूर्यकान्तं च तुलसी सूर्यभक्ता तथैव च ।
एतैस्तु[170] मर्दितः सूतो पुनर्जन्म न विद्यते ।।३९६।।

।। इत्यपुनर्जन्मकवर्गः ।।

Rambhā, cakrā (guḍūcī), milky latex of *snuhī, kañcukī, vidārī, gorambhā, matsyākṣī, somā, balā, niśā, sūrya-kānta, tulasī* and *sūrya-bhaktā* — if mercury [*bhasma*] is triturated with these drugs, then it does not come back to its original form (becomes unretrievable).

DIVYAUṢADHI-VARGA (GROUP OF CELESTIAL DRUGS)

उच्चटा क्षीरिणी वीरा रक्तवज्री तथैव च ।
कटुहुंची च मुसली काकवल्ली समोहनी ।।३९७।।
तारा[171] कुमारी मुद्राक्षी चाण्डाली स्थलपद्मिनी ।
सूरणं वृद्धदारश्च तथा दग्धरुहा मता ।।३९८।।
नीलज्योतिस्तृणज्योतिः कीटघ्नी रक्तकंचुकी ।
आभिः प्रबध्यते सूतो जारयेत्सारयेत्तथा ।।३९९।।

।। इति दिव्यौषधिवर्गः ।।

Uccaṭā, kṣīriṇī, vīrā, rakta-vajrī, kaṭuhuñcī, musalī, kāka-vallī, samohanī, tārā, kumārī, mudrākṣī, cāṇḍālī, sthala-padminī, sūraṇa, vṛddha-dāra, dagdha-ruhā, nīla-jyoti, tṛṇa-jyoti, kīṭaghnī and *rakta-kañcukī*—these are the *divyauṣadhi-s* (celestial drugs). These are useful for the *bandhana* (solidification and making thermostable), *jāraṇa* (inciting the power of digestion) and *sāraṇa* (increasing permeability) of mercury.

महाभागं गंगयमुनयोः पश्चिमायां दिशि ।
मरुदेशं समाश्रित्य स्थलेषु जायते सदा ।।४००।।
अङ्गुल्या समकीलका ।।४०१।।
वर्षासु शुष्यते सा च हेमन्ते संप्ररोहति ।
क्षिप्रं तु वर्धते सा तु गौश्चैतां तु न भक्षयेत् ।।४०२।।

भग्नेषु प्रस्रवेत्क्षीरं शुभ्रं चातिमनोहरम् ।
पत्रैर्विगतपर्वेयं बोद्धव्या सा महौषधी ।।४०३।।
देवदालीं च संगृह्य गन्धपाषाणमेव च ।
द्रावयेत्सर्वलोहानि पारदं चैव वेधयेत् ।
विस्तरेणास्य कर्माणि प्रवक्ष्येऽहं रसायने ।।४०४।।

।।क्षीरक्षिप्राणामौषधी।।

Kṣiprā

The celestial drug called *kṣiprā* (or *kṣīra-kṣiprā*) grows in the land of the arid zone (desert) in the west of the rivers Ganges and Yamunā. It appears like nails of the size and shape of fingers. It gets dried up in rainy season and grows very fast in the early winter season. Cows do not eat this plant. When broken, milky latex which is white and beautiful comes out of the broken surface. It has no leaves and is in the form of reeds with knots.

This *kṣiprā* (also called *devadālī*) should be added with sulphur (*gandha-pāṣāṇa*) and used for melting all metals. It also helps in the transmutation of mercury into gold. The datails about this drug will be described in the *rasāyana* chapter (of another book).

वक्ष्ये दग्धरुहा ग्राह्या रसबन्धविधायिनी ।
दिव्यौषधी तु सा ज्ञेया सर्वकार्यार्थसाधिनी ।।४०५।।
शस्त्रछिन्नेषु दग्धेषु क्षणमात्रं प्ररोहति ।
'रक्तं[७२] पीतं तथा कृष्णं तस्याः पुष्पं प्रजायते ।।४०६।।
चणकस्येव पत्राणि संप्रभूतं [?] विलक्षयेत्'।
सा स्थिता गोमतीतीरे गंगायां चार्बुदे गिरौ ।
जयन्त्या दक्षिणे भागे न चान्यत्र प्रदृश्यते ।।४०७।।

।।दंग्धरुहालक्षणम्।।

Dagdha-ruhā

Dagdha-ruhā which causes *rasa-bandhana* (solidification and thermostability of mercury) is a very useful drug of celestial origin.

Application of this instantaneously heals ulcers (wounds) caused by weapons and by burn.

Its flowers are red, yellow and black in colour. Its leaves are like those of *caṇaka*. It grows in the bank of the river Gomatī, the Ganges, the Mount Ābu and the south of Jayantī (?). It is not found in other places.

पद्मिनीसदृशैः[१७३] पत्रैः पुष्पेणापि च तादृशी ।
भग्ने चैव स्रवेत्क्षीरं रक्तवर्णं सुशोभनम् ।।४०८।।
आलेप्य वामपादेन पश्येद्गगनमण्डलम् ।
लक्षयोजनतो दृष्टिं सा ज्ञेया स्थलपद्मिनी ।
रसबन्धकरी श्रेष्ठा शस्त्रसंघातरोहिणी ।।४०९।।

।। स्थलपद्मिनीलक्षणम् ।।

Sthala-Padminī

Its leaves and flowers are like those of the lotus. When broken, the stem produces red colour latex which looks beautiful. If the paste of this plant is smeared in the sole of the left, a person looking towards the sky can see objects located one lakh *yojana*. away. It is called *sthala-padminī* and it is an excellent drug for the *rasa-bandhana* (solidifying mercury and making it thermostable). It heals wounds caused by weapons.

नागस्य दमनी नाम विख्याता भुवि दुर्लभा ।
लक्षणं च प्रवक्ष्यामि नालपत्रैश्च सुन्दरी ।।४१०।।
कृष्णनाला भवेत्कान्ता पत्रैस्ताम्बूलसन्निभैः ।
पुष्पैः काञ्चनवत्पीता लक्षणैरभिलक्षिता ।।४११।।
दरिद्रेश्वरो येन तेन सा ईश्वरी मता ।
नागानां दमनी यस्मात्तस्मान्नागदमनी मता ।।४१२।।
तस्या[१७४] रसेन संपिष्टो नष्टपिष्टो भवेद्रसः ।
रणे राजकुले द्यूते व्यवहारे तथैव च ।।४१३।।
मर्त्यानां विघ्नशमनी यत्र तिष्टति सा गृहे ।
बाहुभ्यां मुद्रिकयां वा कक्षायां[१७५] धारयेत्तु ताम् ।।४१४।।

।। नागदमनीलक्षणम् ।।

Nāga-Damanī

The plant popularly known as *nāga-damanī* is very rare. The characteristics of its stem and leaf will now be described. Its tender stem is black in colour and leaves are like betel-leaf. Its flowers are yellow like gold.

Use of this plant makes a poor-man wealthy *(īśvara)* because of which it is called *īśvarī* (giver of wealth). Since it destroys (*damana*) cobra snake (*nāga*), it is called *nāga-damanī*.

Mercury, triturated with the juice of this plant, gets reduced to particles. It annihilates dangers to human beings during war, in the presence of the king, in gambling and in day to day affairs, if kept inside the house. It can also be used as a talisman in the arms or in the form of ring or carried in the axillary fossa.

कूर्माभकंदांकुरितैकनाला ग्रीष्मे सुपुष्पा शुकतुण्डतुल्या ।
एषोघटाकंदरसेन वैद्यो देहानि लोहानि च साधयेद्ध्रुवम्[१७६] ।।४१५ ।।
क्षयं रक्तपित्तं कुष्टं ज्वरं त्रिदोषोत्थं नाशयति[१७७] ।।४१६ ।।

।। उच्चटालक्षणम् ।।

Uccaṭā

Uccaṭā has a tuber like a tortoise. It sprouts in the form of one tubular stalk. It flowers in summer and the flower is like parrot's beak. It is also called *ghaṭā-kanda*. The juice of its tuber helps the physician to attain *deha-siddhi* (rejuvenation of the body) and *loha-siddhi* (transmutation of base metals into noble ones).

It cures phthisis, *rakta-pitta* (an ailment characterised by bleeding from different parts of the body), *kuṣṭha* (obstinate skin diseases including leprosy) and fever caused by the simultaneous aggravation of all the three *doṣa-s*.

क्षीरयुक्ता बहुफला ग्रन्थियुक्ता च या भवेत् ।
एषा वर्तुलपर्णी च मन्यते रसबन्धने ।
हस्तिमेहे शुक्रमेहे योजयेच्छोषिणां हिता ।।४१७।।

।। इति वर्त्तुलपर्णीलक्षणम् ।।

Varttula-parṇī

Varttula-parṇī has milky latex. It has many fruits and several nodes in its stalk. It is used in *bandhana* (causing solidification and thermo-stability) of mercury. It is useful in the treatment of *hasti-meha* (a type of polyuria), *śukra-meha* (spermatorrhea) and consumption.

सर्वौषधीनां प्रवरा रुदन्ती रक्तादिभेदात्क्रमशश्चतुर्धा[७८] ।
तीर्थेषु दृश्या चणकाभपत्रा मूले तथोर्द्धं जलविन्दुयुक्ता ।।४१८।।
रोदितीव जनान् दृष्ट्वा जरया जर्जरीकृतान् ।
येन (मां) जानन्ति यत्नेन मूढाः कालवशं गताः ।।४१९।।
रसायनी त्रिदोषघ्नी प्रेमहार्शोज्वरापहा ।
सूतकार्ये तु सा[७९] प्रेष्टा रुदन्ती परिकीर्तिता ।।४२०।।

।। इति रुदन्तीलक्षणम् ।।

Rudantī

Rudantī is an excellent drug and it is of four types, viz; red, etc. It grows in sacred places. It is called *rudantī* because it provides solace to crying (*roditīva*) human beings because of ailments of old age and who because of their ignorance are destined to die. It causes rejuvenation of the body, alleviates all the three *doṣa-s* and cures *prameha* (obstinate urinary diseases including diabetes), piles and fever. *Rudantī* is useful in processing mercury.

रसार्णवात्

"चित्रकस्त्रिविधो ज्ञेयः कृष्णो रक्तो रसायने ।
शुक्लो व्याधिप्रशमने श्रेष्टो मध्यः कनीयसः ।।४२१।।
कृष्णं चित्रं समुत्पाट्य गोभिरघ्रातमीश्वरि[८०] ।
क्षीरमध्ये[८१] क्षिपेत्कृष्णं क्षीरं कृष्णं प्रजायते ।।४२२।।
तस्य पञ्चाङ्गचूर्णेन पारदं सह मर्दयेत् ।
धमेच्च मूकमूषायां खोटो भवति तत्क्षणात् ।।४२३।।
कृष्णपक्षे[८२] तु पञ्चम्यां रक्तांबरधरो भवेत् ।
रक्तमाल्यानुलिप्ताङ्गो[८३] रक्तशाल्योदनेन वै ।।४२४।।
बलिं दत्वा महादेवि! रक्तचित्रकमुद्धरेत् ।
रक्तचित्रकमन्त्रेण[८४] वंगावापैस्त्रिभिस्त्रिभिः ।।४२५।।
सर्वदोषविनिर्मुक्तः स्तम्भो[८५] भवति तत्क्षणात्" ।

[रसार्णव : द्वादशपटल : १३३-१३८]

केशाः कृष्णाः प्रजायन्ते रक्तचित्रकभक्षणात् ।।४२६ ।।

।। चित्रकत्रयगुणाः ।।

Citraka

According to Rasārṇava

Citraka is of three types, viz., black, red and white. The black and red varieties are useful for the purpose of rejuvenation. The white variety of *citraka* is used for curing diseases. The black variety is superior, the red variety is medium and the white variety is of inferior quality.

The black variety of *citraka,* which is not smelt by cows, should be uprooted and used. If this black *citraka* is added to milk, then the latter becomes black in colour.

With the powder of the five parts (leaf, stem, root, flower and fruit) of black *citraka*, mercury should be triturated and keeping in *mūka mūṣā* over fire it should be blown by which the merc instantaneously becomes *khoṭa* (liquefied).

Red variety of *citraka* should be uprooted on the fifth day of the dark fortnight of lunar month while wearing red cloth and garland and paste of red flowers and after offering the preparations of the red variety of *śāli*-rice in sacred ritual. If *vaṅga* (tin) is wrapped with the leaves of this red-*citraka* and immersed in water for three times, then it becomes free from *doṣa-s* (gets purified) and thermo-stable (*stambha*) instantaneously.

Intake of red *citraka* makes the hair black.

"ज्योतिष्मती नाम लता या च कांचनसन्निभा ।
वल्लीवितानबहुला[१८६] हेमवर्णफला शुभा ।।४२७ ।।
आषाढपूर्वपक्षेऽस्या[१८७] गृह्णीयाद्बीजमुत्तमम् ।
तस्य तैलं समाहृत्य[१८८] ताम्रकुम्भे विनिक्षिपेत् ।।४२८ ।।
तापयेद्भूगतं कुंभं क्रमादूर्ध्वं तुषाग्निना ।
षण्मासे तु व्यतिक्रान्ते तत्कुंभं[१८९] काञ्चनं भवेत् ।।४२९ ।।
'ताम्रं'[१९०] हेममयं कृत्वा तैलमाक्षिकमिश्रितम् ।

प्रतिवापे निषिंचेत्तद्धेमताम्रसमं भवेत्' ।।४३०।।
तथा च शतवेधी स्यात्सत्यं सत्यं मम प्रिये"।
[रसार्णव: द्वादशपटल: १४४-१४७]
भूतोन्मादमपस्मारं तत्तैलेनैव साधयेत् ।।४३१।।

।। इति ज्योतिष्मतीगुणाः ।।

Jyotiṣmatī

The creeper of *jyotiṣmatī* is like gold in colour. It has several branches. Its fruit is golden in colour and auspicious. In the first fortnight of the month of *āṣāḍha*, good quality seeds of this plant should be collected. The oil extracted from these seeds should be kept in a copper jar. The jar should be kept in a pit dug in the earth. Husk of paddy should be kept over it and ignited. This process should be continuously done for six months after which the copper jar becomes gold.

If copper smeared with gold-leaf is heated and immersed into the mixture of *jyotiṣmatī* and ghee or if the mixture of *jyotiṣmatī* oil and ghee is sprinkled over this copper, then it becomes gold. This *jyotiṣmatī* oil makes mercury *śatavedhī* (which helps in the transmutation of one hundred times of base metals into noble ones). It also cures insanity caused by the seizure of evil spirits and epilepsy.

कल्पप्रदीपात्[११]
विषोपविषविख्याता उमा देव्या स्वयंभुवा ।
कथिता सादरे सा तु महेशेनैव पूजिता ।।४३२।।
एरण्डसदृशैः पत्रैः फलैश्चैव तु तादृशैः ।
तस्य पत्राणि[१२] निक्षिप्य पारदेन विलेपयेत् ।।४३३।
द्रावयेत्सर्वलोहानि अभ्रकं च विशेषतः ।
तत्तैलं वा रसं वापि पिबेन्मृत्युहरं परम् ।।४३४।।

।। उमागुणाः ।।

Properties of Umā
According to Kalpa-pradīpa

[There are many errors in the verse no. 432, hence left untranslated.]

The leaves and fruits of *umā* are like those of *eraṇḍa*. Its leaves should be triturated with mercury. By smearing this paste and cooking, all metals and minerals, specially mica, get liquefied. Its oil or juice is excellent for preventing [untimely] death.

शृणु छायाद्रुमस्याथ लक्षणं परमेश्वरि ।
छाया न चलते तेषां छायावृक्षास्ततः स्मृताः ।।४३५।।
नानारूपधरास्ते च बहुप्रत्ययकारकाः ।
अञ्जनस्य प्रभावेण दृश्यन्ते ते न संशयः ।।४३६।।
पत्रं[१९३] जीरकसादृश्यैर्गात्रैर्बिल्वसमप्रभैः ।
शिखास्या ज्वलते नित्यं तस्य[१९४] छाया सुनिश्चला ।।४३७।।
तथा स्कन्धपलाशाभैः [?] पत्रैः[१९५] पुष्पैः फलैः सदा ।
अञ्जनेन भवेद् दृश्यो छायावृक्षो महाद्रुमः ।।४३८।।
लक्षणं तस्य वक्ष्यामि येनोपायेन लक्ष्यते ।
हत्वा कुठारघातेन संतिष्ठेत्तु[१९६] पराङ्मुखम् ।
तत्क्षणाद्रोहमायाति तद्व्रणं नैव दृश्यते ।।४३९।।
वृक्षे दत्वा करं वामं गगनं चावलोकयेत् ।
दिवापि दृश्यते रात्रि रात्रौ पश्येद्दिवा यथा ।।४४०।।
अथ तस्मिन्समारुह्य ऊर्ध्वमस्यावलोकयेत् ।
पश्येत्तारागणं सर्वं यथा रात्रौ तथा दिवा ।।४४१।।
एवं तु प्रत्ययं ज्ञात्वा तस्य पत्राणि गृह्य च ।
अग्नौ क्षिप्तं भवेन्मत्स्यो मत्स्यैकं भक्षयेद्बुधः ।।४४२।।
मूर्छितः पतते तूर्णं पुनरुत्तिष्ठते क्षणात् ।
दृश्यते मेदिनीछिद्रं सिद्धद्रव्यविभूषितम् ।।४४३।।
सिद्धद्रव्यं रसं चैव सिद्धैः संख्यापितं भुवि ।
सिद्धानां सिद्ध्यते सर्वं सिद्धद्रव्यं तदुच्यते ।।४४४।।
अस्य वृक्षस्य यत्स्थानं येनोपायेन गृह्यते ।
यत्र यत्र प्रयोक्तव्यो वक्ष्येऽहं तद्रसायने ।।४४५।।

Chāyā-Druma

The characteristics of the tree called *chāyā-druma* will now be described. The shadow (*chāyā*) of these trees does not move [according to the movement of the sun] because of which it is called *chāyā-drumā*. These are of different types and they have different characteristic features which could be visualised by the application of collyrium [impregnated with *mantra-s* in the eyes]. Its leaves are like those of *jīraka* and the structure of the tree is like that of *bilva*. Its top is always with flame and its shadow is always stable. Its trunk is like that of *palāśa*. It is always with leaves, flowers and fruits. This big tree becomes visible only to a person who applies collyrium [impregnated with *mantra-s* in his eyes]. If it is cut by an axe, it remains stable. The injury to the tree by the axe gets healed up instantaneously and cut surface does not become visible. Keeping the left hand on this tree, if a person looks to the sky, he will see darkness (*rātri*) during the day time and light (*divā*) during night time. If climbing over this tree, a person looks to the sky, he will have the vision of stars both during the night and day time. Having ascertained all these characteristic features, its leaves should be collected and thrown over fire which turn into a fish. One such fish should be ingested by which the man becomes unconscious. But he regains his consciousness instantaneously. He visualises holes in the earth in which *siddhadravya-s* (material which help in attaining physical, mental and spiritual perfection) are stored.

These *siddha dravya-s* and mercury are stored in the earth by *siddha-s* (those who have attained spiritual perfection) for helping the *siddha-s* (aspirants of spiritual persons) to attain *siddhi* (spiritual perfection). Because of this, the material is called *siddha-dravya*.

The habitat of this tree, the method of its collection and its usage will be discussed in the chapter dealing with rejuvenation therapy (of another book).

कटुतुम्बीति विख्याता देवि दिव्यौषधी शृणु ।
तिक्तानि तस्य बीजानि सूक्ष्मचूर्णानि कारयेत् ।।४४६।।
एकविंशतिवाराणि भाव्यं धात्रीरसेन वै ।
पयसा सह तेनैव विश्वभेषजसंयुतम् ।।४४७।।
बीजं यंत्रे[११७] विनिक्षिप्य तैलं संगृह्य पंडितः ।
रसं मूर्च्छायते तेन चक्रमर्देन मर्दयेत् ।।४४८।।

।। इति तिक्ततुम्बी ।।

Kaṭu-Tumbī

A celestial drug called *kaṭu-tumbī* is well known and it will be described hereafter. Its seeds which are bitter in taste should be made to a fine powder and impregnated with the juice of *āmalakī* for twenty one times. It should be added with milk and the powder of ginger. These seeds should be placed in oil-pressing machine and the oil should be extracted. By triturating with this oil, mercury succumbs to *mūrcchā* (lit. swoon) by which the metals remain in small particle form and in a coherent mass form. Thereafter, mercury should be triturated with *cakra marda*.

क्षीरकन्दविधिं वक्ष्ये सर्वसिद्धिकरं परम् ।
चतुर्वर्णविधं तत्र[१९८] रक्तकन्दः प्रशस्यते ।।४४९ ।।
भग्ने चैव स्रवेत्क्षीरं रक्तवर्णं सुशोभनम् ।
मेघानां तु निनादेन संजातैरुपशोभितम् ।।४५० ।।
पत्रैः सेहुण्डसंकाशैः सप्तभिर्हेमसुप्रभैः[१९९] ।
बन्धनं रसराजस्य सर्वसत्वान्वशं नयेत् ।।४५१ ।।

।। इति क्षीरकन्दगुणाः ।।

Kṣīra-Kanda

Now the process of using *kṣīra-kanda* which is very useful, will be discussed. *Kṣīra-kanda* is of four types on the basis of their colours. The red variety of the *kanda* (tuber) of this plant is very useful. If broken, this exudes milky latex of red colour which is beautiful. By the thundering sound of the clouds it becomes endowed with leaves like those of *snuhī*.

These leaves are seven in number and golden in colour. It helps mercury to be solidified and to become non-volatile. It also helps mercury to assimilate all the *sattva-s* (metallic essence) added to it during processing.

देवदाल्याः महौषध्याः[२००] विधिं वक्ष्याम्यतः परम् ।
सा श्वेता व्याधिशमने कृष्णा पीता रसायने ।।४५२ ।।
पौर्णमास्यां त्रयोदश्यां राहुग्रस्ते दिवाकरे ।
अथवा कृष्णपञ्चम्यामिमां विधिवदुद्धरेत् ।।४५३ ।।

देवदालीरसं देवि विष्णुक्रान्ता च सूतकम् ।
मूर्छयेद्वेधयेत्क्षिप्रं[२०१] शुल्वं हेमं करोति च ।।४५४।।

।। इति देवदालीगुणाः ।।

Devadālī

Hereafter, the method of using the celestial drug *devadālī* will be described. It is of three types, viz., white, black and yellow. The white variety is useful in the treatment of diseases and the black as well as yellow varieties are useful in rejuvenation therapies. It should be collected after performing sacred rituals on a full-moon day or on the thirteenth day of the fortnight (according to lunar calender), or on the day of solar ecplise or on the fifth day of the black fortnight of the lunar calender.

The juice of *devadālī* and *viṣṇu-krāntā* makes mercury swooned (reduced to small particle form) and instantaneously makes it capable of *deha-vedha* (rejuvenation of the body) and *lauha-vedha* (transmutation of base metals into noble ones). It transmutes copper into gold.

तृणज्योतिरिति ख्याता शृणु दिव्यौषधिः प्रिये! ।
निशासु प्रज्वलेन्नित्यं नाह्नि ज्वलति पार्वति ।।४५५।।
तस्य मूलेपि निक्षिप्ते क्षीरं रक्तं भवेत्प्रिये ।
तन्मूलरसगन्धाभ्रैर्मातुलुंगाम्लपेषितैः ।
शुल्वपत्रं विलिप्तं तु भवेद्धेमपुटत्रयात् ।।४५६।।

।। तृणज्योतिगुणाः ।।

Tṛṇa-Jyoti

The celestial drug called *tṛṇa-jyoti* will now be described. It dazzles (with flames) at night and does not dazzle during the day time. If milk is poured at its root then it (the milk) becomes red in colour. Root of this plant, mercury, sulphur and mica should be triturated by adding the sour juice of *mātuluṅga*. Thin sheets of copper should be smeared with this paste and cooked in *puta* for three times by which copper gets transmuted into gold.

"अतः परं प्रवक्ष्यामि श्वेतगुंजाविधिं प्रिये ।
कृष्णपक्षे चतुर्दश्यामष्टम्यां च महेश्वरि[२०२]! ।।४५७।।

क्ष्माले मृत्तिकां न्यस्य सेचयेत्सलिलेन च ।
बीजानि श्वेतगुंजायाः पुष्पयोगेन वापयेत् ।
वक्ष्यमाणेन मन्त्रेण कुर्यात्संग्रहणं तथा ।।४५८।।
"ॐ नमो भगवति श्वेतवल्लि श्वेतपर्वतवासिनि
सर्वकार्याणि कुरु-कुरु[२०३] अप्रतिहते नमः स्वाहा" ।।४५९।।
शुद्धशुल्वं च संगृह्य मूषामध्ये तु संस्थिते[२०४] ।
त्रिपंचपलसंख्यातं कर्षार्द्धं सितगुञ्जया ।।४६०।।
सहैकत्र भवेत्तारं तस्य गन्धविवर्जितम्" ।
[रसार्णव : १२ : १८३-१८८]
विधानेन गृहीत्वा तु स्थित्वा[२०५] चैवोच्चटा गृहे ।
यस्य तस्य भवेद् वृद्धिर्धनस्य च सुतस्य च ।।४६१।।
।। इति श्वेतगुंजागुणाः ।।

Śveta-Guñjā

Now the method of using white variety of *guñjā* will be described.

On the fourteenth or eighth day of the black fortnight (of lunar month), when there is *puṣya* (name of a constellation through which the moon passes) asterism in the sky, seeds of the white variety of *guñjā* should be sown on earth kept in an earthen plate. Its seeds should be collected while reciting the following *mantra* :

Oṃ namo Bhagavati śveta-valli śveta-parvata-vāsini, sarva-kāryāṇi kuru kuru apratihate namaḥ svāhā.

Three to five *pala-s* of purified copper should be added with half a *karṣa* of *śveta-guñjā*, triturated, kept inside a *mūṣā* (crucible) and cooked by which the copper gets transmuted into silver without any bad odour.

Sveta-guñjā collected according to the above mentioned method and *uccaṭā* kept in the house help in the promotion of wealth and progeny.

"शुक्लपक्षे पौर्णमास्यां दृष्ट्वा पूर्णेन्दुमण्डलम् ।
निर्गच्छन्ति महीं भित्वा चन्द्रतोयान्यनेकधा ।।४६२।।

कानिचिन्मूत्रतुल्यानि व्योमाभानि[२०६] च कानिचित् ।
चन्द्रवृद्ध्याभिवर्धन्ते क्षीयन्ते तत्क्षयेन हि ।।४६३।।
चतुर्दश्यां च दिग्बन्धं कृत्वा संपूजयेद्[२०७] हरिम् ।
कृत्वा व्रतं पौर्णमास्यां[२०८] रात्रौ तदुदकं ग्रहेत् ।
आलोड्य मधुसर्पिभ्यां पिबेन्मंत्रेण मंत्रितम् ।।४६४।।
दिग्बंधनमन्त्रः[२०९]
'ॐ नमो[२१०] दंष्ट्रोत्कटाय विघ्ननाशाय दिशाम् रक्ष-रक्ष
विदिशां रक्ष-रक्ष रुद्रो ज्ञापयति हुं फट् स्वाहा' ।।४६५।।
पानमन्त्रः
'ॐ नमो भगवते रुद्राय त्रिशूलहस्ताय अमृतोद्भवाय
रक्ष-रक्ष हुं फट् स्वाहा' ।।४६६।।
पीतमात्रेण तोयेन मूर्छा भवति तत्क्षणात् ।
चन्द्रोदये तदा[२११] देवि क्षीरं तस्यानुपाययेत् ।।४६७।।
सप्तरात्रप्रयोगेण चन्द्रवन्निर्मलो भवेत् ।
एकविंशतिरात्रेण जीवेद्ब्रह्मदिनत्रयम्" ।
[द्रष्टव्यम् : रसार्णव १२ : १८९-१९६]
चन्द्रोदकेन देवेशि गुटिकां कारयेद्वराम् ।।४६८।।
।। चन्द्रोदकगुणाः ।।

Candrodaka (Moon-Water)

On the full-moon day of the bright fortnight (of lunar calender), because of the vision of the aura of full-moon, different types of *candrodaka* (moon-water) spring out of the earth by penetration. Some of these are like urine and some others have blue colour like the sky. The water of these springs increases in quantity as the moon increases in size [during the bright fortnight] and decreases in quantity as the moon decreases in size [during the dark fortnight].

On the fourteenth day of the [bright] fort-night, prayer should be offered to Lord Hari, having done the ritual (recited the *mantra*) of *digbandha* (protection from all the ten directions) and having practised penance, one should collect this water (*candrodaka*) at the night of full-moon day and mixed with honey and ghee it should be impregnated (sanctified) with the *mantra* and taken. The *mantra* for *digbandha* is as follows :

"Oṃ namo daṃṣṭrotkaṭāya, vighna nāśāya diśām rakṣa rakṣa vidiśām rakṣa rakṣa rudro jñāpayati huṃ phaṭ svāhā."

The *mantra* for drinking this water is as follows :

Oṃ namo bhagvate Rudrāya triśūlahastāya amṛto-dbhavāya rakṣa rakṣa huṃ phaṭ svāhā.''

Immediately after drinking the water, the person gets fainted. After moon-rise, he should be given milk to drink. By using this water for seven days, the person becomes clean like the moon. If he takes the water for twenty one days (nights) then he lives for three days of Lord Brahmā (*Brahma-dina*).

With the help of this *candrodaka* (moon-water) the mercury tablet should be prepared which is very useful.

अतः परं प्रवक्ष्यामि कर्त्तरीतोयमुत्तमम् ।
असुराणां समायोगात्क्रोधाविष्टेन चेतसा ।।४६९।।
सुदर्शनं महाचक्रं प्रेरितं मुरवैरिणा ।
भालपट्टे ततस्तस्य निपेतुः स्वेदविन्दवः[212] ।।४७०।।
ते भूमौ पतिता जाता कर्त्तरीरससंज्ञिताः ।
रक्षार्थं स्थापितं तत्र विष्णुना च सुदर्शनम् ।।४७१।।
चक्रतुल्यं भवेदेतदायुधानि निकृन्तति ।
कुरुते गर्ज्जनं तादृक् धूमज्वालां विमुञ्चति ।।४७२।।
कर्त्तरीदृष्टिमात्रेण तथान्या[213] शब्दकर्त्तरी ।
[रसार्णव : १२ : २०१-२०५]
तस्य संयोगमात्रेण रसो बद्धो भवेद् ध्रुवम् ।।४७३।।

।। इति कर्त्तरीतोयगुणाः ।।

Karttari-Toya

Hereafter, *karttari-toya* will be described. In the days of yore, Lord Viṣṇu, the enemy of the demon Mura, became very angry during the conflict with the demons and impelled his *Sudarśana-cakra* as a result of which sweat drops appeared in His forehead. These sweat drops fell upon the earth which gave rise to *karttarī-rasa*. For the protection of this *karttarī rasa*, Lord Viṣṇu has kept the *Sudarśana cakra* because of which it whirls and cuts down any weapon placed near it. It also produces roaring sound and smoky flame like *sudarśana-cakra*. Coming in contact with *karttarī* another substance called *śabda-karttarī* is produced. [The meaning of this line is not clear.] Mercury undoubtedly becomes *baddha* (solid) by the addition of this *karttarī rasa*.

विषोदकं विषसमं घृतवच्च घृतोदकम् ।
सितपीतादिवर्णाढ्यं तच्च देवि! रसोत्तमम् ।।४७४।।
केशाः क्षिप्ताः स्फुटन्त्यस्मिन्नात्मछाया प्रदृश्यते ।
तैलं च गोलकाकारं घृतं चैव विसर्पति ।।४७५।।
गन्धकस्य हरेद् गन्धं लवणं कललायते ।
आप्त्वा पलाशपत्रेण कटुकालाबुकं क्षिपेत् ।।४७६।।
[रसार्णव : १२ : २१३-२१६]

विषपानीयमादाय वंगमावर्तितं शुभम् ।
निषिक्तं तच्च तत्तोये तारं भवति शोभनम् ।।४७७।।
सूतकर्मणि सर्वत्र योजयेच्च विषोदकम् ।।४७८।।
।। इति विषोदकगुणाः ।।

Viṣodaka, Etc.

Viṣodaka (poisonous water) is like poison. Similarly, *ghṛtodaka* (ghee-water) is like ghee. These waters are of different types on the basis of their colours, viz, white, yellow, etc. These are useful for processing mercury. When hair is thrown into this water, it cracks. A person can not see his own shadow in this water. When oil is dropped over the surface of this water it does not spread but remains in its round shape. Ghee dropped over it, however, spreads. It takes away the smell of sulphur, and salt added with this water becomes soft. In a cup made of the leaves of *palāśa*, this *viṣodaka* (poisonous water) should be kept. To this, the juice of *kaṭukālābu* (bitter variety of *alābu*) should be added. Melted tin should be sprinkled with this liquid. Thus, the tin gets transmuted into beautiful silver. For processing mercury, *viṣodaka* should always be used.

"अस्ति मर्त्ये महापुण्या पवित्रा पापनाशिनी।
नदी गोदावरी नाम प्रसिद्धा जाह्नवी यथा ।।४७९।।
दक्षिणे च तटे तस्याः पंपली (कदली)नगरं वरम्।
तस्य दक्षिणतः शैलः सर्वलोकेषु विश्रुतः।।४८०।।
नाम्ना कृष्णगिरिश्चेति दृश्यते[२१४] सर्वमङ्गलः ।
सुप्रसिद्धाम्बिका[२१५] नाम ग्रामस्तस्यास्ति सन्निधौ।।४८१।।
तत्र संजीवनं जलम् ।।४८२।।
तिष्ठते तत्परीक्षार्थं शुष्कवंशं परिक्षिपेत् ।
जायते हरितं स्निग्धं दिनरात्रैकयोगतः ।।४८३।।
भवत्यंकुर[२१६]पत्राणि दृश्यतेऽतिमनोहरम् ।
क्षेत्राधिपं महेशं च योगिनीं तृप्य चाहरेत्" ।।४८४।।
[रसार्णव : १२ : २३६-२४१]

रसमारणकार्यार्थे बन्धनार्थे सुरेश्वरि ! ।
धातुवादे देहवादे जलमेतत्प्रयोजयेत् ।
इतिकर्त्तव्यता चास्य प्रवक्ष्येऽहं रसायने ।।४८५।।
।। इति संजीवनोदकम् ।।

Sañjīvana Jala (Life-Giving Water)

On the earth, there is a great sacred river called Godāvarī which annihilates all sins like the Ganges. In its southern bank, there is a beautiful township called Pampalī (Kadalī). At the south of this township, there is a mountain called Kṛṣṇagiri which is auspicious. Near this mountain there is a famous village called Ambikā. *Sañjīvana* water is available there.

To test the genuineness of this water, one should throw a piece of dried bamboo into it. In one day and night, this bamboo becomes green with sprouts and leaves, and looks beautiful. This water should be collected after propitiating the tutelary deity of the locality, Maheśa and Yoginī.

This water should be used for the calcination (*māraṇa*) and *bandhana* (solidification and making thermo-stable) of mercury. It is also useful in *dhātu-vāda* (transmutation of base metals into gold) and *deha-vāda* (rejuvenation of the body). The method of its administration will be described in the chapter dealing with rejuvenation therapy (of another book).

महीं समुद्धृतवतो[२१७] वाराहस्य क्लेवरात् ।
यः स्वेदः पतितस्तस्माज्जातं[२१८] शैलोदकंवरम् ।।४८६।।
कर्दमाभो मही[२१९] शैलं चौलं चेति चतुर्विधम् ।
तन्मुखे क्षणिके जाते काण्डदेशे तु वासरान् ।।४८७।।
बाहुभ्यां त्र्यहवेधी स्यान्मासवेधी तु पार्श्वयोः ।
षण्मासमपरागोत्थं[२२०] सर्वं समफलं भवेत् ।।४८८।।
काष्ठं वा यदि वा पत्रं चर्मशंखादिकं तथा ।
क्षिप्तं शिला भवेद्यत्र तच्छैलोदकमुच्यते ।।४८९।।
गन्धकं तालकं चैव तोयपूर्णे घटे क्षिपेत् ।
यदा तद्बुद्बुदाकारं तदा शैलोदकं भवेत् ।।४९०।।
अन्यथा वेष्टकं तच्च यदग्राह्यं निरर्थकम् ।
वासरं माल्यवन्ते तु क्षणवेधी तु तत्र तु ।।४९१।।
श्रीशैले[२२१] श्रीवनप्रांते पर्यंकाख्ये शिलातले ।
तत्रस्थं क्षणवेधी स्यान्नद्यां भगवतीतटे ।।४९२।।
एकाहे वेधकं तत्र गोकर्णे तु दिनत्रयम् ।
भद्रांगे क्षणवेधी च त्रिस्थल्यांते[२२२] त्रिवासरम् ।।४९३।।
तारेश्वरे पाक्षिकं स्याद्वर्षापुर्यां दिनैकतः ।
ब्रह्मेश्वरे मासिकं स्यात् व्याघ्रपूरे तु वासरम् ।।४९४।।
अघोरेशे मासिकं तु सिंहद्वीपे तथा पुनः ।
दिनमेकं ब्रह्मगिरौ विन्ध्यैकक्षणवेधकम् ।।४९५।।

Śailodaka (Water from Mountain Spring)

When Vārāha (one of the incarnation of Lord Viṣṇu) was retrieving the earth from delusion, the sweat of it which fell down on the earth gave rise to *śailodaka* (mountain-water) which is very useful.

It is of four types, viz, *kardamābha*, *mahī*, *śaila* and *caula*.

In the mouth (opening) of this spring *rasa-vedha* takes place in one moment, in its branches *rasa-vedha* takes place in one day, in its tributaries (arms) *rasa-vedha* takes place in three days, in its sides *rasa-vedha* takes place in one month and in its head *rasa- vedha* takes place in six months. All of them have, however, the same effect.

If a piece of wood or a leaf or skin or conch-shell, etc., are thrown into this water, they change into pieces of stone.

If in a jar containing this water, sulphur or orpiment is thrown in, then bubbles appear.

If the water does not stand to these tests, then it should not be used as it is ineffective.

In the *śailodaka* collected from the mountain called Mālyavanta, *rasa-vedha* takes place in one moment.

In the mountain Śrīśaila near the forest Śrīvana, the *śailodaka* available below the stone called Paryaṅka causes *rasa-vedha* in one moment. In the *śailodaka* available at the bank of the river Bhagavatī, *rasa-vedha* takes place in one day. In the *śailodaka* available in Gokarṇa, *rasa-vedha* takes place in three days. In the *śailodaka* available at Bhadrāṅga, *rasa-vedha* takes place in one moment. In the *śailodaka* available at Tristhalī, *rasa-vedha* takes place in three days. In the *śailodaka* available at Tāreśvara, *rasa-vedha* takes place in one fort-night. In the *śailodaka* available in Varṣa-purī, *rasa vedha* takes place in one day. In the *śailodaka* available at Brahma-pura, *rasa-vedha* takes place in one month. In the *śailodaka* available at Vyāghra-pūra, *rasa-vedha* takes place in one day. In the *śailodaka* available at Aghoreśa and Siṃha dvīpa, *rasa vedha* takes place in one month. In the *śailodaka* available at Brahma-giri, *rasa-vedha* takes place in one day. In the *śailodaka* available in the Vindhya mountain, *rasa-vedha* takes place in one moment.

किष्किन्ध्यापर्वते रम्ये पंपातीरे तृणोदकम् ।
शोणभद्रनदे देवि तिष्ठते चार्धवार्षिकम् ।।४९६।।
शरद्ग्रीष्मवसन्तेषु हेमन्ते ग्राहयेद्बुधः ।
आयसे ताम्रपात्रे वा पात्रेऽलाबुमयेऽथवा ।।४९७।।
अघोरेण[२१] हि मन्त्रेण रक्षां कृत्वा दिशाबलिम् ।
दत्वा लक्षं जपित्वाऽथ गृह्णीयादमृतोपमम् ।।४९८।।

कुलत्थाष्टगुणं वारि पचेदष्टावशेषितम् ।
चतुर्गुणेन तेनाज्यं पाचयेद्धृतशेषितम् ॥४९९॥
लिह्यान्मधुसमोपेतं त्रिसप्ताहादृहस्पतिः ।
द्विरष्टवर्षकक्करः सहस्रायुर्न संशयः ॥५००॥
अवशिष्टं कुलत्थं तु पादांशं मधुसर्पिषा ।
भक्षयेत्कर्षमेकं तु मासेनायुतजीवति ॥५०१॥
तत्सिद्धतैलेनाभ्यङ्गं भक्षणं[२२४] वापि कारयेत् ।
पामाविचर्चिकादद्रुकुष्टादीन्[२२५] सहसा जयेत् ॥५०२॥
शैलतोयादिभिर्बद्धो जलबद्धः स उच्यते[२२६] ।
स राजरोगमृत्युघ्नः कल्पोक्तफलदायकः ॥५०३॥
[द्रष्टव्यम् : रसार्णव १२ : २७७-२९९]

Tṛṇodaka (Grass-Water)

In the mount Kiṣkindhyā, there is a lake called Pampā. In the bank of this lake *tṛṇodaka* (grass-water) remains for six months. It should be collected during autumn, summer, spring or early winter and stored in a vessel of iron or copper or made of the outer-shell of the fruit of *alābu*. It should be protected (sanctified) with *Aghora-mantra*. After offering oblation to the ten directions and reciting *Aghora-mantra* for one lakh times, this water should be used and it is like ambrosia.

One part of *kulattha* and eight parts of this water should be boiled till one eighth of water remains. To this, four times of ghee should be added and cooked till one fourth remains. This medicated ghee should be mixed with equal quantity of honey and taken for three weeks which makes a person intelligent like Bṛhaspati. If it is taken for sixteen years then the person lives for thousand years. If the *kulattha* which is filtered out is taken in the dose of one *karṣa* added with one fourth in quantity of honey and ghee for one month then the person lives for *ayuta* (ten thousand) years.

Oil cooked with it should be used externally for massage and internally which instantaneously cures scabies, eczema, ring-worm, *kuṣṭha* (obstinate skin diseases including leprosy) and tuberculosis. It prevents death and rejuvenates body. Mercury solidified and made non-volatile with *śailodaka* and *uṣṇodaka* (water of hot springs) is called *jala-baddha*.

शैलतोयोष्णतोयस्य कर्म वक्ष्ये[२७] रसायने ।
गन्धाकरोपरिस्थं च भवेदुष्णोदकं प्रिये ।।५०४।।
उष्णोदकं भवेद्यत्र वसेत्तत्रैव योगवित् ।
उष्णोदपाचितं खादेत्कुलत्थं क्षीरपो भवेत् ।
स्नानमुष्णाम्बुना कुर्याज्जीवेद्वर्षशतत्रयम् ।।५०५।।

।। इति चन्द्रोदककर्त्तरीविषसंजीवनशैलोष्णोदकनां लक्षणम् ।।

Uṣṇodaka (Water of Hot Springs)

The actions of *śailatoya* (water from mountain springs) and *uṣṇa toya* (water of hot-springs) will be described in the chapter dealing with rejuvenation therapy (of another book).

The water-spring which is located above a sulphur mine is called *uṣṇodaka* (hot-spring). A yogi should inhabit the locality of hot spring. He should eat *kulattha* cooked with the water of hot spring and drink milk. He should take bath in the hot spring. By doing so, he lives for three hundred years.

Thus, ends the description of the characteristics of *candrodaka, karttari-toya, viṣodaka, sañjīvana toya, śailodaka* and *uṣṇodaka.*

AHIPHENA (OPIUM)

समुद्रे चैव जायन्ते विषमत्स्याश्चतुर्विधाः ।
तेभ्यः फेनं समुद्भूतमहिफेनं चतुर्विधम् ।।५०६।।
केचिद्वदन्ति सर्पाणां फेनं स्यादहिफेनकम् ।
चारणे श्वेतवर्णं च कृष्णवर्णं च मारणे ।।५०७।।
सारणे पीतवर्णं च रक्तवर्णं च जारणे ।
विषवद्ध्युत्तमं फेनं युज्यते रसकर्मणि ।।५०८।।

Controversy About Source of Ahiphena

In the sea, there are four types of poisonous fish from the froth of which four types of *ahiphena* take their origin.

According to some, the froth of snakes is called *ahiphena.*

In the *cāraṇa saṃskāra* of mercury, white type of *ahiphena* is useful. In the *mārana, sārana* and *jārana samskāra-s* of mercury black, yellow and red types of *ahiphena* is useful respectively. Like a poison, good quality of *ahiphena* should be used in processing mercury.

अथापरः
मिश्रदेशे भवेत्कृष्णं खसखससमुद्भवम् ।
सारणं मारणं चैव चारणं जारणं तथा ।
दीपाग्रे रोपणात्तस्य भातीव[२२८] स्यात्तु नान्यथा ।।५०९।।

Another View

In the country of Miśra (Egypt), black type of *ahiphena* is extracted from the plant called *khasa-khasa*, and it is useful in *sārana, mārana, cārana* and *jārana samskāra-s* of mercury. If [with the help of a stick] this *ahiphena* is placed in the flame of a lamp, it dazzles; otherwise it is not of genuine quality.

शाल्मलीमूलतोयेन भावितः शुद्धिमृच्छति[२२९] ।।५१०।।
।। अहिफेनजातिशोधनम् ।।

Purification of Ahiphena

Ahiphena, impregnated with the juice of the root of *śālmalī*, becomes purified.

MALINA (INTOXICANTS)

कक्षापुटिः
भंगाहिफेनधुत्तूरमिलितं मलिनं विदुः ।
शीतज्वरहरं ज्ञेयं रसशुद्धिप्रदायकम् ।।५११।।
।। इति मलिनगुणाः ।।

According to Kakṣāpuṭi

Bhaṅgā, ahiphena and *dhuttūra*, these three taken together are called *malina* (group of intoxicants). They cure *śīta-jvara* (fever with cold) and help in the purification of mercury.

विषाणि हालाहलवत्सनागं
तथा च पीतासितशुक्लकानि ।
स्युर्मुस्तकाश्वशर्ययसंज्ञकं
चेत्यष्टौ रसादावुपयोजितानि ।।५१२।।

[There are errors in this verse; hence left untranslated.]

कालकूटं मेषशृङ्गी दर्दुरं च हलाहलम् ।
कर्कटं[२३०] ग्रन्थिः हारिद्रं रक्तशृङ्गी च केसरम् ।।५१३।।
यमदंष्ट्रेति दशधा महाविषमिति स्मृतम् ।
तथा त्रीण्यपराण्याहुर्नागारबुश्वाच्च[२३१] फेनकम् ।।५१४।।

Mahā-Viṣa-s (Strong Poisons)

Kālakūṭa, meṣaśṛṅgī, dardura, halāhala, karkaṭa, granthi, hāridra, rakta-śṛṅgī, kesara and *yama-daṃṣṭrā*these are the ten strongly poisonous ingredients.

The other three strong poisons are the *phena* (frothy saliva) of snake, rat and rabid dog.

रसराजलक्ष्मीतः
'गरलं[२३२] वत्सनाभं च लाङ्गलीकन्दमेव च ।
छागलं माहिषं पित्तं पञ्चामृतमितीरितम् ।।५१५।।
सन्निपातोदरं श्वासं कुष्ठं जयति योजितम् ।
ताम्रादिदोषशान्त्यर्थं शोधनाय प्रयोजयेत्' ।।५१६।।

।। पंचामृत[२३३] परम् ।।

Pañcāmṛta (Five Nectars)
According to Rasa-rāja-lakṣmī

Garala (snake venom), *vatsa-nābha, lāṅgalī-kanda,* bile of goat and bile of buffalo — these five ingredients taken together are also called *pancāmṛta* (five-nectars). These are useful in *sānnipātika* type of *udara* (abdominal diseases), asthma and *kuṣṭha* (obstinate skin diseases including leprosy). These are also useful in counter-acting the adverse effects of metals like copper, etc., and for their purification.

मृतसूताभ्रकं लोहं विषं यत्तुल्यवीर्यकम् ।
तस्माद्विषं योगवाहि रसे[२३४] योज्यं रसायने ॥५१७॥

Properties

The *bhasma* of mercury, the *bhasma* of mica and poisons mentioned above are of similar potency (attributes). Therefore, like the former two ingredients, these poisons are *yogavāhī* (which enhance the properties of other drugs). These poisons should be used for processing metals (specially mercury) and in the preparation of rejuvenating recipes.

यवाष्टकं भक्षयेत्तस्मादभ्यस्तं[२३५] तिलमात्रया ।
सर्वरोगप्रशमनं पुष्टिदृष्टिबलप्रदम्[२३६] ॥५१८॥

Mode of Administration

Eight *yava-s* (weight of barley grains) of these poisons should be regularly used in the dose of one *tila* (grain of sesame) each time. It cures all diseases and promotes nourishment as well as eye-sight.

शृंगी च वत्सनाभं च कालकूटमिति त्रिधा ।
महाविषं समाख्यातं अन्ये चोपविषाः स्मृताः ॥५१९॥

Three Types of Mahā-Viṣa

Śṛṅgī, vatsa-nābha and *kālakūṭa*--these are the *mahā-viṣa-s* (strong-poisons). The remaining poisonous ingredients are called *upaviṣa-s* (subsidiary poisons).

विषं शृङ्गाभिसंज्ञेयं रक्तं पीतं च मेचकम् ॥५२०॥

Śṛṅgī-Viṣa

Śṛṅgī-viṣa is of three types, viz., red, yellow and muddy-coloured

अथ रससिन्धुः
गोशृङ्गवद्विद्रुधा कन्दः श्वेतः स्याद्बहिरन्तरे ।
सा श्वेतशृङ्गी विज्ञेया योज्या सर्वत्र कर्मणि ॥५२१॥
गोशृङ्गाग्रेऽथ संलिप्ते नासयासृक् प्रवर्तते ।
कंदो लघु गोस्तनवद्रक्तशृङ्गीति तद्विषम् ॥५२२॥

According to Rasasindhu

Śṛṅgī-viṣa is like the horn of cows. It is tuber. It is of two types, viz., white and red. The white variety is called *śveta-śṛṅgī* and the tuber of it is white both externally and internally. It is useful in all types of recipes. If the paste of it is applied over the horn of the cows, then it causes bleeding from the nose.

The tuber of the *rakta-śṛṅgī* is red in colour, it is light and it looks like the nipple of cows.

ग्रन्थान्तरात्

रक्तं सर्वोत्तमं मध्यं पीतं कृष्णं तथाऽधमम् ।
रसायने रक्तशृङ्गी अजरामरकारका ।
तस्य संस्पर्शने दुग्धं सफेनं घनतां व्रजेत् ।।५२३।।
पीतशृङ्गी च विज्ञेया[२३७] रक्तशृङ्गीवदेव हि ।
रक्तिकामानतो हन्ति सन्निपातं ध्रुवं वचः ।
कृष्णशृङ्गी सूतबन्धं कुर्यादिव न संशयम् ।।५२४।।

।। इति शृङ्गीविषम् ।।

According to Another Text

Śṛṅgī-viṣa is of three types, viz., red which is the best; yellow which is of medium quality; and black which is of inferior quality.

Red variety of *śṛṅgī* is useful in rejuvenation therapy. It prevents ageing and [premature] death. If milk comes in contact with it, the former becomes frothy and dense.

Yellow variety of *śṛṅgī* is like *rakta-śṛṅgī*. If taken in the dose of one *rattī* it certainly cures diseases (fever) caused by *sannipāta* (simultaneous aggravation of all the three *doṣa-s)*.

The black variety of *śṛṅgī* causes *bandhana* (solidification and making thermo-stable) of mercury.

मेषशृङ्गाकृतिः कन्दो मेषशृङ्गीति सोच्यते ।
उदरेषु च देया स्यात्तथा सूतप्रबन्धने ।।५२५।।

।। इति मेषशृङ्गी विषम् ।।

Meṣa-śṛṅgī

Meṣa-śṛṅgī is like the horn of a sheep. It is useful in *udara* —

(obstinate abdominal diseases including ascites). It helps in the *bandhana* (solidification and making thermo-stable) of mercury.

रससिन्धुः
सक्तुकं[२३८] मौष्टिकं कौर्मं दार्वीकं सार्षपं तथा[२३९] ।
सैक्तं वत्सनाभं च श्वेतशृंगी तथाऽष्टमी ।
योज्यमित्यष्टभिर्विधैर्विषं[२४०] च रसकर्मणि ।।५२६ ।।

Eight Types of Poison According to Rasasindhu

Saktuka, mauṣṭika, kaurma, dārvīka, sārṣapa, saikata, vatsanābha and *śveta-śṛṅgī* -- these are the eight types of poison to be used in processing mercury.

अङ्गुष्टाङ्गुलियोगेन पिष्टं भवति यद्विषम् ।
सक्तुकं तद्विजानीयाद्दीर्घवेगं[२४१] महोल्वणम् ।।५२७ ।।

Saktuka-Viṣa

The poisonous drug which when pressed between the thumb and finger becomes like a paste is called *saktuka-viṣa*. It has long lasting and acute effects.

मुष्टिकासदृशाकारं गर्भे रोमावलीवृतम् ।
ह्रस्ववेगं च रोगघ्नं उत्तमं[२४२] मौष्टिकं विषम् ।।५२८ ।।

Mauṣṭika-Viṣa

The poisonous drug which looks like a *muṣṭi* (fist), which has hairs in the centre, which has slow effect and which cures diseases is called *mauṣṭika-viṣa*.

कूर्माकृतिर्भवेत्कन्दो मद्यवत्स्तब्धकारकः[२४३] ।
चिराच्छरीरे क्रमते कौर्मं तद्विषमुच्यते ।।५२९ ।।

Kaurma-Viṣa

The poisonous drug, the tuber of which looks like a tortoise, which causes stiffness (intoxication) like alcohol and which takes a long time to spread over the body after ingestion is called *kaurma-viṣa*.

दीर्घसर्पफणाकारो[२४४] गर्भे पीतः सुकन्दकः ।
बहिः पाण्डुशिरानद्धो विषं दार्वीकमुच्यते ।।५३०।।

Dārvika-Viṣa

The poisonous drug which is like the elongated hood of a snake, which is yellow inside, whose tuber is beautiful and which is yellowish outside having prominent veins is called *dārvika-viṣa*.

सर्षपाकारकणिकाचितः कन्दस्तु रोमवान् ।
तद्विषं सार्षपं ज्ञेयं शीघ्रं ज्वरं विनाशयेत्[२४५] ।।५३१।।

।। सार्षपविषम् ।।

Sārṣapa-Viṣa

The poisonous drug, whose tuber is studded with mustard (*sarṣapa*) like pigments and which is hairy is called *sārṣapa-viṣa.* It instantaneously cures fever.

स्थूलसूक्ष्मैः कणैर्युक्तः श्वेतं पीतं[२४६] विरोमकः ।
ज्वरादिसर्वरोगघ्नः कंदः सैकत उच्यते ।।५३२।।

।। सैकतं विषम्[२४७] ।।

Saikata-Viṣa

The poisonous drug whose tuber is studded with small and big nodules, which is white and yellow in colour, which is without any hair root and which cures all diseases like fever, etc. is called *saikata-viṣa.*

न स्थूलो गोस्तनादूदूर्ध्वः द्विविधो वत्सनाभकः ।
आयुष्करी[२४८] लघुत्यागी[?] शुक्लः कृष्णोऽन्यथा भवेत् ।।५३३।।
प्रयोज्यो दोषहरणे जारणाय रसायने ।
कुष्टादिरोगिणां श्रेष्ठो जेता भवति नान्यथा ।।५३४।।

।। इति वत्सनाभविषम् ।।

Vatsanābha-Viṣa

The poisonous drug, whose root is like the nipple of cows in shape, [which is not longer than five *aṅgula-s*] and which is not thicker than the nipple of the cows is called *vatsanābha*. It promotes longevity and it is light. It is also of two types, viz., white and black. It is useful in alleviation of *doṣa-s*, in *jāraṇa* (which helps in digestion) of mercury, and in rejuvenating recipes. It is an excellent drug for the treatment of *kuṣṭha* (obstinate skin diseases including leprosy), etc.

वृत्तः कन्दो भवेत्कृष्णो जंबीरफलवच्च[२४१] यः ।
प्रयोज्यो दोषहरणे जंबीरफलवच्च यः [?] ।
तत्कालकूटं जानीयात् घ्रातमात्रं मृतिप्रदम् ।।५३५।।

।। इति कालकूटविषम् ।।

Kālakūṭa-Viṣa

The poisonous drug whose tuber is round, black and like the fruit of *jambīra* and which alleviates *doṣa-s* is called *kālakūṭa*. If just inhaled, it leads to death.

अन्तर्नीलो बहिः शुक्लः कंदस्तच्च हलाहलम् ।
भित्वा चर्म च शस्त्रेण सन्निपाते विषं न्यसेत् ।।५३६।।

।। इति हलाहलविषम् ।।

Halāhala-Viṣa

The poisonous drug whose tuber is blue inside and white outside is called *halāhala-viṣa*. In *sannipāta* (when all the three *doṣa-s* are simultaneously vitiated), it should be applied by incising the skin.

मूलाग्रयोः सवृत्तः स्यादायतः पीतवर्णकः ।
कंचुकाढ्यः स्निग्धपर्वा हारिद्रो धातुवादकृत्तम् ।।५३७।।

।। हारिद्रविषलक्षणम् ।।

Hāridra-Viṣa

The poisonous drug whose tuber is round at the bottom and top, which is gross in size, which is yellow in colour, which is full of scales and whose nodes are greasy is called *hāridra-viṣa*. It is useful in *dhātu-vāda* (processing of mercury for transmutation of base metals into noble ones).

श्वादंष्ट्रा रूपसंस्थाना यमदंष्ट्रा च सोच्यते ।
रसवादे धातुवादे विषवादं क्वचिद्भवेत् ।
दशैतानि प्रपूज्यन्ते भैषज्येन रसायने ।।५३८।।

।। इति श्वदंष्ट्राविषम् ।।

Yama(śva)daṃṣṭrā-Viṣa

The poisonous drug which is like the canine teeth of dog is called *yama-daṃṣṭrā*. It is very useful in *rasa-vāda* (processing of mercury), *dhātu-vāda* (transmutation of base metals into noble ones) and *viṣa-vāda* (treatment with poisons).

All the above mentioned ten drugs are useful in the preparation of rejuvenating recipes.

विषभागांश्चणकवत्स्थूलान्कृत्वा तु भाजने ।
तत्र गोमूत्रकं क्षिप्त्वा प्रत्यहं नित्यनूतनम् ।।५३९।।
शोषयेत्त्रिदिनादूर्ध्वं धृत्वा तीव्रातपे ततः ।
प्रयोगेषु प्रयुञ्जीत भागमानेन तद्विषम् ।।५४०।।

Purification of Viṣa (Poisonous Drugs)

Poisonous drugs should be cut into small pieces of the shape and size of *caṇaka* (pea or chick-pea) and soaked in cow's urine for three days. Every day fresh cow's urine should be added to it. After three days, it should be exposed to and dried in hot sun-rays. Then in appropriate dosage it should be used in recipes.

सप्ताहोरात्रमुषितं गोमूत्रे वा विषं नवम् ।
ततस्तु घर्मसंशुष्कं योगयुक्तं भवेद् ध्रुवम् ।।५४१।।

Second Method of Viṣa-Purification

Freshly collected poisonous drugs should be soaked in cow's urine for seven days and nights. Thereafter, it should be dried in sun and used in recipes.

भंडीरस्वरसेनापि स्वेदयेद्घटिकात्रयम् ।
तथा छागलदुग्धेन घटिकाद्वितयेन वै ।

दोलायन्त्रेण संशुद्धो यथोक्तगुणदो भवेत् ।।५४२।।

।। इति विषशोधनम् ।।

Third Method of Viṣa-Purification

The poisonous drug should be steam-boiled [in *dolā-yantra*] along with the juice of *bhaṇḍīra* for three *ghaṭikā-s*. Thereafter, it should be boiled in *dolā-yantra* by adding goat-milk for two *ghaṭikā-s*. Thus, it becomes purified and produces the prescribed therapeutic effects.

Thus, ends the description of the method of purifying poisonous drugs.

गन्धक-मरिच-यवानी-घनोग्राजीरतंडुलीमूलैः ।
एकैकशः प्रयुक्तैः विषवेगं जयति किं चित्रम् ।।५४३।।

Reducing Poisonous Effects

Processing poisonous drugs with each one of *gandhaka*, *marica*, *yavānī*, *ghana* (*mustā*), *ugrā* (*vacā*), *jīraka* and root of *taṇḍulīyaka* reduces their toxic effects.

समटंकणसंमिश्रं[250] तद्विषं मृतमुच्यते ।।५४४।।

।। इति विषमारणम् ।।

Māraṇa (Calcination) of Poisonous Drugs

Viṣa, added with *taṅkaṇa* in equal quantity and cooked in *puṭa* is reduced to *bhasma* form.

कुष्ठोदरज्वरहरं सन्निपातरोगापहम् ।
वलीपलितखालित्यहरं चाशु रसायनम् ।।५४५।।

।। इति विषगुणाः ।।

Properties of Viṣa (Poisons)

Viṣa cures *kuṣṭha* (obstinate skin diseases including leprosy), *udara* (obstinate abdominal diseases including ascites), fever, diseases caused by *sannipāta* (simultaneous vitiation of all the three *doṣa-s*), wrinkling, graying of hair and baldness. It instantaneously rejuvenates the body.

'अतिमात्रं[251] यदा भुक्तं वमनं कारयेत्तदा' ।
नृणां यावदजादुग्धं स्थिरीभवति कोष्ठके ।।५४६।।

विषवेगं तदोत्तीर्णं जानीयात्कुशलो भिषक् ।
विषवेगप्रतीकारं लिख्यते विषचिकित्सिते ।।५४७।।

Treatment of the Toxicity of Poisons

If the poisonous drug is taken in excess dose, then the physician should administer emesis. When goat's milk remains stable (does not come out by vomiting) in the gastro-intestinal-tract, then it should be known that the toxicity of the poison is subsided.

Treatment of different stages of toxicity will be described in the chapter dealing with the treatment of different types of poison.

अथ रसरत्नाकरात्

क्षिप्त्वा 'तक्रघटे[५२] पाच्या कांचनीपलपंचकम्' ।
तक्रे जीर्णे समुद्धृत्य ततः क्षीरघटे पचेत् ।।५४८।।
क्षीरे जीर्णे समुद्धृत्य क्षालयित्वा प्रशोधयेत् ।
स्वर्णक्षीरी भवेत्शुद्धा अथवा छागमूत्रके[५३] ।
कुष्ठार्शोगरशोफं[५४] च विषमांश्च ज्वराञ्जयेत् ।।५४९।।

।। इति चोकशुद्धिः ।।

Purification of Coka (Svarṇa-Kṣīri)
According to Rasaratnākara

In a jar containing butter-milk, five *pala-s* of *svarṇa-kṣīrī* should be kept and cooked. When the butter-milk gets evaporated, the *svarṇa-kṣīrī* should be taken out, placed in a jar containing milk and cooked. Thereafter, it should be washed in water. Thus, *svarṇa-kṣīrī* gets purified.

Alternatively, *svarṇa-kṣīrī* can be purified by boiling with goat's urine.

It cures *kuṣṭha* (obstinate skin diseases including leprosy), piles, poisoning, oedema and *viṣama jvara* (irregular fever).

दोलायन्त्रेणारनाले[२५५] विषमुष्टिं दिनत्रयम् ।
विपक्वं शोधितं[५६] चूर्णं शुद्धं सर्वत्र योजयेत् ।।५५०।।

।। इति कुचलाशुद्धिः ।।

Purification of Viṣamuṣṭi

Seeds of *viṣa-muṣṭi* should be cooked in *dolā-yantra* along with *āranāla* (vinegar) for three days. Thus, it gets purified and its powder should be used in all recipes.

जेपालकस्तु[२५७] गोक्षीरैः क्रमात् पक्वं विशुद्ध्यति।
फलं कनकसंज्ञं तु योगयुक्तं भवेद्[२५८] ध्रुवम्।। ५५१।।

।। इति जयपालशुद्धिः।।

Purification of Jayapāla & Kanaka

Jayapāla, gradually cooked in cow's milk gets purified. Similarly, the fruit of *kanaka* (*dhustūra*) gets purified. Thereafter, these ingredients can be used in recipes.

रसचिन्तामणिः[२५९]
स्वर्जिका षट्पला देया[२६०] पर्णचूर्णं च षट्पलम्।
जलं शतपलं दत्त्वा तद् द्वयं[२६१] च जले क्षिपेत्।।५५२।।
त्रिभागं तज्जलं नीत्वा तस्मिन्केशान्विनिक्षिपेत्।
कृतसूक्ष्माश्च कृष्णाश्च पलद्वादशसंख्यया।।५५३।।
मंदं मंदं पचेद्वह्नौ जलशेषं गते सति।
ग्राहयेत्केशतैलं च साधयेत्स्वसमाहितम्।
अथवा [२६२]नलिकायन्त्रे केशतैलं समुद्धरेत्।।५५४।।

।। केशतैलग्रहणोपायः।।

Collection of Oil From Hair
According to Rasacintāmaṇi

In one hundred *pala-s* of water, six *pala-s* of *svarjikā* and six *pala-s* of the powder of betel-leaf should be added and boiled till one third of water remains. In this water, twelve *pala-s* of the fine powder of black hair should be added and cooked over mild fire till the water gets evaporated. Thus, the oil of hair is collected.

Alternatively, oil of hair can be extracted through *nalikā-yantra*.

प्रस्थं कुमारीस्वरसमभयात्कुडवोन्मितम्[२६३]।
'विचूर्णिता[२६४] वस्त्रपूता कुर्यादिकत्र तद्द्वयं।।५५५।।
प्रमर्द्य लोहभाण्डेन विपचेन्मंदवह्निना।
दर्व्या विघट्टयेत्तावद्यावदेकत्वमागतम्'।।५५६।।

पुनः प्रघट्टयेत्तावद्यावद्गाढतरं भवेत् ।
उत्तार्य लोहजे भाण्डे स्थापयेत्तत्प्रयत्नतः ।।५५७।।
शूलाध्मानानाहगुल्मेषु[२६५] कृमिदोषेषु योजयेत् ।
बोलपिण्ड इति ख्यातो रसशोधनकर्मसु ।।५५८।।

।। इति बोल [पिण्ड][२६६] करणम् ।।

Preparation of Bola-Piṇḍa

One *kuḍava* of the powder of *abhayā* should be strained through a cloth. To this, one *prastha* of the juice of *kumārī* should be added and triturated together. This should be kept in an iron pan and cooked over mild fire. It should be stirred well with the help of a spoon till both these ingredients get well mixed. The stirring should be continued till it becomes thicker. After taking out of the oven, it should be carefully stored in an iron jar. It is called *Bola-piṇḍa* (bolus of *bola*) which is useful in processing mercury. It cures colic pain, flatulance, constipation, *gulma* (phantom tumour) and parasitic infestation.

तोत्तलात्
दलितकुमारीदलतः शिवाचूर्णावचूर्णितात् ।
धृतो वेणुमये पात्रे स्रवति प्रवरो रसः ।।५५९।।

।। इति कुमारीरसग्रहणम् ।।

Extraction of Kumārī-Juice
According to Tottala

Leaves of *kumārī* should be crushed and powder of *harītakī* should be sprinkled over it. Then the paste should be kept in a pot prepared of bamboo and squeezed by which the juice of *kumārī* comes out.

शाल्मलीखदिरादीनां वृक्षं वर्षोद्भवं शुभम् ।
स्निग्धमजन्तुजुष्टं[२६७] च स्निग्धभूमिसमुत्थितम् ।।५६०।।
तस्याग्रे वा दक्षिणे वा वामे वा पृष्ठतोपि वा ।
भूमौ प्रणालीं किष्क्वर्द्धमिती वा किष्कुसंमितम् ।।५६१।।
अधोमुखी सुदीर्घा[२६८] च खनयत्राप्यते यथा ।
मुशलाभा तदाख्या च जटा चाथ भिषक्तमः ।।५६२।।

छेदयेदेकघातेन यथायं[२६९] जायते द्विधा ।
घातद्वये चापि[२७०] रसं न स्रवेत्पूर्ववद् ध्रुवम् ।।५६३।।
वृक्षाद्भिन्नतरं[२७१] यच्च जातं तन्मुशलं त्यजेत् ।
अपरं विन्यसेत्कुम्भे मुखं सम्यक् निरुन्धयेत् ।।५६४।।
यथा न धूलिसंसर्गो[२७२] न वातातपयोस्तथा ।
तथा यत्नेन तत्कुंभं भूमौ सम्यङ्निखानयेत्[२७३] ।।५६५।।
तत्प्रणाली च मृत्स्नाभिः[२७४] पूरयित्वा तु[२७५] यत्नतः ।
मधूकसारवत्स्थूलकाष्ठैर्वृक्षसमन्ततः ।।५६६।।
भूमौ प्रज्वालयेदग्निं यथा किञ्चित् दहेत्तरुः ।
स्वांगशीतं परिज्ञाय ततः कुंभं समुद्धरेत् ।
ग्राहयेद्वृक्षजं सत्वं सर्वकार्यप्रसाधकम्[२७७] ।।५६७।।

।। वृक्षसत्त्वम् ।।

Vṛkṣa-Sattva (Extraction of Essence from Trees)

Śālmalī, *khadira* and such other trees should be selected for the extraction of *sattva* (essence). These trees should be one year old, auspicious, unctuous, not infested with parasites and grown over unctuous soil. In its front, right, left or back side, a tunnel of the size of half *kiṣka* (cubit) or one *kiṣka* should be dug downwards deep into the soil till one reaches one of the strong tap roots of the tree. This tap root should be cut in one stroke into two pieces. Cutting it by two (more than one) strokes does not make the sap to come out of this root as before. The distant part of the cut root should be rejected and the cut piece of the root connected with the tree should be put into a jar and the remaining space in the mouth of the jar should be carefully sealed so that dust, wind and sun-rays do not enter into the jar. Thus, the jar should be properly kept stable on the ground and the pit should be filled with earth. Around the base of this tree, pieces of heart-wood of *madhūka* etc., should be kept and ignited till the tree gets slightly burnt. When it becomes cool of its own, the jar should be taken out. The *sattva* (essence) of the tree exudes into this jar and it is used in recipes.

वृक्षमूलोत्थरसस्थाः[२७८] कतकफलाश्चातिकठिनतराः यामद्वयेन
मृदुतां प्रयान्ति[२७९] निर्दोषतां यान्ति ।।५६८।।

Properties of Vṛkṣa-Sattva

If hard substances like the fruits of *kataka* are kept in the *vṛkṣa-sattva* described above for two *yāma-s,* then they become soft and purified.

PREPARATION OF DRUTI (METALS IN LIQUID FORM)

रसदर्पणात्

अभ्रकद्रुतिमज्ञातुः कुतोऽस्ति रससाधनम् ।
लोहरत्नद्रुतिं[२८०] हित्वा कुतोऽस्ति रससाधनम् ।।५६९।।
द्रुतिरभ्रकसंज्ञाता त्रिषु लोकेषु दुर्लभा ।
सा पुनः सुलभा पुंसि सुप्रसन्ने महेश्वरे ।।५७०।।
अभ्रकं द्रावितं येन पारदं च वशीकृतम् ।
कपाटोद्घाटितं तेन स्वर्गस्य धनदस्य वा[२८१] ।।५७१।।
अभ्रकसत्वं[२८२] पूर्वं शास्त्रोक्तं क्रमशः आदाय
तप्ते स्विन्नावापो देयस्तस्माद्द्रुतिर्भवति ।।५७२।।

Preparation of Mica-Druti
According to Rasa-darpaṇa

A physician, not acquainted with the process of making *abhraka-druti* (liquefied mica), is not capable of processing mercury. Similarly, without the *druti* (liquefaction) of *loha* (metals) and gems, processing of mercury is not possible. *Abhraka-druti* (liquefied mica) is rare in the three worlds. This could be achieved only if a person has the blessings of Lord Maheśvara.

A person, who has liquefied mica and who has controlled (effectively processed) mercury, has opened the doors of the heaven and the house of Kubera i.e. he attains salvation and great-wealth.

Abhraka-sattva (metallic essence of mica) should be prepared according to the procedure prescribed in the text before. This should be heated and immersed in prescribed liquids by which it gets liquefied.

स्वरसेन वज्रवल्ल्याः गगनः सौवर्चलान्वितो भवति[२८३] ।
'पक्वं[२८४] स हि लावपुटे निर्लेपं भवति रसरूपम् ।
वज्रवल्लीअस्थि।।५७३।।

Preparation of Abhraka-Druti with Vajra-vallī

Mica with *sauvarcala* salt should be cooked in the juice of *vajra-vallī* (stem). Thereafter, keeping in a crucible, it should be cooked in *lāva-puṭa* by which it becomes non-sticky and liquid like mercury.

मुनिकुसुमं सलिलपिष्टं सूरणकंदोदरेषु निक्षिप्तम् ।
नीरसमं भवति धनं निक्षिप्तं गोष्टगोमये मासम् ।।५७४ ।।

Second Method of Preparing Abhraka-Druti

Flowers of *agastya* should be made to a paste by triturating with water. Mica should be added to this paste and kept inside a tuber of *sūraṇa* and covered with cow-dung cakes for one month by which mica becomes liquefied and looks like water.

नरचिकुरपिष्टतैलं पिष्टं तल्लेपः कुलिशमूषायाम् ।
अचिरेण जलौकाभं घनसत्वं स्याद्दृढं ध्मातम्' ।।५७५ ।।

Third Method of Preparing Abhraka-Druti

Abhraka-sattva should be triturated with oil of human hair. This should be kept in *vajra-mūṣā* and over fire by which the *abhraka-sattva* becomes soft like a leech immediately.

सौवर्चलं सैन्धवं च विडमौद्भिदपांशुजम् ।
नवसारं यवक्षारं तुत्थं तुल्यं विचूर्णयेत्' ।।५७६ ।।
'केशतैलेन[२८५] संमिश्र्य नालीयंत्रे विनिक्षिपेत् ।
षोडशांगुलमुत्सेधा दातव्या नालिका शुभा ।।५७७ ।।
दृढं संरोधयेदास्यं ध्रुवं स्वेदाः स्रवेत्ततः ।
तेन शंखादयः सर्वे द्रवन्ति सलिलं यथा ।
तथैव संप्रजायेत क्षुधावान्पारदो भवेत्' ।।५७८ ।।

।। इति क्षारद्रुतिः ।।

Fourth Method of Preparing Abhraka-Druti by Alkalies

Sauvarcala, saindhava, viḍa, audbhida, pāṃśuja, navasāra, yavakṣāra and *tuttha,* taken in equal quantities, should be made to a powder and triturated with *Keśa-taila* (oil extracted from human-hair). This should be kept in a *nālī-yantra* having a tube which is sixteen *aṅgula-s* in length. Its opening (mouth) should be strongly sealed. From this tube, exudation of liquid like sweat, takes place. If *śaṅkha*, [mica], etc., are triturated with this liquid, they become liquefied like water. Adding this liquid to mercury promotes the digestive power of the latter.

त्रिफला च त्रिकटुकं त्रिक्षारं पटुपंचकम् ।
बला चातिबला चैव तृतीया च महाबला ॥५७९॥
अश्वगन्धा च दीनारी भूलता मातृवाहकः ।
गोपेन्द्रमण्डली चैव षड्बिन्दु विमुखी तथा ॥५८०॥
वीरा सूरणकन्दश्च कंचुकी च पुनर्नवा ।
स्नुह्यर्कोन्मत्तहलिनी पाठा चोत्तरवारुणी ॥५८१॥
अयस्कान्तो गोक्षुरश्च भृंगदूर्वाम्लवेतसम् ।
शिलाजतुश्च सौवीरं विषगन्धकटंकणम् ॥५८२॥
पृथग्दशपलं सर्वं सूक्ष्मचूर्णं तु कारयेत् ।
कुम्भद्वयं कुलत्थानां काष्ठेन तिमिरस्य च ॥५८३॥
क्वाथयेन्मृदुतापेन यावत्कुम्भांशशोषितम् ।
तेन क्वाथेन तच्चूर्णं भावयेदेकविंशतिः ॥५८४॥
रत्नानि तेन लिप्तानि तत्क्वाथे स्वेदयेत्पुनः ।
अहोरात्रेण तान्याशु द्रवन्ति सलिलं यथा ॥५८५॥
अभ्रकादीनि लोहानि द्रवन्ति ह्यचिरात्ततः[२८६] ।
निर्लेपानि[२८७] च जायन्ते हरबीजोपमानि च ॥५८६॥

Fifth Method of Preparing Abhraka-Druti

Triphalā, trikaṭu, tri kṣāra, pañca-lavaṇa, balā, atibalā, mahā balā, aśvagandhā, dīnārī, bhū-latā, mātṛ-vāhaka, gopendra-maṇḍalī, ṣaḍbindu, vimukhī, vīrā, sūraṇa, kañcukī, punarnavā, snuhī, arka, unmatta (dhustura), halinī, pāṭhā, uttara-vāruṇī, ayaskānta, gokṣura, bhṛṅga-rāja, dūrvā, amla-vetasa, śilājatu, sauvīra-añjana, viṣa, gandhaka and *ṭaṅkaṇa,* ten *pala-s* of each of these ingredients should be made to fine powder.

Two *kumbha-s* of *kulattha* should be boiled over mild fire of the wood of *timira* (*dāru-haridrā*) till one *kumbha* of water remains. In this decoction, the powder mentioned above should be impregnated for twenty one times. Gems should be smeared with this paste and boiled [in *dolā-yantra*] by adding the same decoction for one day and night by which these gems get liquefied and become like water [in consistency]. With this method, mica and other metals also get liquefied quickly. These metals thus become non-sticky and fluid like mercury.

रसालंकारात्

अभ्रादिसर्वलोहानां महालोहस्य सर्वतः ।
रसोपरसकादीनि[२८८] सत्त्वानां द्रावणं शृणु ।।५८७।।
यथोदितैश्च संस्कारैः संस्कृतं गगनादिकम् ।
द्रुतित्वं जात्यसंदेहो नान्यथा तद्द्रुतिर्भवेत् ।।५८८।।
निश्चन्द्रकाभ्रकं कृत्वा छागलाद्यैः पलैः समम् ।
निष्पिष्य कलशान्तस्थं कृत्वा तत्र विनिक्षिपेत् ।।५८९।।
षड्बिन्दून् शतशश्चैव खादयेत्तं पलाभ्रकम् ।
पिधाय जीर्णवस्त्रेण घटवक्त्रं विधारयेत् ।।५९०।।
यावद्यत्नादेकविंशद्वारान्खादेत्पुनः[२८९] पुनः ।
गृह्णीयाच्च तद्विष्णुकीटेन[२९०] सह ता [?] धमेत् ।।५९१।।
वज्रमूषान्तरस्थां च तद्बिन्दूगगनद्रुतिः[२९१] ।
सा द्रुति पारदप्रख्या द्रवरूपा स्थिरा भवेत् ।।५९२।।

Sixth Method of Preparing Abhraka-Druti According to Rasālaṅkāra

Now the *drāvaṇa* (liquefaction) of all *loha-s* (metals including minerals) including mica, etc., of *mahārasa-s* (*loha-s*), *rasa-s, uparasa-s* and *sattva-s* (metallic essence) will be described.

Mica, etc., should be purified, according to the method prescribed before, for their *drāvaṇa* (liquefaction). Without such purification, liquefaction of these metals, etc., does not take place. Mica *bhasma* (one *pala*), free from dazzling particles should be triturated with one *pala* of *chāgala-pañcaka* (urine, milk, curd, ghee and stool of goat) and kept in a jar. To this, one hundred *ṣaḍ-bindu-s* should be thrown.

These insects will eat away the mica. The mouth of the jar should be covered with an old piece of cloth. This process should be done for twenty one times. These insects should be kept in a *vajra-mūṣā* and blown ove fire. Thus, these insects (*bindu*) and mica eaten by them get liquefied and remain stable like mercury in a liquid form.

अग्निजारं समाहृत्य नवे कुम्भे विनिक्षिपेत् ।
अधरोत्तरभावेन[२१२] व्योमचूर्णं विनिक्षिपेत् ।।५९३।।
मुखं सम्यग्मृदा वस्त्रैः पिधान्याच्छादयेद् दृढम् ।
धान्यराशौ भूमिष्टं च तदङ्कं विनिपातयेत्[२१३] ।।५९४।।
द्वाविंशतिदिनादूर्ध्वं घटं यत्नात्समुद्धरेत् ।
उद्घाट्य वक्त्रं गृह्णीयात् द्रुतिं मुक्ताफलप्रभाम् ।।५९५।।

Seventh Method of Preparing Mica-Druti

Agnijāra should be kept in a new jar. Above and below this, the *bhasma* of mica should be placed. The mouth (opening) of the jar should be covered with a lid and the joint between the mouth of the jar and the lid should be sealed with mud-smeared cloth. The jar should be kept in a pit on the earth covered with a heap of grains. After twenty two days, the jar should be carefully removed from the heap of grains and its mouth should be opened. The mica which is liquefied and which looks like pearls should then be collected.

वज्राभ्रकं विचूर्ण्याथ लोहखल्वे विनिक्षिपेत् ।
दृढे कृष्णशिलाजे वा मर्दयेत्तदहर्निशम् ।।५९६।।
लोहितागस्तिसुमनोद्भवैश्च सलिलैस्ततः ।
मासमात्रं प्रयत्नेन पश्चात्कल्कं समुद्धरेत् ।।५९७।।
अर्शोरिपुभवं कन्दं वर्षत्रितयसंभवम्[२१४] ।
आदाय कुर्यात्तन्मध्ये गर्त्तां कल्कोचितां तथा ।।५९८।।
तदन्तः स्थापयेत्कल्कं व्योमजं तं पिधापयेत् ।।
पिधान्या कन्दभवया[२१५] लिंपेत् पटमृदा ततः ।।५९९।।
पुटत्रयं ततो गर्त्ते व्योमविस्तारकं विधेत् ।
पुरुषद्वयं [?] दध्नं च [?] गोशकृद्विनियोजयेत् ।।६००।।

यावच्च कीटजघ्नं स्यात्तत्र कंदं विधापयेत् ।
उपरिष्टात्क्षिपेत्प्राग्वद्यावद्गर्तः प्रपूर्यते ।
गोपयसा ततः सम्यक् कुट्टयेत् काष्टपट्टकैः ।।६०१।।
गर्तोपरिष्टात्संदद्यात्कीटदध्नं च गोमयम् ।
मासत्रितयपर्यन्तं स्थापयेत्तत्तथा बुधः ।।६०२।।
त्रिमासानन्तरं पश्चाद्गर्तात्कन्दं समुद्धरेत् ।
उद्धृत्य कन्दं निर्भिद्य गृह्णीयात् गगनद्रुतिम् ।
विशुद्धपारदप्रख्यामपुनः कठिनात्मिकाम् ।।६०३।।

Eighth Method of Preparing Mica-Druti

The powder of *vajra* type of mica should be kept in a mortar of iron or strong black-stone and triturated for one day and night continuously. Thereafter, the flower-juice of the red variety of *agastya* should be added to it, triturated for one month and made to a paste.

A tuber of three years old plant of *sūraṇa* should be collected. In the middle of this tuber, a hole should be made the size of which should be adequate for the paste. The paste of mica mentioned above should be kept inside this hole. The hole should then be packed with the cut piece of *sūraṇa* which should be wrapped with mud-smeared cloth. Then, three *puṭa-s* should be given.

Thereafter, a pit of the size of mica containing *sūraṇa* should be dug on the earth. The depth of the pit should be about 12 feet (*puruṣa-dvaya*). This pit should be filled with curd and cowdung till maggots appear in it. Then the tuber of *sūraṇa* [containing mica] should be placed in the pit. Over this, curd and cowdung should be placed to fill up the remaining space of the pit. Over this, cow's milk should be poured and with the help of an wooden-plank, the surface of the pit should be hammered. Over this pit, maggot infested curd and cow-dung should be placed and kept as such for three months. Thereafter, the tuber of *sūraṇa* should be taken out of the pit and incised to collect the *druti* (liquid) of mica which looks like mercury and which never becomes hard again.

रक्तछागभवैर्मूत्रैश्चूर्णमर्कटतिन्दुजम् ।
भावयेत्छतवारांस्तु[११] भूयो भूयः प्रपिष्य च ।।६०४।।

दत्त्वा धमेत्खराङ्गारैश्चिरं भस्राद्वयेन वै ।
खसत्त्वं तद् द्रवं ज्ञात्वा तच्चूर्णं योजयेत्पुनः ।।६०५।।
खसत्त्वं वज्रमूषायां तच्चूर्णमधरोत्तरम् ।
एवं त्रिवारं कर्त्तव्यं रसरूपं प्रजायते ।।६०६।।

Ninth Method of Preparing Mica-Druti

The powder of *markaṭa-tinduka* should be impregnated with the urine of a red goat for one hundred times and triturated repeatedly to make a powder. The *sattva* of mica should be kept in *vajra-mūṣā* and above and below this, the above mentioned powder should be kept. Keeping the crucible over strongly hot charcoal it should be blown with the help of two blowers. When the mica-*sattva* gets liquefied the above mentioned powder should be placed below it. This process should be done for three times by which the *sattva* of mica turns to a liquid form and looks like mercury.

इन्द्रगोपकचूर्णानि पीतवेणीफलानि च ।
चूर्णितानि समांशानि पीतवेणीफलोद्भवैः ।।६०७।।
रसैः संशोषयेद्वारान्[१७] शतं पिष्ट्वा पुनः पुनः ।
मूषामध्ये द्रवेद्धेम्नि तच्चूर्णं प्रवपेद्बुधः [?] ।।६०८।।
तच्चूर्णं याममात्रेण द्रुतित्वं कनकं व्रजेत् ।
भूयः कठिनतां नैति कल्पान्तेऽपि च पार्वति ।।६०९।।

Method of Preparing Gold-Druti

The powders of *indra-gopa* and fruit of *pīta-veṇī*, taken in equal quantities should be impregnated with the juice of the fruit of *pīta-veṇī* for one hundred times and triturated each time. In a crucible, gold should be kept and melted. Over this, the above mentioned powder should be sprinkled. Thus, in one *yāma*, the gold gets liquefied. This liquefied gold never becomes solid even after several years.

पीतवेणीभवं चूर्णं भावयेन्नरवारिणा ।
शतवारान्मर्दयित्वा पुनः पुनरतन्द्रितः ।।६१०।।
ततः संद्रावयेद्धेम द्रवरूपं यदा भवेत् ।

तदा तस्मिन्क्षिपेच्चूर्णं रसरूपं भवेद् ध्रुवम् ।।६११।।

Second Method of Preparing Gold-Druti

The powder of *pīta-veṇī* should be impregnated with human-urine and triturated each time for one hundred times. The gold should be melted and made to a liquid form. To this, the above mentioned powder should be added by which the gold becomes in permanent liquid form like mercury.

दग्धा पीता देवदाली पञ्चाङ्गी भस्मितां ततः ।
रक्तार्जुनीभवे मूत्रे शतवारं कुसुम्भवत् ।।६१२।।
स्रावयित्वा जलं नीत्वा भस्मं तत्र पुनः क्षिपेत्[298] ।
नवं नवं क्षिपेद् भस्म एकविंशतिवारकम् ।।६१३।।
क्षारवद् स्रावणं[299] कार्यं कारयेल्लवणं ततः ।
आतपे शोष्य मतिमानथवा लवणं ततः[300] ।।६१४।।
कारयेत्प्रद्रुते हेम्नि योजयेन्नात्र संशयः ।
हेमं जलनिभं स्वच्छं संततं जायते ध्रुवम् ।।६१५।।
तीक्ष्णमेव तथा ताम्रं तारं वंगं भुजङ्गमम् ।
द्रुतिः सर्वं भवत्येव सर्वथा शिवभाषितम् ।।६१६।।

Third Method of Preparing Gold-Druti

All the five parts of the yellow variety of *devadālī* should be burnt and reduced to ash. It should be percolated like *kusumbha* by adding the urine of *raktārjunī* (?). To this water, the ash should be added again and percolated. This process should be performed for twenty one times by adding fresh ash. The process of percolation should be done as suggested for the preparation of *kṣāra* (alkalies). Then, from the sediment, salt like substance should be collected and dried in the sun. This salt should be added to melted-gold by which the latter becomes liquefied and clean like water.

According to the same process *tīkṣṇa* type of iron, copper, silver, tin, lead, etc., get liquefied.

द्रवन्ती-एरण्डवत्पत्रं [विटपारसेनैव] व्योमचूर्णं प्रमर्दयेत् [?]।
घस्रैकविंशतिर्यावत्सुतश्रेणीरसैस्ततः ।।६१७।।

पचेद् व्योमं यथा सर्वं नवनीतं समं भवेत् ।
तदादाय सुतश्रेणीक्षीरैः पश्चात्प्रमर्दयेत् ।
ततो रंडासमुद्भूतनिजतैलेन मर्दयेत् ॥६१९॥
ऊनविंशद्दिनं यावत्महापटमथाहरेत् ।
तत्पेटन[301] तु लिंपेत् पश्चाद्वर्ति प्रकारयेत् ॥६२०॥
रंडासम्भूतबीजोत्थरसेनैव[302] विभावयेत् ।
बहुवारं ततो धृत्वा संदंशेनाथ[303] वर्तिकाम् ॥६२१॥
सिञ्चत्तद्राजतैलेन[304] ज्वालयेद्वर्तिकां[305] बुधः ।
अधस्तात्स्थापयेत्पात्रं कांतजं कांस्यजं च वा ॥६२२॥
वर्त्या सज्वाल्यमानापि[306] द्रुतिः पतति निश्चितम् ।
सुनिर्मलरसप्रख्या द्रव्यसिद्धिकरी परा ॥६२३॥

Tenth Method of Preparing Mica-Druti

With the juice of *dravantī* (which has leaves like those of *eraṇḍa*), the *bhasma* of mica should be triturated for twenty one times. Thereafter, mica should be cooked in the juice of *suta-śreṇī* by which it becomes soft like butter.

Thereafter, this mica should be triturated with the milky latex of *suta-śreṇī.* Then this should be triturated with castor-oil for ninteen days. This paste should be kept in a long piece of cloth and rolled to make a wick. This should be soaked in the oil of castor-seed for several times. Then this wick should be grasped with a forceps and after sprinkling *rāja-taila* (castor oil) it should be ignited. Below it, a pot made of *kānta-lauha* or bronze should be kept. When the wick burns, the *druti* (liquefied mica) falls down from it. It is like pure mercury and is very useful in *dhātu-vāda* (transmutation of base metals into noble ones).

कूर्मास्थीनि समादाय मेषशृङ्गसमन्वितम् ।
चूर्णयित्वा[307] भावयेत्ताच्छिलाजतुभिः सहतः ॥६२४॥
अम्लवेतससंयुक्तैः[308] वारांस्त्रिःसप्तकान्ततः ।
तद्वापणाद् क्षणेनैव माक्षिकं जलवद्भवेत् ॥६२५॥

Preparation of Mākṣika-Druti

The bone of tortoise and the horn of sheep should be made to a powder and impregnated with *śilājatu*. Thereafter, it should be impregnated with the juice of *amla-vetasa* for twenty one times. If *mākṣika* (chalco pyrite), triturated with this powder is heated in a crucible, then instantaneously, *mākṣika* gets liquefied (*druti*).

दैत्येन्द्रनिहितं शुल्वं तीक्ष्णं दरदमारितम् ।
दरदं[309] ताप्यनिहतं सुवर्णं करिमारितम् ।।६२६।।
एवं मन्यतमं भस्मं कन्दचूर्णैः समांशकम् ।
बलक्षकंचुकीव्रातै[?]रेकीकृत्य[310] प्रमर्दयेत् ।।६२७।।
[311]तद्द्रवैरेव शतशो वेणीफलरसैस्ततः ।
पीतवेणीभवैः क्षीरैः समायुक्तं[312] प्रमर्दयेत् ।।६२८।।
शतवारांस्ततो[313] वज्रमूषायां[314] सकलं क्षिपेत् ।
धमेच्च खदिराङ्गारैस्तद्रसं प्रद्रुतिं[315] व्रजेत् ।
सर्वसत्त्वानि जायन्ते द्रुतान्यत्र न संशयः ।।६२९।।

Preparation of Druti of Metals

Bhasma of copper prepared with sulphur, *bhasma* of *tīkṣṇa* type of iron prepared with cinnabar, *bhasma* of cinnabar prepared with copper pyrite, *bhasma* of gold prepared with lead and similar *bhasma-s* of other metals are to be processed for *druti* (liquefaction). These *bhasma-s* should be added with equal quantity of the powder of the *sūraṇa-kanda* and triturated by adding the juice of *balakṣa-kañcukī-vrāta* for one hundred times. Thereafter, it should be triturated with the juice of the fruit of *pīta-veṇī* and with the milky latex of *pīta-veṇī* for one hundred times. Then this should be kept in *vajra-mūṣā* and placing over the hot charcoal of *khadira*, it should be blown by which the *sattva-s* of all metals become liquefied.

पनसफलरसे[316] तु भावितमातिमृदितान्यम्लवर्गतोयेन ।
लिपिलेखनयोग्यानि स्वच्छानि भवन्ति लोहानि ।।६३०।।

Second Method of Preparing Druti of Metals

All the metals should be impregnated with the juice of the fruit of *panasa* and strongly triturated by adding the juice of drugs belonging to *amla-varga* (group of sour drugs). Thus, transparent liquids like ink (suitable of writing) of each of these metals are prepared.

केतकीस्वरसं कांक्षी मणिमंथं सखेचरम् ।
चतुर्भिः स्वेदनादेतैः वैक्रान्तं रसवद्भवेत् ।।६३१।।
सुवर्णमभ्रकं[17] ताम्रं कान्तं लोहितवाजरम् ।
अनेन स्वेदविधिना द्रवति[18] सलिलं यथा ।।६३२।।

Preparation of Vaikrānta-Druti

Vaikrānta (tourmaline), fomented [in a *dolā-yantra*] with four drugs, viz., the juice of *ketakī, kāṅkṣī, maṇi-mantha* and *khecara* becomes liquid like mercury.

Gold, mica, copper, *kānta-lauha* and *lohita-vājara* (?), if fomented according to the above mentioned method, become liquefied like water.

मुक्ताफलं च सप्ताहं वेतसाम्लेन भावितम् ।
जंबीरोदरमध्यस्थं धान्यराशौ निधापयेत् ।।६३३।।
पुटपाकेन तच्चूर्णं द्रवते सलिलं यथा ।
कुरुते योगराजोऽयं रत्नानां द्रावणं परम् ।।६३४।।

Preparation of Pearl-Druti

Pearl should be impregnated with *vetasāmla* for seven days, kept inside the fruit of *jambīra* and then kept inside a heap of grains. Then it should be made to a powder and cooked in *puṭa* by which it gets liquefied like water.

According to this method all the gems can be liquefied.

MIXTURE OF DRUTI-S (LIQUEFIED METALS)

मेलनं चाथ वक्ष्येऽहं रसद्रुत्योर्यथा भवेत् ।
सैन्धवं निंबपत्राणि बाकुची द्वे फणिज्जके ।
द्रुत्यभ्रक[19]रसेन्द्रेण मेलनं परमं मतम् ।।६३५।।

Now the methods of mixing of liquefied metals with mercury will be described.

First Method of Preparing Mixture

Saindhava, leaves of *nimba*, *bākucī* and two types of *phaṇijjhaka* are the excellent drugs for mixing the mica-*druti* with mercury.

कृष्णागुरुसितनाभिरसोनसितं रामठम् ।
द्रुतिरेतास्तप्तखल्वे रसेन सह मर्दयेत् ॥६३६॥
नारीकुसुमसंयुक्तैर्ब्रह्मबीजरसैः समम् ।
सद्यो मिलति[120] सूतेन नात्र कार्या विचारणा[121] ॥६३७॥

Second Method of Preparing Mixture

Druti (liquid) of metals and mercury should be kept in a hot mortar and triturated by adding *kṛṣṇāguru*, *sita-nābhi*, white garlic and *rāmaṭha* (*hiṅgu* or rock-salt). Then it should be triturated by adding the menstrual blood of women and the juice of *brahma-bīja*. Thus, these metal-*druti-s* get mixed up with mercury instantaneously.

रसालंकारात्
एतद्बद्धं रसं खादेद्द्रुतीनां च कदाचन[122] ।
गुंजामात्रं पलं यावद् दिवसे दिवसे बुधः ॥६३८॥
ततः पूर्णपले जग्धे कल्पायुः स्यान्नरो भवेत् ।
इति संपादितो मार्गो द्रुतीनां पातनं स्फुटम् ॥६३९॥
साक्षादनुभवैर्दृष्टो न श्रुतो गुरुदर्शितः ।
रत्नानि चैव लोहानि द्रावणं[123] चाभ्रकस्य च ॥६४०॥

Dosage of Mixed Druti and Mercury According to Rasālaṅkāra

The mixture of metallic *druti* (liquid) and mercury may at times be administered in the dose starting from one *guñjā* to one *pala* by gradually increasing the dosage every day. When a person takes this recipe in the dosage of full one *pala*, then he lives for one *kalpa* (several years).

These methods of preparing and administering *druti* of gems and metals including mica described above are just not heard only but experienced and instructed by the preceptors.

GEMS AND COSTLY STONES

अथ रसदर्पणात्

राजावर्तं च तुत्थं मौक्तिकं विद्रुमं तथा।
वैक्रान्तकसमायुक्ता एते मणिरसाः स्मृताः ।।६४१ ।।

।। इति मणिरसाः ।।

Rejuvenating Gems (Maṇi-Rasa)

Rājāvarta (lapis lazuli), tuttha (copper sulphate), *muktā* (pearl), *vidruma* (coral) and *vaikrānta* (tourmaline)—these taken together are called *maṇi-rasa* (rejuvenating gems).

वैक्रान्तः सूर्यकान्तश्च हीरकं मौक्तिकं तथा ।
चन्द्रकांतं[१२४] तथा चैव राजावर्तस्तथैव च ।।६४२ ।।
पुष्परागं तथा नीलं पद्मरागं प्रवालकम् ।
वैडूर्यनीलमित्येव[१२५] मणयो रसबन्धकाः ।।६४३ ।।

।। इति मणिवर्गः ।।

Group of Gems (Maṇi-Varga)

Vaikrānta (tourmaline), *sūryakānta* (sun stone), *hīraka* (diamond), *mauktika* (pearl), *candra-kānta* (moon-stone), *rājāvarta* (lapis lazuli), *puṣpa-rāga* (topaz), *nīla* (sapphire), *padma-rāga* (ruby), *pravāla* (coral), *vaiḍūrya* (cat's eye) and *nīla*—these gems are used for *rasa-bandhana* (making mercury solid and heat-resistant).

रससिन्धुः

पुंवज्रं गरुडोद्गारं माणिक्यं वासवोपलम् ।
वैडूर्यं पुष्पं गोमेदं मौक्तिकं सप्रवालकम्।
एतानि नवरत्नानि सदृशानि सुधारसैः ।।६४४।।

Nine Gems
According to Rasa-sindhu

Puṃ-vajra (male diamond), *garuḍodgāra* (emerald), *māṇikya* (ruby), *vāsavopala* (diamond), *vaiḍūrya* (cat's eye), *puṣpa* (topaz), *gomeda* (cinnamon stone), *mauktika* (pearl) and *pravāla* (coral)—these are the nine gems which are like ambrosia.

रत्नदीपिकायाम्
उपरत्नानि चत्वारि महारत्नानि पञ्चधा ।
प्रवालं गरुडोद्गारं वैडूर्यं पुष्परागकम् ।
उपरत्नं समाख्यातं रत्नशास्त्रार्थकोविदैः ।।६४५।।

।। इति उपरत्नानि ।।

***Uparatna-s* (Subsidiary Gems)**
According to Ratna-dīpikā

Uparatna-s are four in number and *mahāratna-s* (important gems) are five in number. The four *uparatna-s* are *pravāla* (coral), *garuḍodgāra* (emerald), *vaiḍūrya* (cat's eye) and *puṣparāga* (topaz).

रससिन्धुः
माणिक्यमुक्ताफलविद्रुमाणि तार्क्ष्यं च पुष्पं भिदुरं च नीलम् ।
गोमेदकंचाथ विदूरकंच क्रमेण रत्नानि नवग्रहाणाम् ।।६४६ ।।
क्रमेण मुद्राधृतमिष्टसिद्धये, द्विपाठः[?] ।।६४७।।

Nine Gems to Propitiate Nine Planets
According to Rasa-sindhu

Māṇikya (ruby), *muktā-phala* (pearl), *vidruma* (coral), *tārkṣya* (emerald), *puṣpa-rāga* (topaz), *bhidura* (diamond), *nīla* (sapphire), *gomedaka* (cinnamon stone) and *vidūraka* (cat's eye)—these are the nine gems to propitiate nine *graha-s* (planets), viz., *ravi* (sun), *candra* (moon), *maṅgala* (mars), *budha* (mercury), *bṛhaspati* (jupitor), *śukra* (venus), *śani* (saturn), *rāhu* (Dragon's head) and *ketu* (Dragon's tail) respectively. These gems are to be worn in a ring.

रसे रसायने दाने धारणे देवतार्चने ।
सुलक्ष्याणि सुजातीनि रत्नान्युक्तानि संग्रहेत् ।।६४८।।

Selection of Gems

For the purpose of alchemy, rejuvenation, donation (gift), wearing and propitiating the gods, one should select these gems having *sulakṣaṇa* (auspicious characteristic features) and being of *sujāti* (proper variety).

MĀṆIKYA (RUBY)

रसदर्पणात्

माणिक्यं पद्मरागाख्यं द्वितीयं नीलगन्धि च।
माणिक्यं चैव विज्ञेयं ब्राह्मणादिक्रमेण च ।।६४९।।

Varieties

Māṇikya is of two types, viz., (1) *padma-rāga*, and (2) *nīla-gandhi*.

Māṇikya is also divided into four categories, viz., *brāhmaṇa-māṇikya*, *kṣatriya-māṇikya*, *vaiśya-māṇikya* and *śūdra-māṇikya*.

कुशेशयं यदछायं[३२६] स्वच्छं स्निग्धं गुरु स्फुटम् ।
वृत्तायतं समं गात्रं माणिक्यं श्रेष्ठमुच्यते ।।६५०।।

Characteristics of Good Quality of Māṇikya

Ruby which has no shadow (black spot) and which is clean, unctuous, heavy, dazzling, round, big in size and uniform in shape is excellent in quality.

ग्रन्थान्तरात्

निर्धूमखदिराङ्गारमिन्द्रगोपसमं प्रभम् ।
गुंजरागप्रतीकाशं बाह्याभ्यन्तरतस्तथा ।
गंभीरं चैकवर्णं च माणिक्यं सर्वकर्मणि ।।६५१।।

Ruby Useful for All Purposes
According to Another Text

Ruby which is not smoky in colour, which dazzles like red hot charcoal of *khadira* or like *indragopa*, which is of the colour of *guñjā* both externally and internally, which has deep coloration and which has uniform coloration is useful for all purposes.

स्फुटं गात्रं गुरु स्निग्धं स्वच्छं रागाधिकं[३२७] समम् ।
भग्नमस्तकपिण्डाङ्गं माणिक्यं रसकर्मणि ।।६५२।।

Ruby Useful for Processing Mercury

Ruby whose body is cracked, which is heavy, unctuous, transparent and deep coloured, and whose head (top) or body is broken is useful for alchemy (processing mercury).

रन्ध्रकर्कश्य-मालिन्य-रौक्ष्य-वैशद्यसंयुतम् ।
चिपिटं लघुवक्रं च माणिक्यं दुष्टमष्टशः[२२८] ॥६५३॥

Eight Defects in Ruby

Ruby which has (1) holes, which is (2) rough, (3) dirty, (4) ununctuous and (5) non-slimy, which is (6) pressed like scales, which is (7) light in weight and which is (8) curved—these eight are the defects of ruby.

माणिक्यं दीपनं रुच्यं कफवातक्षयार्तिनुत् ।
भूतवेतालपापघ्नं कर्मजव्याधिनाशनम् ॥६५४॥

॥ इति माणिक्यगुणाः ॥

Properties of Ruby

Ruby stimulates the power of digestion, promotes appetite and cures diseases caused by *kapha* and *vāyu* and consumption. It annihilates seizures by evil spirits and *vetāla-s* (vampire) and counteracts sinful acts. It cures diseases caused by the sinful acts of the past life *(karmaja)*.

MUKTĀ (PEARL)

मेघानामथ शंखानां वराहस्य च दन्तिनः ।
मीनजं वंशजं चैव खनिजं शुक्तिजं तथा ॥६५५॥
अष्टौ मुक्ताफलान्येव सर्वदा रसकर्मणि ।
गुणयुक्तानि संगृह्य दोषयुक्तानि वर्जयेत् ॥६५६॥

Varieties

Pearls (*muktā*) are of eight types, viz.,

(1) which originates from cloud;
(2) which is taken out of conch-shell;
(3)-(6) which is extracted from boar, elephants, fish and bamboo;
(7) which is taken out of mines; and

(8) which comes out of pearl oyester (*śukti*).

These eight varieties of *muktā* (pearl) are always useful for processing mercury.

Pearls having auspicious characteristics should be used and faulty ones should be rejected.

ह्लादि श्वेतं लघु स्निग्धं रश्मिवन्निर्मलं महत् ।
सजलं चञ्चलं वृत्तं मौक्तिकं[329] रसकर्म्मणि ।।६५७।।

Pearl Useful for Processing Mercury

Pearl which is pleasing to look at, which is white, light and unctuous, which has rays emanating, which is free from dirt, which is big in size, which has water particles in the centre, whch is of fickle nature and which is round, is useful for processing mercury.

रूक्षाङ्गं समलं श्यामं ताम्राभं लवणोपमम् ।
अर्द्धशुद्धं च विकटं ग्रन्थिलं मौक्तिकं मतम् ।।६५८।।

Defects in Pearl

The pearl which is ununctuous, dirty, brownish black and coppery coloured, which is like salt, which has auspicious qualities only in half (the other half of the pearl being defective), which is unpleasing in look and which has knots, is not useful.

मौक्तिकंसुमधुरं[330] सुशीतलं दृष्टिरोगशमनं विषापहम् ।
राजयक्ष्मपरिक्षेपनाशनं[?] भेदकं भवति पुष्टिदम् ।।६५९।।

।। इति मौक्तिकगुणाः ।।

Properties of Pearl

Pearl is sweet in taste and excessively cooling. It cures eye-diseases, poisoning and tuberculosis. It is laxative and nourishing.

PRAVĀLA (CORAL)

पक्वबिम्बफलच्छायं वृत्तायतमवक्रकम् ।
स्निग्धमव्रणकं स्थूलं प्रवालं सप्रभं[331] शुभम् ।।६६०।।

Characteristics of Good Pravāla

The coral which has the colour like that of the ripe fruit of *bimba*, which is round and large in size, which is not curved, which is unctuous, which is free from cracks, which is thick and which is lusturous, is auspicious.

पाण्डुरं धूसरं रूक्षं सव्रणं कोटरान्वितम् ।
निर्भरं ताम्रवर्णं च प्रवालं नेष्यतेऽष्टधा ॥६६१॥

Characteristics of Bad Pravāla

The coral which is yellowish, brown, ununctuous, with cracks & holes, light & coppery in colour is to be rejected. [In the text, these characteristic features are described to be eight in number; but actually seven features are enumerated].

वीर्यवृद्धौ तथा पुष्टौ यस्येच्छा वर्त्तते परा ।
विद्रुमं[112] शोधितं तेन सेवनीयं गुणप्रदम् ॥६६२॥

Need For Purification

If a person wants promotion of semen and nourishment of the body, then he should use coral after purification.

रससिन्धुः
विद्रुमं सर्वदोषघ्नं दीपनं रुचिपुष्टिकृत् ।
क्षयपाण्डुज्वरश्वासकासमेहगदाञ्जयेत् ॥६६३॥
पाचनं रक्तपित्तघ्नं नेत्र्यं विषगरापहम् ।
भूतोन्मादहरं ज्ञेयं प्रवालं लघुपाचनम्[?] ॥६६४॥

॥ इति प्रवालगुणाः ॥

Properties of Coral
According to Rasasindhu

Coral alleviates all *doṣa*-s. It stimulates the power of digestion and relish for food. It promotes nourishment of the body. It cures consumption, anemia, fever, asthma, bronchitis and *meha* (obstinate urinary disorders including diabetes). It is carminative. It cures *rakta-*

pitta (a disease characterised by bleeding from different parts of the body). It promotes eye-sight. It cures poisoning, affliction by evil spirits and insanity. It is light for digestion.

रससिन्धुः

प्रवालमञ्जरी सार्द्रा कामपुष्टिकरी नृणाम् ।
सेविता संततं देहवीर्यस्तंभं करोति च ।।६६५।।

।।आर्द्रप्रवालमञ्जरीगुणाः।।

Property of Freshly Collected Coral
According to Rasasindhu

Freshly collected (not dried) coral stems promote sexual desires, and when regularly used, it stops ageing process and helps in the retention of semen.

GARUḌODGĀRA (EMERALD)

भवानीमतात्

विज्ञेयो गरुडोद्गारः कीटपक्षसमद्युतिः ।
द्वितीयः शिखिकंठाभस्तृतीयो माषपत्रवत्[३३३] ।
धूलिधूसरवज्ज्ञेयश्चतुर्थश्चातिनिन्दितः[३३४] ।।६६६।।

Varieties of Emerald
According to Bhavānī

Emerald is of four types as follows :

(1) The first variety has lustre like that of the wings of the insect (glow-worm).
(2) The second variety is like the throat of pea-cock in colour.
(3) The third variety is like the leaves of *māṣa* in colour.
(4) The fourth variety is brown like dust, and it is of inferior quality.

खद्योतद्युतिसंकाशः शिखिकण्ठनिभस्तथा[३३५] ।
कोमलश्च चतुर्णां च रसकर्मणि शस्यते ।।६६७।।

Characteristics of Useful Emerald

Emerald which has lustre like that of glow-worm (first type) or the neck of peak-cock (second type) and which is soft (among the four varieties) is useful in processing mercury.

TĀRKṢYA (A TYPE OF EMERALD)

रसदर्पणात्

हरिद्वर्णं[336] गुरु स्निग्धं स्फुटद्रश्मिरयं शुभम् ।
मसृणं[337] भासुरं गात्रं तार्क्ष्यं सप्तगुणं स्मृतम् ।।६६८।।

Characteristics of Useful Tārkṣya

The seven attributes of good emerald are — greenish colour, heaviness, unctuousness, emanation of rays, auspicious look, smoothness and dazzling body.

कपिलं कर्कशं नीलं पाण्डु कृष्णं सलाघवम् ।
चिपिटं विकटं कृष्णं [?] रसे [?] तार्क्ष्यं[338] न शस्यते ।।६६९।।

Characteristics of Tārkṣya of Inferior Quality

Tārkṣya which is brownish, rough, blue, yellowish, black, light, pressed and ferocious in look is not useful.

ज्वरं छर्दिं विषं श्वासं सन्निपाताग्निमान्द्यनुत् ।
दुर्नामपाण्डुशोथघ्नं तार्क्ष्यमोजोविवर्धनम् ।।६७०।।

Properties of Tārkṣya

Tārkṣya cures fever, vomiting, poisoning, asthma, *agnimāndya* (suppression of the power of digestion) caused by *sannipāta* (simultaneous vitiation of all the three *doṣa-s*), piles, anemia and oedema. It promotes *ojas* (vital essence).

PUṢPARĀGA (TOPAZ)

पुष्परागं गुरु स्निग्धं स्वच्छं स्थूलं समं मृदुः ।
कर्णिकारप्रसूनाभं प्रमसृणं शुभमष्टधा ।।६७१।।

Characteristics of Good Topaz

Heaviness, unctuousness, transparency, large-size, uniformity, softness, colour like that of the flower of *karṇikāra* and smoothness—these are the eight attributes of topaz of good quality.

निष्प्रभं कर्कशं रूक्षं पीतं श्यामं[१११] तनोन्नतम् ।
कपिलं कललं पाण्डुं पुष्परागं परित्यजेत् ।।६७२।।

Characteristics of Bad Topaz

Lack of lustre, roughness, ununctuousness, yellow & bluish colouration, having elevation in the body, grayishness, jelly like feeling in touch and yellowishness—the topaz having these characteristic features should be rejected.

पुष्परागं महाछर्दिकफवाताग्निमान्द्यनुत् ।
[रसामृत : रत्नविज्ञानीय ८:३]
दाहकुष्ठश्रमहरं दीपनं लघुपाचनम् ।।६७३।।

।। पुष्परागगुणाः ।।

Properties of Topaz

Topaz cures serious type of vomiting, *agnimāndya* (suppression of the power of digestion) caused by *kapha* and *vāta*, burning syndrome, *kuṣṭha* (obstinate skin diseases including leprosy) and fatigue. It stimulates the power of digestion. It is light and carminative.

NĪLA (SAPPHIRE)

जलनीलेन्द्रनीलश्च शुक्रनीलस्तयोर्वरम् ।
सैत्यगर्भितं तोयाभं लघु तज्जलनीलकम् ।
कार्ष्ण्यगर्भितं नीलाभं सभारं शक्रनीलकम् ।।६७४।।

Varieties of Sapphire

Nīla is of two types, viz., *jala-nīla* and *indra-nīla*. Of these two, the latter is better in quality.

Jala-nīla is white in the center and blue out side. It is lighter.

Indra-nīla is black in the center and blue out side. It is heavier.

मेघछायं गुरुस्निग्धं स्वच्छं पिण्डितविग्रहम् ।
मृदुमध्योल्लसदूज्योतिः सप्तधा नीलमुत्तमम् ।।६७५।।

Properties of Good Sapphire

Good sapphire is like cloud in lustre, heavy, unctuous, transparent, solid and soft. Rays emanate from its centre. These are the seven attributes of good sapphire.

अतसीपुष्पसंकाशं नीलजीमूतसन्निभम् ।
यः करोति पयो नीलं महानीलः स उच्यते ।।६७६ ।।

Mahā-Nīla

The sapphire which is like the flower of *atasī* or blue cloud and which makes the water blue is called *mahā-nīla*.

कोमलं विहितं रूक्षं निर्भारं रक्तगन्धि च ।
चिपिटाभं सरूक्षं [?] च त्याज्यं नीलं च सप्तधा ।।६७७ ।।
कोमलमित्यनिष्पन्नवर्णम्[३४०] ।विहितमित्यर्धभागेन
सम्पूर्णवर्णाभम्[३४१] ।।६७८ ।।

Properties of Bad Sapphire

Sapphire which is *komala* (unmanifested colour), *vihita* (having proper colour only in half), ununctuous and light in weight, which smells like blood, which is pressed and which is *sarūkṣa* (?), is useless. Sapphire having the above mentioned seven attributes should be rejected.

कासश्वासहरं वृष्यं त्रिदोषघ्नं सुदीपनम् ।
विषमज्वरदुर्नामपापघ्नं नीलमीरितम् ।।६७९ ।।

।इति नीलगुणाः ।।

Properties of Sapphire

Sapphire cures bronchitis and asthma. It is aphrodisiac. It alleviates all the three *doṣa-s*. It is an excellent stimulant of digestion. It cures *viṣama-jvara* (irregular fever) and piles. It annihilates sinful acts.

GOMEDA (CINNAMON STONE)

गोमेदं गोजलछायं गवां[३४२] मेदः समुद्भवम् ।

सुस्वच्छं मसृणं स्निग्धं संभारं निलदं तथा ।
दीप्तगात्रं च निःसारं गोमेदं शुभमष्टधा ।।६८१।।

Characteristics of Gomeda

Gomeda is prepared of the fat (*meda-s*) of the cow (*go*). Colour like that of the cow's urine, transparency, smoothness, unctuousness, heaviness, *nilada* (?), dazzling body, free from any hard substance in the centre—these are the eight attributes of good *gomeda*.

विच्छायं लघु रूक्षाङ्गं चिपिटं पटलान्वितम् ।
निष्प्रभं पीतकाभं च गोमेदं न सुखावहम्[३४३] ।।६८२।।

Characteristics of Bad Gomeda

Gomeda which has bad complexion, which is light, ununctuous, pressed and having layers, which is free from any lustre and which is yellowish is not useful.

गोमेदं कफपित्तघ्नं क्षयपाण्डुज्वरापहम् ।
मेहघ्नं पाचनं रुच्यं त्वच्यं बुद्धिप्रबोधनम् ।।६८३।।

।। इति गोमेदगुणाः ।।

Properties of Gomeda

Gomeda alleviates *kapha* and *pitta*. It cures consumption, anemia, fever and *meha* (obstinate urinary disorders including diabetes). It is carminative, appetiser, wholesome for skin and stimulant of wisdom.

MARAKATA (ANOTHER TYPE OF EMERALD)

पिण्डरागामलं गात्रं कीटपक्षसमं गुरु ।
सुवर्णाभं मृदुस्निग्धं ज्ञेया मारक्ते गुणाः ।।६८४।।

Characteristics of Good Marakata

Marakata of good quality is like a solid mass with colour but transparency. It is like the wings of an insect (glow-worm). It is heavy in weight, like gold in colour, soft and unctuous.

कर्करं कपिलं स्निग्धं[?] रेखारागाद्यं भागकम् ।
रक्षारूक्षमलत्रासं दोषाः मरक्ते मतः ।।६८५।।

Characteristics of Bad Marakata

Marakata which is rough, graying brown, unctuous (?) and having lines and colour spots, which is cracked, ununctuous, rough and dirty and which is fierceful is faulty and defective.

शोफघ्न[४४]शूलप्रमेहघ्नं महाप्रदरनाशनम् ।
प्रलेपाख्यज्वरहरं मेध्यं मरक्तं मतम् ।।६८६।।

।। इति मरक्तगुणाः ।।

Properties of Marakata

Marakata cures oedema, colic pain, *prameha* (obstinate urinary disorders including diabetes), serious type of menorrhagia and *pralepaka* (hectic) type of fever. It promotes intellect.

VAIḌŪRYA (CAT'S EYE)

विडालनेत्रसंकाशं नीलं[४५] पीतं सुनिर्मलम् ।।६८७।।

Characteristics of Good Vaiḍūrya

Vaiḍūrya is like cat's eye. It is blue and yellow and exceedingly clean (transparent).

"वैडूर्यं रक्तपित्तघ्नं[४६] प्रज्ञायुर्बलवर्धनम् ।
पित्तप्रधानरोगघ्नं दीपनं ग्रहमोचनम्" ।।६८८।।

[रसामृत : रत्नविज्ञानीय ८ : ५]

Properties of Vaiḍūrya

Vaiḍūrya cures *rakta-pitta* (a disease characterised by bleeding from different parts of the body). It promotes intellect, longevity and strength. It cures diseases caused by the aggravation of *pitta*. It stimulates the power of digestion. It alleviates ailments caused by the afflictions by evil planets.

श्यामं तोयसमच्छायं विकटं लघुकर्कशम् ।
यस्तु गर्भोत्तरीयं च वैडूर्यं नेष्यते रसे ।।६८९।।

।। वैडूर्यगुणाः ।।

Characteristics of Bad Vaiḍūrya

Vaiḍūrya which is bluish, which has lustre like that of water, which looks fierceful, which is light and rough and which has a mark of *uttarīya* (sacred thread) inside is not useful in processing mercury.

RASONIKĀ (A TYPE OF CAT'S EYE)

गोरक्षमतात्
रसोनरससंकाशा सुस्निग्धा मलवर्जिता ।
चलत्सूत्रैर्गर्भितया श्रेष्ठा स्यात्सा[३४७] रसोनिका ।।६९०।।

Characteristics of Rasonikā
According to Gorakṣa

Rasonikā (*lahasunīyā*) is like the juice of garlic (*rasona*) in colour. It is unctuous and free from dirt. It has a moving thread-like substance inside. This type of *rasonikā* is the best.

दुश्चिकित्स्यामयहरी नेत्र्या वृष्या रसोनिका ।।६९१।।

।। इति रसोनिकागुणाः ।।

Properties of Rasonikā

Rasonikā cures obstinate and otherwise incurable types of diseases. It promotes eye-sight and virility.

GARUḌODGĀRA PĀṢĀṆA (RAW EMERALD)

गरुडोद्गारपाषाणं हरित्पीतं प्रजायते ।
निंबकल्के विनिक्षिप्तो निंबस्तु मधुरायते ।
भाजने रुधिरं कृत्वा विषं पिष्ट्वा च निक्षिपेत् ।
रुधिरं जलतां याति[३४८] परीक्षां तत्र कारयेत् ।।६९२।।
वारिणा गरुडोद्गारं घर्षयित्वा विनिःक्षिपेत्[३४९] ।
तज्जलं स्वबलेनैव करोति रुधिरं पुनः ।।६९३।।

Characteristics and Test

Garuḍodgāra stone is green and yellow in colour. If placed in the paste of *nimba*, the latter becomes sweet in taste.

In a pot blood should be kept and the paste of aconite (*viṣa*) should be added to it by which the blood turns into water. To this water, if the rubbed powder of *garuḍodgāra* is added then it becomes blood again.

अमूल्यं तद्भवेद्रत्नं नृपाणामति दुर्लभम् ।
विषं दूषीविषं चैव तथा चाशीविषं जयेत् ।।६९४।।

Properties of Garuḍodgāra

Garuḍodgāra is a priceless gem and even kings find it difficult to procure. It cures poisons, artificially prepared poisons and snake poisons (*āśī-viṣa*).

अथ रससिन्धुः
मुक्तादिष्वसिद्धेषु न दोषः स्याच्च शास्त्रतः ।
तथापि गुणवृद्धिः स्याच्छोधनेन विशेषतः ।।६९५।।

।। इति मुक्तादिशुद्धिः ।।

Purification of Pearl, Etc.
According to Rasasindhu

According to scriptures, pearl, etc., can be used in recipes without purification and unpurified gems do not produce any adverse effects. Even then, these gems should be purified for the enhancement of their therapeutic value.

रसदर्पणात्[१५०]
शुध्यन्तेऽम्लेन माणिक्यं जयन्त्या मौक्तिकं तथा ।
विद्रुमं क्षारवर्गेण तार्क्ष्यं गोदुग्धतस्तथा ।।६९६।।
पुष्परागं च सन्धानैः कुलत्थक्वाथसंयुतैः ।
नीलं नीलीरसेनैव वैडूर्यं त्रिफलाजलैः ।
रोचनाभिश्च गोमेदं दोलायन्त्रेण शोधयेत् ।।६९७।।

।। इति माणिक्यादिशुद्धिः[३५१] ।।

Method of Purifying Different Gems According to Rasa-darpaṇa

Māṇikya (ruby) gets purified [by boiling] with sour-juice. *Mauktika* (pearl) gets purified by [boiling with the juice of] *jayantī*. *Vidruma* gets purified by [boiling with] drugs belonging to *kṣāra-varga* (group of alkalies). *Tārkṣya* (emerald) gets purified by [boiling with] milk. *Puṣparāga* (topaz) gets purified by [boiling with] *sandhāna* (vinegar prepared by fermenting grains=*dhānyāmla*) and the decoction of *kulattha*. *Nīla* (sapphire) gets purified by [boiling with] the juice of *nīla* (indigo). *Vaiḍūrya* (cat's eye) gets purified by [boiling with] the decoction of *triphalā*. *Gomeda* (cinnamon stone) gets purified by [boiling with] the solution of *gorocanā*. The boiling (cooking) of all these gems should be performed in *dolā-yantra*.

अथ रसांकुशात्[३५२]

स्वेदयेद्दोलिकायन्त्रे जयन्त्याः स्वरसेन च ।
मणिमुक्ताप्रवालानि म्रियन्ते नात्र संशयः ।।६९८।।

Purification and Calcination of Gems According to Rasāṅkuśa

Gems including pearl and coral should be boiled in *dolā-yantra* by adding the juice of *jayantī* [and then cooked in *puṭa*]. By this they get [purified and] calcinated.

कुमार्यास्तण्डुलीयस्य रसेन परिषेचनात् ।
क्षणाद्विविधवर्णानि म्रियन्ते नात्र संशयः ।।६९९।।

If gems are heated and then sprinkled with the juices of *kumārī* and *taṇḍulīyaka* then these gems having different colours get calcinated.

अथ माक्षिकवन्मुक्ताप्रवालदीनि मारयेत् ।
वज्रवत्सर्वरत्नानि शोधयेन्मारयेत्तथा ।।७००।।

Pearl, coral, etc., should be calcinated according to the processes prescribed for the calcination of *mākṣika* (copper pyrite). All the gems and costly stones can be purified and calcinated on the lines suggested for the purification and calcination of diamond.

रसार्णवात्

"लकुचद्रवसंपिष्टैः[३५३] शिलागन्धकतालकैः ।
वज्रं विनान्यरत्नानि म्रियन्तेऽष्टपुटैः खलु" ।।७०१।।
[रसकामधेनु : पृष्ठ २२३]

Calcination of Gems
According to Rasārṇava

Gems should be made to a paste by triturating with the juice of *lakuca*. To this, *manaḥ śilā* (realgar), sulphur and *tāla* (orpiment) should be added and triturated. By giving eight *puṭa-s* all gems except diamond get calcinated.

TAILA-S (OILS)

रसरत्नाकरात्

"तैलानां पातनं वक्ष्ये सूर्यपाकादियोगतः ।
यस्मिन्योगे[३५४] तु यत्तैलं योजनीयं भवेद्ध्रुवम् ।।७०२।।

According to Rasaratnākara

In different recipes (processes), different types of oil are described to be used. Hereafter, the methods of extracting oil from different ingredients according to *sūrya pāka* (exposure to sun-rays), etc., will be described.

धत्तूरबीजचूर्णानि वस्त्रपूतानि कारयेत् ।
समूलोत्तरवारुण्याः कषायेण च भावयेत्[३५५] ।।७०३।।
आलिप्य कांस्यपात्रं[३५६] तु धारयेदातपे खरे ।
संतप्तं कांस्यपात्रस्थं[३५७] पीडनात्तैलमाहरेत् ।।७०४।।

Extraction of Oil from Dhattūra-Seeds

Seeds of *dhattūra* should be made to a fine powder by straining through a cloth. This should be impregnated with the decoction of *uttara-vāruṇī*. The paste should be smeared on the wall of a bronze pot and exposed to hot rays of the sun. When the paste becomes hot, it should be squeezed into the bronze-pot by which oil of *dhattūra* comes out.

सुपक्वानि समानीय हेमबीजानि यत्नतः ।
निस्तुषानि समं तानि कृत्वा तैलं समाहरेत् ।
तिलपीडनयन्त्रेण तैलमेवं च निःसरेत् ।।७०५।।

Second Method of Extracting Oil from Dhattūra-Seeds

Matured seeds of *dhuttūra* should be dehusked and pressed in an oil-press by which oil will ooze out.

शिग्रुमुष्कककार्पासमपामार्गपलाशजम् ।
ग्राह्यं धत्तूरवत्तैलं एकैकस्य पृथक् पृथक् ।।७०६।।

Extraction of Oil from Other Seeds

The oil from each of the seeds of *śigru*, *muṣkaka*, *kārpāsa*, *apāmārga* and *palāśa* may also be extracted according to the methods described above for the extraction of oil from *dhuttūra*-seeds.

यथा धत्तूरजं तैलं क्वाथाद्धर्मे समुद्धरेत् ।
तथा सर्वाणि तैलानि ग्रह्येन्मतिमान्भिषक् ।।७०७।।

As the oil of *dhuttūra*-seeds is extracted by impregnating with decoctions and exposing to sun-rays (described earlier in verse nos. 703-704), in the same way oil of all the other seeds can be extracted.

अंकोलस्यापि तैलं च काकतुण्ड्यास्तथैव च ।
बाकुची-देवदाल्योश्च अर्कमूलेन भावयेत् ।।७०८।।

For the extraction of oil from the seeds of *aṅkola*, *kāka-tuṇḍī*, *bākucī* and *devadālī*, these seeds should be impregnated with the decoction of the root of *arka*.

अपामार्गकषायेण तैलं स्याद्विषमुष्टिजम् ।
मूलक्वाथैः कुमार्याश्च तैलं जैपालजं भवेत् ।।७०९।।

The oil of *viṣa-muṣṭi* can be extracted by impregnating its seeds with the decoction of *apāmārga*. The oil of *jayapāla* can be extracted by impregnating its seeds with the decoction of the roots of *kumārī*.

क्वाथेन चेन्द्रवारुण्यास्तैलमारग्वधं भवेत् ।।७१०।।

The oil of *āragvadha* can be extracted by impregnating with the of decoction of *indra-vāruṇī*.

कटुतुम्बी देवदाली पटोली चेन्द्रवारुणी ।
तिक्तकोशातकी तासां शुष्कबीजानि चूर्णयेत् ।
काकतुण्ड्यपामार्गक्वाथे तैलं समाहरेत् ।।७११।।

The dried seeds of *kaṭu-tumbī*, *deva-dālī*, *paṭola*, *indra-vāruṇī* and *tikta-kośātakī* should be made to powders and impregnated with the decoctions of *kāka-tuṇḍī* and *apāmārga* for the extraction of oil.

बीजानि कटुतुम्ब्याश्च गोमयेन विलोड्यते ।
निस्त्वग्मज्जां विचूर्ण्याथ भृङ्गराजरसैः सह ।
मर्दयित्वातपे तैलं गृह्णीयात्पीडनेन हि ।।७१२।।

The seeds of *kaṭu-tumbī* should be boiled with cow-dung and dehusked. The pulp of these seeds should be made to a powder, impregnated with the juice of *bhṛṅgarāja* and triturated in hot sun. Then by squeezing this pulp, the oil should be extracted.

महाकालस्य बीजानि चूर्णितानि विलोडयेत् ।
धात्रीफलरसेनैव भावयेच्च[३५८] पुनः पुनः ।।७१३।।
शोषं कृत्वा तु तत्तैलं ग्रहेद् धत्तूरतैलवत् ।
अथवा तैलयन्त्रेण ग्राहयेद्योगवद्द्विजः ।।७१४।।

Extraction of Mahākāla Oil

Seeds of *mahākāla* should be made to a powder and repeatedly impregnated with the juice of *āmalakī*. Thereafter, this powder should be dried, and from this powder oil should be extracted according to the procedure suggested earlier for the extraction of oil from *dhuttūra*-

seeds. Alternatively, oil of *mahākāla* seeds should be extracted by pressing in an oil-press.

कृष्णायाः काकतुण्ड्याश्च बीजचूर्णानि कारयेत् ।
कान्तपाषाणचूर्णानि[३५९] एकीकृत्य निरोधयेत् ।
धान्यराशिगतं पक्षादुद्धृते तैलमाहरेत् ।।७१५।।

Pippalī and seeds of *kāka-tuṇḍī* should be made to a powder and mixed with the *bhasma* of *kānta-pāṣāṇa* and covered with heap of grains. After fifteen days, the powder should be taken out and oil should be extracted from it.

चूर्णं करञ्जबीजोत्थं भृङ्गराजरसैः सह ।
समालोड्यातपे तप्तं पीडनात्तैलमाहरेत् ।।७१६।।

Extraction of Karañja-Oil

The powder of the seeds of *karañja* should be boiled with the juice of *bhṛṅgarāja* and dried in the sun. By pressing this powder in an oil-press, oil of *karañja* should be extracted.

धात्रीफलरसैर्भाव्यं चूर्णं पालाशबीजजम् ।
ततः[३६०] पातालयन्त्रेण ग्राहयेत्तैलमुत्तमम् ।।७१७।।

Extraction of Palāśa-Oil

The powder of the seeds of *palāśa* should be impregnated with the juice of *āmalakī* and keeping (cooking) this powder in *pātāla-yantra*, oil should be extracted.

गुंजां त्वग्वर्जितं चूर्णं नरमूत्रेण भावयेत् ।
सप्तवारं ततो घर्मे तैलं पतति नान्यथा ।।७१८।।

Extraction of Guñjā-Oil

The outer coating of the seeds of *guñjā* should be removed and the pulp should be made to a powder. This should be impregnated with human urine for seven times. By exposing it to sun-rays, its oil should be extracted. There is no alternative.

रत्नमालारनालेन[३६१] पिष्ट्वा चूर्णं विभावयेत् ।
ज्योतिष्मत्युत्थबीजानामातपे तैलमाहरेत् ।।७१९।।

Extraction of Jyotiṣmatī-Oil

Powder of the seeds of *jyotiṣmatī* should be impregnated with the vinegar called *ratnamālā* (?) and exposed to sun-rays. From this powder, oil should be extracted.

चूर्णं बदरबीजोत्थं[३६२] शिवाबीजं त्वचान्वितम् ।
नालिकेराम्बुनालोड्य घर्मे तत्स्थापयेत्क्षणम् ।
पीडयेन्निज[३६३]पाणिभ्यां तैलं पतति तद्द्रुतम् ।।७२०।।

Powder of the seed of *badara* and the powder of the seed and pulp of *harītakī* should be boiled in coconut-water and kept for sometime exposed to the sun-rays. Pressing this powder with hands results in the exudation of oil.

आम्राडबीजचूर्णं च दशांशं चित्रमूलकम् ।
नालिकेराम्बुना पिष्टं घर्मे तैलं समाहरेत् ।।७२१।।

Extraction of Āmrāḍa-Oil

Powder of the seeds of *āmrāḍa* should be added with one tenth in quantity of the powder of the root of *citraka* and triturated by adding coconut-water. By exposing it to sun-rays, oil should be extracted.

पुत्रंजीवस्य बीजोत्थं अथवा रक्तबीजजम् ।
आम्राडवत्प्रकर्त्तव्यं तयोस्तैलं पृथक् पृथक् ।।७२२।।

Extraction of Putrañjīva-Oil

The seeds of *putrañjīva* or *rakta-bīja* should be made to powders. Their oils should be extracted on the lines suggested above for the extraction of oil from *āmrāḍa*.

नालिकेराम्बुना भाव्यं बिल्वबीजस्य चूर्णकम् ।
दिनैकं तैलयन्त्रेण तैलमाहृत्य योजयेत् ।।७२३।।

Extraction of Bilva-Oil

Powder of the seeds of *bilva* should be impregnated with coconut-water for one day. Then by pressing in an oil-press, oil should be extracted.

निस्त्वचकोलबीजानां किंचिदुद्घाटयेन्मुखम् ।
प्ररोहयेत्कांस्यपात्रे पिष्ट्वा चणकलेपिते ।।७२४।।
तन्मुखे टंकणं चूर्णं किञ्चित्किञ्चित्प्रलेपयेत् ।
धारयेदातपे तीव्रे मुखात्तैलं समाहरेत् ।।७२५।।
अथवा कांस्यपात्रे तु घर्मे धार्यमधोमुखम् ।
अधःस्थे कांस्यपात्रे च तैलं पतति निश्चितम् ।।७२६।।

Extraction of Kola-Oil

Fruits of *kola* should be scrapped out of their pulp and the mouth of their seeds should be slightly opened. In a bronze pot smeared with the paste of *caṇaka*, these seeds should be kept and their mouths (openings) should be smeared with the powder of borax. The pot should then be exposed to strong rays of the sun by which from the mouth (openings) of these seeds, oil comes out which is to be collected.

Alternatively, the bronze pot should be held with its mouth downwards over another bronze pot. Oil from the seeds kept in the upper pot will fall down and get collected in the lower bronze pot.

सुखवर्चसजं क्षारं वृषादिसंभवम् ।
चतुर्गुणं नृकेशं च कुट्टितं सूक्ष्मकारितम् ।।७२७।।
जलेन सेचयेत्सर्वं स्थाप्यं पातालयन्त्रके ।
तत्क्षणाद् द्रवरूपं च केशतैलं स्रवेद् ध्रुवम् ।।७२८।।

Extraction of Oil From Hair

Sauvarcala, *sarji-kṣāra* and *kṣāra-s* (alkali preparations) of *vāsaka*, etc. should be added with four times of human hair and pounded to make a fine powder. This powder should be sprinkled with water and kept in *pātāla-yantra*. By cooking, liquid oil from the hair will instantaneously comes out.

सुपक्वभानुपत्राणां रसमादाय भावयेत् ।
समस्तबीजचूर्णं च उत्तानंतं [?] पृथक् पृथक् ।
आतपान्मुञ्चते तैलं साध्यासाध्यं न संशयः ।।७२९।।

Extraction of Oil From All Types of Seed

Powders of different types of seed should be impregnated with the juice of the matured leaves of *arka* separately and exposed to sun rays by which oil comes out of these seeds.

तथैवोत्तरवारुण्याः कषायेण समाहरेत् ।
खरातपेन तैलानि यत्नतः तत्वधीर्भिषक् ।।७३०।।
सर्वबीजास्थिमांसानां[३६४] शुष्केष्वेवं[३६५] ह्यनेकधा ।
सर्वबीजेषु वा तैलं ग्राह्यं पातालयन्त्रके ।।७३१।।
[रसकामधेनु : पृष्ठ ५५-५७]

Similarly, oils from different types of seeds can be extracted by impregnating them separately with the decoction of *uttara-vāruṇī* and exposing to hot sun. Similarly, different types of oil from the stones and pulp of different fruits (seeds) can be extracted. Alternatively, oil of all these seeds can be extracted with the help of *pātāla-yantra*.

रसरत्नाकरात्
वंशादिसर्वकाष्ठानां नारिकेरकपालिके[३६६] ।
तुषधान्यादिबीजानि गर्भयन्त्रेण तैलकम् ।
ग्राहयेत्सर्वमूलानां तैलं चापि प्रयत्नतः[३६७] ।।७३२।।
[रसरत्नाकर : रसखण्ड : १० : २६-२७]

According to Rasa-ratnākara

Oil from all types of wood including bamboo, outer hard shell of the coconut, husks, seeds of cereals and roots can be extracted with the help of *garbha-yantra*.

इति श्रीमहाराजाधिराजटोडरमल्लविरचिते टोडरानन्दे
आयुर्वेदसौख्ये रसोपरसमहारसमणिरत्नशोधनमारणसत्त्वपातन-

सत्त्वमारण-द्रुतिकरणगुणागुणविषलक्षणदिव्योषधादि-लक्षण-वह्निलक्षण-तैलपातनकथनं नामैकादशो हर्षः।।

Thus, ends the eleventh chapter of *Āyurveda-saukhya* in *Ṭoḍarānanda* composed by the Great King Ṭoḍaramalla dealing with purification, calcination, *sattva*-extraction, calcination of *sattva, druti*, good and bad qualities of *rasa-s, uparasa-s, mahārasa-s, maṇi-s* and *ratna-s* and description of *viṣa-s, divyauṣadhi-s*, different types of *agni* and methods of oil-extraction.

NOTES AND REFERENCES

1. (क) This is the beginning of the eleventh chapter of *Āyurveda-saukhya* in *Ṭoḍarānanda* and the invocation reads as follows :

श्यामाकृतिः कान्तिमयी प्रसिद्धा विधुन्वती स्वाततमो नराणाम्।
आनन्दवल्लीविपिने नरेन्द्रे श्रीटोडराख्ये शिवमातनोतु।।

(ख) "श्यामाकृतिः .... शिवमातनोतु" पाठोऽयं चतुर्थपुस्तके नोपलभ्यते।

२. विज्ञेयोष्टेन इति चतुर्थपुस्तके पाठः।
३. याष्टमं इति प्रथमपुस्तके पाठः।
४. केचिद्रसविदुः इति चतुर्थपुस्तके पाठः।
५. पाठोऽयं द्वितीयपुस्तके नोपलभ्यते।
६. श्रुत्वा इति आकरे पाठः।
७. पादतले इति आकरे पाठः।
८. (क) स्तेन इति प्रथमपुस्तके पाठः।
(ख) स्वेत इति द्वितीयपुस्तके पाठः।
९. पीतशुक्लविभागतः इति आकरे पाठः।
१०. सुवर्णतः इति प्रथमचतुर्थपुस्तकयोः पाठः।
११. क्षीरं इति प्रथमपुस्तके पाठः।
१२. संज्ञितम् इति प्रथमचतुर्थपुस्तकयोः पाठः।
१३. संहसाव्यपक्वः इति प्रथमपुस्तके पाठः।

१४. निःक्वाथयेद्दशं इति प्रथमपुस्तके पाठः।

१५. कुलत्थजे इति प्रथमचतुर्थपुस्तकयोः पाठः।

१६. वरपुष्टिमेति इति प्रथमपुस्तके पाठः।

१७. मेखशृंग्युच्छैर्द्रवै० इति प्रथमपुस्तके पाठः।

१८. ०सुदीपनः इति प्रथमपुस्तके पाठः।

१९. व्रध्मातं इति प्रथमपुस्तके पाठः।

२०. तैलाभ्यां इति प्रथमचतुर्थपुस्तकयोः पाठः।

२१. माक्षिक्यं इति प्रथमपुस्तके पाठः।

२२. वाहक इति द्वितीयपुस्तके पाठः।

२३. ध्यापितं इति आकरे पाठः।

२४. ज्ञयव्रणहरं परं इति प्रथमपुस्तके पाठः।

२५. विमलारसायनसत्वपातनगुणाः इति चतुर्थपुस्तकेपाठः।

२६. 'सत्त्वो०......शोधन' पाठोऽयं चतुर्थपुस्तके नोपलभ्यते।

२७. वर्ण्यते इति प्रथमचतुर्थपुस्तकयोः पाठः।

२८. चक्षुरोगनुत् इति चतुर्थपुस्तके पाठः।

२९. शंखाटकी च कंकुष्ठं इति प्रथमपुस्तके पाठः।

३०. निश्चियम् इति प्रथमचतुर्थपुस्तकयोः पाठः।

३१. ह्यनुष्टं च सुलेखनं इति प्रथमचतुर्थपुस्तकयोः पाठः।

३२. शिलाजतुतुल्यवर्णं इति प्रथमचतुर्थपुस्तकयोः पाठः।

३३. किंचिदुष्णममृतोपमम् इति प्रथमपुस्तके पाठः।

३४. 'शैलं .... यथा' पाठोऽयं द्वितीयपुस्तके नोपलभ्यते।

३५. 'इति .... ०गुणाः' पाठोऽयं चतुर्थपुस्तके नोपलभ्यते।

३६. 'मृत्पाषाण०.... मतः' पाठोऽयं द्वितीयपुस्तके नोपलभ्यते।

३७. कृतमस्तु तत् इति प्रथमपुस्तके पाठः।

३८. ०सप्तभावनाभिश्च इति प्रथमपुस्तकेपाठः।

३९. पाठोऽयं द्वितीयपुस्तके नोपलभ्यते।

४०. पाठोऽयं द्वितीयपुस्तके नोपलभ्यते।

४१. 'मदायतन०... कीर्तिता' पाठोऽयं प्रथमपुस्तके नोपलभ्यते।

४२. तालश्च इति प्रथमपुस्तके पाठः।

४३. पटलाकृति इति प्रथमपुस्तके पाठः।

४४. तापस्फोटोंगसंकोच० इति प्रथमपुस्तके पाठः।

४५. वर्दाली इति चतुर्थपुस्तके पाठः।

४६. दद्याप्लानैः इति चतुर्थपुस्तके पाठः।

४७. (क) मध्येसा इति प्रथमपुस्तके पाठः।
(ख) मध्येस्म भ्राम्यते च क्षणम् इति चतुर्थपुस्तके पाठः।

४८. वाधिकं इति प्रथमचतुर्थपुस्तकयोः पाठः।

४९. सर्वतिक्ता इति द्वितीयपुस्तके पाठः।

५०. रसैस्त्वत्प्रमर्दयेत् इति प्रथमचतुर्थपुस्तकयोः पाठः।

५१. दद्याद्गुडसैंधवसौभाग्यप्रीतिका इति प्रथमपुस्तके पाठः।

५२. क्षिपेज्जंत्रेथ सैकते इति प्रथमपुस्तके पाठः।

५३. षोटिकाभं इति प्रथमचतुर्थपुस्तकयोः पाठः।

५४. 'वा शब्दात् अगस्तियंत्रास्ये ग्राह्याः' पाठोऽयं
चतुर्थपुस्तके अधिकमुपलभ्यते।

५५. 'रसै० .... सरा' पाठोऽयं चतुर्थपुस्तके नोपलभ्यते।

५६. भूतावेशं ज्वरं इति प्रथमचतुर्थपुस्तकयोः पाठः।

५७. ०सत्त्वपातनकथनं इति प्रथमचतुर्थपुस्तकयोः पाठः।

५८. गन्धालाभशिला० इति प्रथमपुस्तकेपाठः।

५९. तेनात्र न मया ख्यातः इति प्रथमपुस्तके पाठः।

६०. (क) शरैः इति प्रथमपुस्तके पाठः।
(ख) सतैः इति चतुर्थपुस्तके पाठः।

६१. षडश्च इति प्रथमपुस्तके पाठः।

६२. विशेषाद् सबन्धक इति प्रथमपुस्तके पाठः।

६३. बलक्षरश्च इति द्वितीयपुस्तके पाठः।

६४. सत्त्वरूपो इति प्रथमपुस्तके पाठः।

६५. चपलो इति प्रथमपुस्तके पाठः।

६६. 'देहवेधं .... मतः' पाठोऽयं प्रथमपुस्तके नोपलभ्यते।

६७. सूतबन्धकरं इति चतुर्थपुस्तके पाठः।

६८. सदृशः इति द्वितीयपुस्तके पाठः ।

६९. देवं इति प्रथमचतुर्थपुस्तकयोः पाठः।

७०. शिवन्नवैक्रान्तः इति प्रथमपुस्तके पाठः।

७१. स्वेदपदेयेत्सप्तवासरान् इति चतुर्थपुस्तके पाठः।

७२. विसायः इति चतुर्थपुस्तके पाठः।

७३. महत्सुसंपहतम् इति प्रथमपुस्तके पाठः।

७४. ज्वरकुष्ठजरापहः इति प्रथमचतुर्थपुस्तकयोः पाठः।

७५. शिफाकल्कलाक्षाटंकणसंयुतम् इति द्वितीयपुस्तके पाठः।

७६. मूखमूषागतं इति प्रथमपुस्तके पाठः।

७७. (क) वज्रातें इति प्रथमपुस्तके पाठः।

(ख) वैक्रान्तं इति चतुर्थपुस्तके आकरे च पाठः।

७८. रससन्निभम् इति प्रथमचतुर्थपुस्तकयोः पाठः।

७९. त्रिवर्गं इति द्वितीयपुस्तके पाठः।

८०. रोगोद्गमो इति चतुर्थपुस्तके पाठः।

८१. कर्षकं इति चतुर्थपुस्तके आकरे च पाठः।

८२. वापयेत्सिद्धं इति प्रथमपुस्तके पाठः।

८३. मदोन्मत्तगजः इति प्रथमचतुर्थपुस्तकयोः पाठः।

८४. यान्य इति प्रथमचतुर्थपुस्तकयोः पाठः।

८५. भाश्वराः इति प्रथमचतुर्थपुस्तकयोः पाठः।

८६. याताः इति द्वितीयपुस्तके पाठः।

८७. रत्नानां इति चतुर्थपुस्तके पाठः।

८८. शूद्राश्चैवं इति प्रथमपुस्तके पाठः।

८९. स्त्रीपुन्नपुंसकमिति त्रिधे वृताः इति प्रथमपुस्तके पाठः।

९०. वृहत्तराः इति प्रथमपुस्तके पाठः।

९१. रेखा इति प्रथमपुस्तके पाठः।

९२. ०रोगहा इति प्रथमचतुर्थपुस्तकयोः पाठः।

९३. तद्ग्राह्यं इति प्रथमपुस्तके पाठः।

९४. ०समं इति प्रथमपुस्तके पाठः।

९५. सत्सुचरोनि इति प्रथमपुस्तके पाठः।

९६. युक्तया इति प्रथमपुस्तके पाठः।

९७. अछेद्योयमदाह्यं इति द्वितीयचतुर्थपुस्तकयोः पाठः।

९८. तत् शुभं इति प्रथमपुस्तके पाठः।

९९. सह इति प्रथमपुस्तके पाठः।

१००. तस्मिन्तु इति प्रथमपुस्तके पाठः।

१०१. अहम् इति चतुर्थपुस्तके पाठः।

१०२. 'जायते ..... स्वेद्यं' पाठोऽयं चतुर्थपुस्तके नोपलभ्यते।

१०३. षाट्टूं इति प्रथमपुस्तके पाठः।

१०४. भवेत्सिद्धसमं इति प्रथमपुस्तके पाठः।

१०५. ताप तापं इति प्रथमचतुर्थपुस्तकयोः पाठः।

१०६. चतुर्याति इति प्रथमपुस्तके पाठः।

१०७. पिष्ट्वा इति प्रथमपुस्तके पाठः।

१०८. क्षिपेत् इति प्रथमपुस्तके पाठः।

१०९. नपुंसदमृतिस्तेषां इति चतुर्थपुस्तके पाठः।

११०. सह इति प्रथमपुस्तके पाठः।

१११. टंकणवत्सुद्धि ।। इति प्रथमपुस्तके पाठः।

११२. निवारणा इति चतुर्थपुस्तके पाठः।

११३. खनिजः इति प्रथमपुस्तके पाठः।

११४. नेकादापहश्च इति प्रथमपुस्तके पाठः।

११५. प्लीहगुल्मास्य इति प्रथमपुस्तके पाठः।

११६. विडग्यं इति प्रथमचतुर्थपुस्तकयोः पाठः।

११७. मतम् इति प्रथमपुस्तके पाठः।

११८. जारणे इति प्रथमपुस्तके पाठः।

११९. पुंवरादास्यु इति प्रथमपुस्तके पाठः।

१२०. ०मवाप्नुयुः इति प्रथमचतुर्थपुस्तकयोः पाठ।

१२१. 'चाल्पी० .... रसबन्धन०' पाठोऽयं चतुर्थपुस्तके नोपलभ्यते।

१२२. (क) जातवेंदरसंज्ञितम् इति प्रथमपुस्तके पाठः।
(ख) जातं वोढरसंज्ञितम् इति चतुर्थपुस्तके पाठः।

१२३. 'रसबंधकं .... ०ग्रिमम्' पाठोऽयं
प्रथमपुस्तके अधिकमुपलभ्यते।

१२४. गात्रदौर्गन्धिं इति प्रथमपुस्तके पाठः।

१२५. रसा इति प्रथमपुस्तके पाठः।

१२६. संशयं इति प्रथमपुस्तके पाठः।

१२७. ०शिषरे इति प्रथमपुस्तके पाठः।

१२८. मदम् इति द्वितीयपुस्तके पाठः।

१२९. वर्चस्तत्स्यामपीताभं इति प्रथमपुस्तके पाठः।

१३०. चित्राणां इति प्रथमपुस्तके पाठः।

१३१. काशीशं इति प्रथमपुस्तके पाठः।

१३२. शुक्लं कृष्णं पीतमिति प्रिये इति आकरे पाठः।
[रसार्णवः ७ : ८१]

१३३. काशीशं इति प्रथमपुस्तके पाठः।

१३४. श्यामं पीतं भवेचान्यदुत्तमा० इति प्रथमपुस्तके पाठः।

१३५. काशीशं इति प्रथमपुस्तके पाठः।

१३६. काशीशं इति प्रथमपुस्तके पाठः।

१३७. काशीसशोधनम् इति प्रथमपुस्तके पाठः।

१३८. हि इति प्रथमपुस्तके पाठः।

१३९. तुंबरैः इति प्रथमपुस्तके पाठः।

१४०. त्रिदिना शुद्धिमिच्छति इति प्रथमपुस्तके पाठः।

१४१. व्रणोरक्तशूलघ्नी इति चतुर्थपुस्तके पाठः।

१४२. स्फटिकीसूतघातिनी इति प्रथमपुस्तके पाठः।

१४३. मुराद्रिकावत्शोधनं इति प्रथमपुस्तके पाठः।

१४४. पाठोऽयं द्वितीयपुस्तके नोपलभ्यते।

१४५. वन्ध्याकंदं इति प्रथमपुस्तके पाठः।

१४६. रसः सम्यक् पटुक्षाराम्लसंयुतैः इति द्वितीयपुस्तके पाठः।

१४७. शुक्रदीप्तः इति प्रथमपुस्तके पाठः।

१४८. काले वह्निलक्षणं लिष्यते इति प्रथमपुस्तके पाठः।

१४९. स्वात्सत्वे इति प्रथमपुस्तके पाठः।

१५०. दृढाङ्गारैः रधा इति प्रथमपुस्तके पाठः।

१५१. चक्रमालं इति प्रथमपुस्तके पाठः।

१५२. पाठोऽयं चतुर्थपुस्तके एव उपलभ्यते।

१५३. 'मारये०...... च' पाठोऽयं द्वितीयपुस्तके नोपलभ्यते।

१५४. एभिस्तु इति प्रथमपुस्तके पाठः।

१५५. 'समुद्र०........ देशजम्' पाठोऽयं
प्रथमपुस्तके अधिकमुपलभ्यते।

१५६. मधुराजसरोयातं इति प्रथमपुस्तके पाठः।

१५७. त्रिदोषघ्नं गरापहं इति प्रथमपुस्तके पाठः।

१५८. दृष्टिजं इति प्रथमपुस्तके पाठः।

१५९. गन्धनादने इति प्रथमपुस्तके पाठः।

१६०. करवीरौ च इति प्रथमपुस्तके पाठः।

१६१. किणही इति प्रथमपुस्तके पाठः।

१६२. ०पञ्चाम्लवर्गमतं इति प्रथमपुस्तके पाठः।

१६३. सितापुष्पास्तथौषध्याः इति प्रथमपुस्तके पाठः।

१६४. परिकीर्तिता इति द्वितीयपुस्तके पाठः।

१६५. कक्काची पनखः इति द्वितीयपुस्तके पाठः।

१६६. क्षीरनीली च कारवेल्लोर्क पत्रिका
इति प्रथमपुस्तके पाठः।

१६७. षड्गारी इति प्रथमपुस्तके पाठः।

१६८. रक्तशृङ्गी दन्ती इति प्रथमपुस्तके पाठः।

१६९. रसमारकवर्गः इति प्रथमपुस्तके पाठः।

१७०. एभिस्तु इति प्रथमपुस्तके पाठः।

१७१. तारां कुक्कुरी च इति प्रथमपुस्तके पाठः।

१७२. 'रक्तं.....विलक्षयेत्' पाठोऽयं प्रथमपुस्तके
नोपलभ्यते।

१७३. सदृशीपत्रैः पुष्पैनापि इति प्रथमपुस्तके पाठः।

१७४. तस्यां इति प्रथमपुस्तके पाठः।

१७५. वाक्यां वा धारयेत्सुभां इति प्रथमपुस्तके पाठः।

१७६. साधये ध्रुवं इति प्रथमपुस्तके पाठः।

१७७. जयति इति प्रथमपुस्तके पाठः।

१७८. श्वेतादि वर्णा क्रमशः चतुर्द्धा इति
प्रथमपुस्तके पाठः।

१७९. योग्या च इति प्रथमपुस्तके पाठः।

१८०. 'गोभिर्नाऽऽघ्रातमीश्वरि' इति
आकरे प्रथमपुस्तके च पाठः।

१८१. 'क्षीरमध्यस्थितं क्षीरं कृष्णवर्णं भवेत् क्षणात्' इति आकरे पाठः।

१८२. रक्ताम्बरधरो भूत्वा रक्तामाल्यानुलेपनः
इति आकरे पाठः।

१८३. कृष्णपक्षे तु पञ्चम्यां रक्तशाल्योदनेन
तु इति आकरे पाठः।

१८४. रक्तचित्रकचूर्णेन वङ्गस्तापैस्त्रिभिः इति आकरे पाठः।

१८५. स्तम्भमायाति इति आकरे पाठः।

१८६. बल्लीवितानबहुला हेमवर्णफला शुभा इति आकरे पाठः।

१८७. तु गृहीत्वा बीजमुत्तमम् इति आकरे पाठः।

१८८. समादाय कुम्भे ताम्रमये क्षिपेत् इति आकरे पाठः।

१८९. स घटः इति आकरे पाठः।

१९०. (क) तं तु इति आकरे पाठः।
(ख) 'ताम्रं .... भवेत्' पाठोऽयं
द्वितीयपुस्तके नोपलभ्यते।

१९१. पाठोऽयं द्वितीयपुस्तके नोपलभ्यते।

१९२. पत्राण्यसंख्यानि परिगृह्य प्रलेपयेत्
इति प्रथमपुस्तके पाठः।

१९३. पत्रैर्जीरक० इति प्रथमपुस्तके पाठः।

१९४. रात्रौ इति प्रथमपुस्तके पाठः।

१९५. पत्रपुष्पफलैः इति प्रथमपुस्तके पाठः।

१९६. स तिष्ठेत्तु इति द्वितीयपुस्तके पाठः।

१९७. यत्र इति द्वितीयपुस्तके पाठः।

१९८. तंत्रं रक्तकन्दं प्रशस्यते इति प्रथमपुस्तके पाठः।

१९९. ०सुप्रभा इति प्रथमपुस्तके पाठः।

२००. महोषध्या इति द्वितीयपुस्तके पाठः।

२०१. मूर्छायेद् वंधयेत्क्षिप्रं इति प्रथमपुस्तके पाठः।

२०२. सुरेश्वरि इति प्रथमपुस्तके पाठः।

२०३. पाठोऽयं द्वितीयपुस्तके नोपलभ्यते।

२०४. संस्थितं इति प्रथमपुस्तके पाठः।

२०५. स्थिता श्वेतोच्चटा इति प्रथमपुस्तके पाठः।

२०६. रसेन लवणानि चन्द्रतुल्यानि व्योमाभानि च
कानिचित् इति प्रथमपुस्तके पाठः।

२०७. पूजयेद्दहम इति प्रथमपुस्तके पाठः।

२०८. पूर्णमांस्यां इति प्रथमपुस्तके पाठः।

२०९. पाठोऽयं द्वितीयपुस्तके नोपलभ्यते।

२१०. 'ॐ.........स्वाहा' पाठोऽयं
द्वितीयपुस्तके नोपलभ्यते।

२११. ततो इति प्रथमपुस्तके पाठः।

२१२. श्वेतविन्दवः इति प्रथमपुस्तकेपाठः।

२१३. तत् इति द्वितीयपुस्तकेपाठः।

२१४. 'दृश्यते सर्वमङ्गलः' पाठोऽयं
प्रथमपुस्तके नोपलभ्यते।

२१५. सुप्रसिद्धो हविष्यक ग्रामस्तस्यास्ति
निकटे तत्र संजीवनं जलम्।।
इति प्रथमपुस्तके पाठः।

२१६. मुंचत्यंकुरपत्राणि इति प्रथमपुस्तके पाठः।

२१७. समुधृतवतो इति प्रथमपुस्तके पाठः।

२१८. पतितस्तस्माद्यातं इति प्रथमपुस्तके पाठः।

२१९. मही शैलशैलं चेति इति प्रथमपुस्तके पाठः।

२२०. षण्मासमपरांगोत्थं इति प्रथमपुस्तके पाठः।

२२१. श्रीशैलशिवनप्रांते इति प्रथमपुस्तके पाठः।

२२२. त्रिस्थल्यं इति प्रथमपुस्तके पाठः।

२२३. अद्योरेशंन इति प्रथमपुस्तके पाठः।

२२४. लक्षणं इति प्रथमपुस्तके पाठः।

२२५. ०कुष्ठात् इति प्रथमपुस्तके पाठः।

२२६. स कथ्यते इति प्रथमपुस्तके पाठः।

२२७. कर्मवक्ष्येद्रसायने इति प्रथमपुस्तके पाठः।

२२८. भातीत स्यात्तु इति प्रथमपुस्तके पाठः।

२२९. शुद्धिमिच्छति इति प्रथमपुस्तके पाठः।

२३०. कर्कटा इति द्वितीयपुस्तके पाठः।

२३१. ०र्नागावुश्वाहिफेनजम् इति प्रथमपुस्तके पाठः।

२३२. 'गरलं... प्रयोजयेत्' पाठोऽयं
प्रथमपुस्तके नोपलभ्यते।

२३३. पाठोऽयं प्रथमपुस्तके अधिकमुपलभ्यते।

२३४. रसि इति प्रथमपुस्तके पाठः।

२३५. भक्षयेत्तमभ्यस्तं इति प्रथमपुस्तके पाठः।

२३६. अब्धिर्जलाग्निं पाठोऽयं प्रथमपुस्तके
अधिकमुपलभ्यते।

२३७. विज्ञेयं इति द्वितीयपुस्तके पाठः।

२३८. शक्तुकं इति प्रथमपुस्तके पाठः।

२३९. ०वाक्म् इति प्रथमपुस्तके पाठः।

२४०. ०भिर्भेदैः विषं इति प्रथमपुस्तके पाठः।

२४१. शक्तुकं तं विजानीया० इति प्रथमपुस्तके पाठः।

२४२. रोगघ्नमुत्तम० इति प्रथमपुस्तके पाठः।

२४३. मद्यवत्स्तब्धताकरः इति प्रथमपुस्तके पाठः।

२४४. दीर्घः इति प्रथमपुस्तके पाठः।

२४५. विमोक्ष्यं इति प्रथमपुस्तके पाठः।

२४६. पीतैर्विरोमक इति प्रथमपुस्तके पाठः।

२४७. 'यः कंद्रो गोस्तनाकारो न दीर्घः पंचमांगुलात्।'
पाठोऽयं प्रथमपुस्तके अधिकमुपलभ्यते।

२४८. आश्च इति प्रथमपुस्तके पाठः।

२४९. पाठोऽयं प्रथमचतुर्थपंचमपुस्तकेषु नोपलभ्यते।

२५०. संपिष्टं इति प्रथमपुस्तके पाठः।

२५१. 'अति...कारयेत्तदा' पाठोऽयं द्वितीयपुस्तके नोपलभ्यते।

२५२. 'तक्रघटे...पलपंचकम्' इति द्वितीयपुस्तके पाठः।

२५३. छागं मूत्रके इति द्वितीयपुस्तके पाठः।

२५४. कुष्ठार्शगरशोफं च इति प्रथमपुस्तके पाठः।

२५५. दोलायन्त्रे सारनाले विषमुष्टिर्दिनत्रयम् इति प्रथमपुस्तके पाठः।

२५६. शोषितं इति प्रथमपुस्तके पाठः।

२५७. तोयारनाल० इति प्रथमपुस्तके पाठः।

२५८. भवेद् भुवम् इति प्रथमपुस्तके पाठः।

२५९. पाठोऽयं प्रथमपुस्तके अधिकमुपलभ्यते।

२६०. षट्पला ग्राह्या इति प्रथमपुस्तके पाठः।

२६१. तद्वयं इति प्रथमपुस्तके पाठः।

२६२. नालिका इति प्रथमपुस्तके पाठः।

२६३. ०कुह्वोन्मिता इति प्रथमपुस्तके पाठः।

२६४. 'विचूर्णिता...वेदकत्वमागतम्' पाठोऽयं द्वितीयपुस्तके नोपलभ्यते।

२६५. शूलाध्मानामगुल्मेषु इति प्रथमपुस्तके पाठः।

२६६. आबोलकरणम् इति प्रथमपुस्तके पाठः।

२६७. स्निग्धमज्जं इति द्वितीयपुस्तके पाठः।

२६८. सुदीर्घां च खणयेत्प्राप्यते इति प्रथमपुस्तके पाठः।

२६९. यथासं इति प्रथमपुस्तके पाठः।

२७०. नापि इति प्रथमपुस्तके पाठः।

२७१. वृक्षोद्भिन्नतरं इति प्रथमपुस्तके पाठः।

२७२. संस्पर्शो इति प्रथमपुस्तके पाठः।

२७३. सम्यगग्नि खातयेत् इति प्रथमपुस्तके पाठः।

२७४. मृत्छ्राभिः इति प्रथमपुस्तके पाठः।

२७५. ति इति प्रथमपुस्तके पाठः।

२७६. साखस्थूल० इति प्रथमपुस्तके पाठः।

२७७. प्रशाधकम् इति प्रथमपुस्तके पाठः।

२७८. क्तकफलाश्चाति कठिनतरा इति प्रथमपुस्तके पाठः।

२७९. प्रयीति निर्दोषतां यांति इति प्रथमपुस्तके पाठः।

२८०. लोहरत्नद्रुतिं हत्वा इति प्रथमपुस्तके पाठः।

२८१. च इति प्रथमपुस्तके पाठः।

२८२. सत्वं पूर्वं इति प्रथमपुस्तके पाठः।

२८३. द्रवति इति प्रथमपुस्तके पाठः।

२८४. 'पक्वं...ध्मातम्' इति प्रथमपुस्तके अधिको पाठः।

२८५. 'केशतैलेन...भवेत्' पाठोऽयं द्वितीयपुस्तके नोपलभ्यते।

२८६. ह्यविचारतः इति प्रथमपुस्तके पाठः।

२८७. निर्लेपिनि इति प्रथमपुस्तके पाठः।

२८८. रसोपरसकादीनां इति प्रथमपुस्तके पाठः।

२८९. विंशद्वार खादेत्पुनः इति प्रथमपुस्तके पाठः।

२९०. तद्विष्णीकीटेन सहती इति प्रथमपुस्तके पाठः।

२९१. तद्विष्णी इति प्रथमपुस्तके पाठः।

२९२. अधरोत्तमभावेन इति प्रथमपुस्तके पाठः।

२९३. विनिघातयेत् इति प्रथमपुस्तके पाठः।

२९४. भवयात् लिंपेत्पटमृद्य ततः इति प्रथमपुस्तके पाठः।

२९५. कंद्रभवयात् लिपेत्पटमृदा तत इति प्रथमपुस्तके पाठः।

२९६. वारीस्तु प्रथमपुस्तके पाठः।

२९७. ढालयेद्वारान् इति प्रथमपुस्तके पाठः।

२९८. स्थिये इति प्रथमपुस्तके पाठः।

२९९. क्षारवत् द्रावणं इति द्वितीयपुस्तके पाठः।

३००. यथा इति प्रथमपुस्तके पाठः।

३०१. तत्पटं तेन सलिंपेत् इति प्रथमपुस्तके पाठः।

३०२. तैलनैव इति प्रथमपुस्तके पाठः।

३०३. संदंसेनाथ वर्तिकाम् इति प्रथमपुस्तके पाठः।

३०४. सिञ्चन्नंद्राजतैलेन इति प्रथमपुस्तके पाठः।

३०५. ०द्वर्तिकी इति प्रथमपुस्तके पाठः।

३०६. मानायी इति प्रथमपुस्तके पाठः।

३०७. चूर्णयित्ता इति प्रथमपुस्तके पाठः।

३०८. ०संयुक्तैश्च वारांस्त्रिःसप्तकांस्ततः इति प्रथमपुस्तके पाठः।

३०९. रजतं इति प्रथमपुस्तके पाठः।

३१०. जातैरेकीकृत्य इति प्रथमपुस्तके पाठः।

३११. तदद्रसैवैरेव इति प्रथमपुस्तके पाठः।

३१२. समं युक्तं इति प्रथमपुस्तकं पाठः।

३१३. शतं वारां इति प्रथमपुस्तके पाठः।

३१४. वज्रमूखायां शक्लं क्षिपेत् इति प्रथमपुस्तके पाठः।

३१५. प्रदुतां इति प्रथमपुस्तके पाठः।

३१६. यवसफलं० इति प्रथमपुस्तके पाठः।

३१७. सुवर्णरजतं ताम्रं कान्तलोहि च वाजरम्
इति प्रथमपुस्तके पाठः।

३१८. द्रवंति इति प्रथमपुस्तके पाठः।

३१९. द्रुत्यभ्रखरसेन्द्रेण इति प्रथमपुस्तके पाठः।

३२०. मिलंति इति प्रथमपुस्तके पाठः।

३२१. विचारणात् इति प्रथमपुस्तके पाठः।

३२२. क्मावनः इति प्रथमपुस्तके पाठः।

३२३. च्यवनं इति द्वितीयपुस्तके पाठः।

३२४. चन्द्रकांतस्तथा इति प्रथमपुस्तके पाठः।

३२५. ०नीलमित्येष इति प्रथमपुस्तके पाठः।

३२६. छायां इति प्रथमपुस्तके पाठः।

३२७. रंगाधिकं इति प्रथमपुस्तके पाठः।

३२८. दुष्टमष्टधा इति प्रथमपुस्तके पाठः।

३२९. मौक्तिक्मणि इति द्वितीयपुस्तके पाठः।

३३०. तु मधुरं इति प्रथमपुस्तके पाठः।

३३१. सप्तधा इति प्रथमपुस्तके पाठः।

३३२. विद्रतं इति प्रथमपुस्तके पाठः।

३३३. वंसपत्रवत् इति प्रथमपुस्तके पाठः।

३३४. ०वहज्ञेयश्च इति प्रथमपुस्तके पाठः।

३३५. क्रठसमस्तथा इति प्रथमपुस्तके पाठः।

३३६. हरिद्वर्णगुरुस्निग्धं इति प्रथमपुस्तके पाठः।

३३७. मश्रिणं इति प्रथमपुस्तके पाठः।

३३८. तक्ष्यं इति प्रथमपुस्तके पाठः।

३३९. पीतश्यामिं इति प्रथमपुस्तके पाठः।

३४०. कोमलमित्यनिःपन्नवर्णम् इति प्रथमपुस्तके पाठः।

३४१. सम्पूर्णवर्णान् इति प्रथमपुस्तके पाठः।

३४२. गवीमेदः इति प्रथमपुस्तके पाठः।

३४३. शुभावहम् इति प्रथमपुस्तके पाठः।

३४४. शोकशूलप्रमेहघ्नं इति प्रथमपुस्तके पाठः।

३४५. पीतं नीलं इति प्रथमपुस्तके पाठः।

३४६. सर्वकार्येषु योजनीयं गुणप्रदम् इति प्रथमपुस्तके पाठः।

३४७. तेजाद्यारसमानिका इति प्रथमपुस्तके पाठः।

३४८. जातं इति प्रथमपुस्तके पाठः।

३४९. विनिक्षिपेत् इति प्रथमपुस्तके पाठः।

३५०. पाठोऽयं द्वितीयपुस्तके नोपलभ्यते।

३५१. पाठोऽयं प्रथमपुस्तके नोलपभ्यते।

३५२. पाठोऽयं द्वितीयपुस्तके नोपलभ्यते।

३५३. कुचलद्रवसपिष्टः इति द्वितीयपुस्तके पाठः।

३५४. क यस्मिन्योगेषु इति प्रथमपुस्तके पाठः।
ख. जलयोगेन तैलं तदग्राह्यं योगेषु योजयेत्।
इति आकरे पाठः।

३५५. विलोडयेत् इति प्रथमपुस्तके पाठः।

३५६. कांसपात्रेण इति प्रथमपुस्तके पाठः।

३५७. क सूक्ष्मवस्त्रस्थं पीडयेत्तैलमाहरेत् इति प्रथमपुस्तके पाठः।
ख. स्वच्छवस्त्रेण इति आकरे पाठः।

३५८. सप्तवारं इति आकरे पाठः।

३५९. ०चूर्णं च इति प्रथमपुस्तके पाठः।

३६०. ततो इति प्रथमपुस्तके पाठः।

३६१. रत्नानमारनालेन इति आकरे पाठः।

३६२. क. तुंबरबीजोत्थं इति प्रथमपुस्तके पाठः।
ख. वरुणबीजोत्थं इति आकरे पाठः।

३६३. पीडयन्निजपाणिभ्यां इति प्रथमपुस्तके पाठः।

३६४. सर्वजीवास्थि० इति प्रथमपुस्तके पाठः।

३६५. शुष्के विष्टे इति प्रथमपुस्तके पाठः।

३६६. नालिकेरकपालिके इति प्रथमपुस्तके पाठः।

३६७. 'नारिकेरी कुट्टयित्वा स्थापयेत्स्थालिकान्तरे।
त्रिपादं हि तदुपरि स्थापयेत्तस्य चोपरि।
कटोरीं च ततः स्थालीमुखं समुद्रये दृढम्।
प्रोक्तानां पालिकीं दत्वा जलं पाल्यां प्रपूरयेत्।
ततश्चुल्यां समारोप्य मंदवह्निं प्रदापयेत्।
ऊर्ध्वं गत्वा पतत्याशु कटोरीं तैलमुत्तमम्।
एवं तुम्बादिबीजानामसाध्यानामपि साधयेत्।
पाली ताम्रमयी कार्या गंभीराथ कटोरिका।
कार्या लोहमयी चाथ त्रिपादी संप्रदापयेत्'।।
प्रमादपूर्णपाठोऽयं आदर्शपुस्तकेषु अधिकमुपलभ्यते।

INDEX - 1
(Authors and Books Quoted in the Book)

INDEX - II
(Names of Recipes Described in the Book)

INDEX III
(Pharmaceutical Processes Described in the Book)

INDEX IV
(List of the Processing - Methods of Minerals, Metals, etc. Described in the Book)

Index-V
(Names of Drugs, etc. Used in the Book)

INDEX-VI
(Glossary of Technical Terms)

Abīja 161
Mercury in which *bīja* or seed is not added.

Abhiṣeka, 42
The substance which is added to melted iron, etc. for further liquefaction.
107
Immersion.

Abhyaṅga, 15
Massage.
86, Massage over head.

Adhaḥ pātana, 117, 152, 154, 155
Downward distillation.

Āḍhaka (-s) 4,16,17,28,49,97
Unit of measurement. Four *prastha-s* make one *āḍhaka;* equivalent to 3.072 kg. or ltrs.

Adhama, 105
Inferior.

Adhimantha, 85
N.of an eye- disease.

Āḍhyavāta, 125
Gout.

Aghora mantra, 413
A specific sacred incantation.

Aghoreśa, 412
N. of a place of ancient time.

Agni, 6, 26 31, 69
Power of digestion.
462
Fire.

Agni doṣa, 153
One of the five *doṣa-s* (defects) of mercury which causes burning sensation.

Agnika, 236
A type of gold obtained from fire of vulçanic eruptions.

Ajīrṇa, 161
Mercury in which *jāraṇa* (a process, meaning digestion) has not been done.

Agnimāndya, 96,125,179,447,448
Suppression of the power of digestion.

Agni nakra, 369
A type of whale.

Akṛta yūṣa, 48
Vegetable soup without addition of fat, salt & pungent spices.

Akṛtrima, 220
Which is not artificially prepared.

Akṣa-s, 4, 14, 33
Unit of weight; Syn. of *karṣa*, approx. 12 gm.

Ākṣiki, 75
An alcoholic preparation.

Akṣi nimeṣa, 88
Twinkling.

Āma, 251, 253, 259, 315, 349, 366-368, 385

Āma doṣa, 38, 251, 255
Product of defective digestion and metabolism. For detail, see page 587 of Basic principles of Ayurveda.

Āmājīrṇa, 255
Indigestion.

Amarṣa mantra, 110
N. of a specific sacred incantation.

Āma śula, 344
Colic pain caused by indigestion of food.

Āmavāta, 219, 243, 272, 274
Rheumatic arthritis.

Amla pitta, 176, 179, 219, 251, 274, 325
Gastritis or hyper-acidity.

Āmra, 4, 16
Unit of weight; Syn. of *pala*; approx. 48 gm. / ml.

Amṛta traya, 294
Three nectars; diamond, gold and mercury, taken together are called *amṛta traya*.

Amṛtikaraṇa, 217
A processing of mica, inculcating the effect of ambrosia.

Andha mūṣā, 181, 182, 213, 215, 282,

Aṣṭhliā, 251
Hard tumour.
Aśvinīkumāra bhāga, 115
A part of medicine given the patient to the physicion.
Audumbara, 336
N. of a type of *kuṣṭha* (obstinate skin-disease).
Avabāhuka, 125
N. of a disease; brachial-nuralgia.
Avagāha, 88, 89
Bath.
Avaleha, 52, 117
Linctus.
Āvāpa, 42, 71, 128
Addition of powdered drugs in the recipe at the end.
Āyata, 381
Depth.
Ayuta, 413
Ten thousand years.
Baddha, 143, 409
Lit. binding; in present context-solid or solidification.
Bala, 6
Strength.
Bāla jāraṇa, 174
Young type of *jāraṇa* in which mercury is digested with same quantity of sulphur.
Bāla - rakṣakara-maṇi, 356
Talisman for protecting foetus.
Balla, 7, 13
Unit of weight; equivalent to three *guñjā-s,* approx. 375 gm./ml.
Bandhana, 159
Prevention of vapourisation.
166, 399, 410, 418, 419
Mercury-solidification and making it thermostable.
Baṅgāla, 247
N. of a state in India.
Basti, 15
Recipe used for medicated enema.
86, 88
Keeping oil over head.
89
Bath.
101
A type of medicated enema. For details, see chapter XIV of 'Five Specialised Therapies Of Ayurveda'.
Bhadra, 179
Endower of blessing.
Bhadrāṅga, 412
N. of a place.
Bhairava yantra, 119, 189
N. of a secret pharmaceutical instrument, used for cooking mercury, etc.
Bhājana, 4, 16
Unit of weight; Syn. of *āḍhaka,* approx. 3.072 kg./ltrs.
Bhājanabhedin, 146
Which penitrates into and causes cracks in the container.
Bhakta, 71
A Fermented liquid distilled properly.
358-360
A process of *māraṇa* by which metal becomes soft and swollen like rice.
Bhāra, 4, 17
Unit of weight; equivalent to two hundred *pala-s* or twenty *tulā-s;* approx. 96kg./ltrs.
Bhasma, 107, 109, 110, 114, 121, 128, 147, 154, 169, 175, 179-182, 186, 189-196, 198-201, 212-220, 238-240, 244, 246, 247, 251-254, 257-259, 261-264, 267, 271, 272, 286-291, 294, 295, 347, 358, 359, 361-364, 367, 382, 383, 395, 417, 431, 432, 436, 437,458
Calcined powder.
145
Lit. *hanyāt* = to kill.
Bhāvanā, 54, 68, 114, 126, 289
Impregnation.
Bhīmavikrānta, 74
An alcoholic drink; Syn. of *mārdvīka.*
Bhūdhara yantra, 119, 159, 162, 180, 185, 191
N. of a pharmaceutical instrument used for special cooking of medicines.
Bhūdoṣa, 144, 145
A defect of mercury because of which mercury causes obstinate skin

diseases.

Bhūta, 314, 376
Parasitic infestation.

Bīja, 118 119, 127, 128, 157, 161, 170, 172, 174, 195, 203, 219, 394
Seed or essence.

Bilva, 4, 16
Unit of weight; Syn. of *pala* and *prakuñca*, approx. 48 gm./ml.

Bindu, 15
Drop.
432
Insect.

Bola piṇḍa, 426
Bolus of *bola*.

Brāhma dina, 408
Day of Lord Brahmā, equivalent to one thousand *caturyuga-s* (four *yuga-s* or ages,namely *sat, tretā dvāpara* abd *kali* yuga), i.e 1, 96, 08,852976 years.

Brahma giri, 412
N. of a place.

Brahma hatyā, 145
Killing a brahmin.

Brahma pura, 412
N. of a place in ancient India.

Bṛhaspati, 441
N. of a planet known as Jupitor

Bṛmhaṇa, 193
Nourishing agent.
243
Which causes nourishment of tissues.

Buddha, 441
N. of planet known as Mercury.

Camas, 84
Spoon.

Cakrikā-s, 213, 313
Round and flat tablets.

Candra, 441
Moon.

Candrodaka, 407, 408, 414
Moon-water.

Capala, 342
Which melts easily or quivering.
146
More fickle.

Cāpalya, 160
Fickleness.

Caraka, 2
Belonging to the school of medicine.

Cāraṇa, 415
- *saṃskāra*, 414
A process of mercury.

Carma dala, 336
N. of a skin-disease.

Cāṣa, 325
N. of a bird, wagtail.

Catuḥ-ṣaṣṭi - pala 4
Unit of weight; Syn. of *āḍhaka*, approx. 3.072 kg./ltrs.

Catuḥ-ṣaṣṭi-śarāvaka, 4
Unit of weight; Syn. of *śūrpa*, approx. 24.576 kg./ltrs.

Caturthikā, 4, 16
Unit of weight; Syn. of *pala* and *prakuñca;* approx. 48 gm./ml.

Chāyā, 403
Shadow.

Citrakūṭa, 110
N. of a place.

Cora, 109
N. of a place.

Cukra, 76
A type of sour vinegar.

Cūrṇa, 27, 36, 49
Powder.

Dadru, 144, 336
Ring-worm or a type of *kuṣṭha* (obstinate skin disease).

Dakṣiṇāvarta, 378
Clock wise.

Damana, 398
Destroy.

Ḍamarū yantra, 180
N. of an instrument used for special cooking of recipe.

Dantī, 280
Elephant.

Darpa doṣa, 145
A defect of mercury because of which latter causes cracking of limbs.

Deha siddhi, 161, 261, 370, 398

Deha vāda, 411

Deha vedha, 344, 405
Rejuvenation of the body

Deśa. 6
Nature of the habitation

Unit of weight, Syn. of *kola;* approx. 6 gm./ml.
Kuḍava, 4-6, 16, 17, 19, 20, 32, 34, 44, 48, 54, 72, 92, 188, 426
Unit of weight; equivalent to four *pala-s;* approx. 192 gm./ml.
Kukkuṭa puṭa, 120, 313
A special process of cooking.
Kumbha, 4, 431
Unit of weight or measurement; Syn. of *śūrpa;* approx. 24.576 kg./ltrs.
Kumbha puṭa, 346
Special process of cooking.
Kuṣṭha, 33, 62, 111, 125, 144, 176, 205, 206, 217, 249, 251, 252, 254, 255, 259, 264, 272, 276, 291, 312, 314, 324, 325, 327, 334, 336, 347, 398, 413, 416, 421, 423, 424, 448.
Obstinate skin diseases including leprosy.
Kusuma, 325
Lit. Flower; in the present context menstrual blood.
Kvāthya, 95
Ingredient for decoction.
Laghu, 314
Light.
Laghu puṭa, 162, 193
Half in size of *gaja puṭa*. Ref. *gaja puṭa*.
Lākṣāmbu, 176
Solution of lac.
Lākṣā rasa, 92, 178
Lac mixed with water.
Lauha siddhi 160, 370
Lauha vedha 405
Transmutation of the base metals into noble ones, like gold.
Lāva puṭa, 429
Special method of cooking.
Leha, 51, 53, 115
Lehya, 126
Linctus.
Lekhana(ī), 79-83
Collyrium which scrapes out dirt, etc. from eyes.
243, 244, 255, 265, 266, 315, 325, 339
Which scrapes out tissues.
Lepa(s), 9, 62
External application of drugs in the form of paste or ointment.
65
Cold ointment.
Likṣā, 12, 17
Unit of weight or measurement; equivalent to six *truṭi-s*.
Liṅga, 276
Phallus.
Loha(s), 124, 126
Iron and other metallic preparations
379, 431
Metals.
Loha-siddhi, 398
Loha vedha, 344
Transmutation of base metals into noble ones.
Lomila, 269
N. of a demon.
Mada, 90
Intoxication.
Madhūlaka, 75
An alcoholic preparation.
Madhu śukta, 77
A type of fermented liquid.
Madhvāsava, 73
An alcoholic preparation made of th decoction of *dhātakī* and honey.
Madhyama, 79
Moderate type of collyrium.
105
Moderate.
Pāka, 102
Moderate cooking.
Magadha, 2
N. of an ancient kingdom of India; at present Bihar in the north India.
Māgadha, 2, 6, 7, 42
Weights and measures prevalent in the ancient state Magadha.
Magna, 88
Keeping the body deeped upto six *aṅgula-s* (three inches) above the umblicus.
Mahā kuṣtha, 144
Major type of obstinate skin-disease.
Mahā loha, 235
Important iron.
Mahāmūrcchā, 202
Great swoon.

Mahā ratna-s, 441
Important gems.
Mahā viṣa-s, 416, 417
Strong poisons.
Maireya, 73, 74
A type of fermented liquid.
Mala(doṣa), 144, 145, 147, 151, 160, 176
One of the defects of mercury because of which mercury causes fainting.
Malina, 415
Intoxicants.
Malla, 157
Arsenic.
Malla mūṣā, 168
A crucible smeared with the two layers of *malla* (arsenic).
Mālyavanta, 412
N. of a mountain.
Maṇa, 17
Unit of weight; equivalent to four *āḍhaka-s;* approx. 12.288 kg./ltrs.
Maṇḍa, 46
A type of gruel prepared of rice by adding fourteen times of water.
Mṛdu cikkaṇa, 101
Mild cooking of oil and ghee in which paste is soft and sticky like wax.
Maṇḍaka, 190
See *maṇḍa* above.
Mandara, 323
N. of a mountain.
Maṅgala, 441
one of the nine planets, known as Mars.
Maṇi-s, 462
Gems.
Māṇikā, 4, 16
Unit of weight; equivalent to two *kuḍava-s;* approx. 394 gm./ml.
Maṇi rasa, 440
Rejuvenating gems.
Manohvā, 338
Which pleases mind.
Mantha, 32
A preparation which is made by stirring the drugs with water.
Mantra-s, 403, 407, 408
Sacred incantations.

Māraka varga, 394
Group of drugs which help in calcination of metals, etc.
Māraṇa, 106, 142, 161, 162, 166, 202, 415
-saṃskāra, 415
Lit. killed; calcination.
Mardana, 159
-saṃskāra, 150
Process of trituration with juice, etc.
Mārdvīka, 74
An alcoholic preparation made out of *mṛdvīkā* (dried grapes).
Marīci, 3
Unit of weight and measurement; equivalent to six *vaṃśī-s*.
Marmaccheda, 144
Damage to the vital organs.
Māṣa-s, 3, 4, 7, 14, 17, 18, 34, 40, 66, 93, 117, 121, 184, 190, 196, 219, 288, 331
Unit of weight; approx. 1 gm./ml.
Mastu, 76, 97
Butter-milk.
Mataṅga, 356
N. of a place in ancient India.
Mātrā(s), 87, -89, 91,-92
Unit of time required to pronounce one short vowel.
Mātṛvāhaka, 360
N. of an animal.
Māyāpura, 110
N. of a desert.
Meda-s 450
Fat.
Medaka, 75
Layer still below alcoholic preparation.
Meha, 90, 191, 219, 243, 244, 254, 260, 324, 325, 327, 333, 371, 445, 450
Obstinate urinary diseases including diabetes.
Miśra, 415
Egypt.
Mitra pañcaka, 288
Five friendly ingredients, namely honey, ghee, *guggulu*, *guñjā* and borax.
Mleccha, 109
-deśa, 248

Nirvāpana, 105
Hot immersions.
268
Making iron hot and immersing in liquid.

Nirvega, 78
Free from bubbles.

Nirvīrya, 195
Type of mercury-*bhasma*.

Niyamana saṃskāra, 159
A process by which fickleness of mercury is reduced.

Niryāsa, 27
Juice.

Niryūha, 27, 46
Decoction prepared by boiling pulses and legumes.

Niṣeka, 42
Further addition of drugs after *prativāpa*.

Niṣka, 7, 368
Unit of weight; approx. 4 gm./ml.

Ojas, 219, 324, 327, 44[illegible]
Vitality or vital essence.

Pācana, 36, 38
Carminative decoction.

Pāda, 28
One-fourth.

Padābhyaṅga, 89
Massage over soles of feet.

Paittika, 45, 57, 65, 83, 85, 206, 219, 274, 367
Diseases caused by the aggravation of *pitta doṣa*.

Pāka, 102
Cooking.

Pakva mūṣā, 168
Strong crucible, burnt well like jar.

Pakvānna, 190
Sweets prepared by frying with ghee.

Pala(-s), 4, 7, 14-18, 21, 28, 29-36, 43-45, 47-50, 52, 54, 59, 60, 67, 69, 71, 97, 104, 105, 108, 109, 119, 129, 178, 180, 181, 188, 216, 241, 250, 268, 279, 282, 406, 424, 425, 430, 431, 439
Unit of weight and measurement; approx. 48 gm./ml. equivalent to two *śukti*-s or two *ardhapala*-s.

Pāmā, 336
Scabies, a skin disease.

Pampā, 413
N. of a lake.

Pampalī, 410
See *Kadalī*.

Pāna, 15, 101
Potion used for drinking or taking internally.

Pañca drāvaka, 392
Five drugs which help metals to melt quickly.

Pañca karma, 240
Collective name for five elimination therapies, viz.; 1) *vamana*, or emetic, 2) *virecana* or purgation, 3) *nasya* or inhalation, 4) *nirūha basti* (a type of medicated enema), and 5) *anuvāsana basti* (another type of medicated enema with oil, etc.)

Pañcakā yantra, 182
N. of an instrument.

Pañcāmla, 390
Five sour drugs.

Pañcāmṛta, 253, 254, 416
Five nectars.

Pañca mṛttikā, 128, 237
Five types of mud, namely ant-hill, house-soot, red ochre, brick and salt

Pañca ratna, 393
Five gems.

Pāṇḍu, 125, 266
Anemia.

Pāṇika, 14

Pāṇimānikā, 4
Unit of weight; Syn. of *karṣa*, approx. 12 gm./ml.

Pāṇi śukti, 15, 66
Unit of measurement; equivalent to 32 drops.

Pāṇitala, 4, 14, 51
Unit of weight, Syn. of *karṣa*; approx 12gm./ml

Pānīya, 68
Potion for drinking.

Paramāṇu-s 3
Atoms.

Paribhāṣā, 130, 162, 170, 174, 192
Explanation of technical terms.

Pariṇāma śūla, 125, 369
Colic pain caused by duodenal ulcer.

Pātra, 4, 16, 17
Unit of weight; Syn. of *āḍhaka*, approx. 3.072 kg./ltrs.

185, 190, 193, 194, 217, 219, 247, 252, 256, 259, 260, 263, 264, 272, 274, 282, 288, 293, 295, 314, 316, 318, 324, 325, 328, 344, 359, 364, 399, 451
Obstinate urinary diseases including diabetes.

Prapurāṇa 69
Very old.

Prasādana, 79
A type of collyrium which provides nourishment to the eye-tissues.

Prasādya, 82
Nourishing.

Prasannā, 75
Upper layer of alcoholic preparation.

Prasṛta(i), 4, 16
Unit of weight; equivalent to two *pala-s;* approx. 96 gm./ml.

Prastha, 4, 5, 17-19, 21, 34, 42, 44, 47, 48, 426
Unit of weight; equivalent to two *śarāva-s;* approx. 768 gm./ml.

Prasthāṣṭaka, 16
Unit of weight; equivalent to four *prastha-s*. This appears erroneons because this term means equivalent to eight *prastha-s*.

Pratisāraṇa 67, 68
Drugs in powder form which is applied over tongue with the help of finger tip.
68
Local application.

Prativāpa, 41
Addition of drugs to the recipe after *āvāpa*.

Pṛthvī kañcuka, 144
One of the five defects of mercury because of which latter causes *kuṣṭha* (obstinate skin-diseases including leprosy).

Puṇḍarīka, 336
A type of *kuṣṭha* (obstinate skin-disease).

Puṇya, 356
Virtuousness.

Puruṣa dvaya, 433
Unit of measurement; about twelve feet.

Puṣya, 406
N. of a constellation through which moon passes.

Puṭa, 126, 157, 164, 195, 212, 214, 216, 219, 237-241, 246, 253, 254, 258, 259, 261-263, 267, 287, 289, 291, 311, 314, 331, 343, 386, 405, 424, 433, 438, 454, 455
Cooking or fire.
-pāka, 82
Pouring juice of specially cooked drugs.
54, 127, 186, 242, 289, 343
Special method of cooking.

Puṭa yantra, 180, 189
An instrument for *puṭa pāka*.

Rāhu, 441
One of the nine *graha-s* (planets); Dragon's head.

Rajas, 13, 49
Unit of weight, Syn. of *vaṃśī* or *trasareṇu* (30 atoms).
162, 203
Menstrual blood.

Rājikā, 3, 120
Unit of weight, equivalent to 6 *marīci-s*

Rakta, 284
Blood.

Rakta gulma, 326
Type of tumour caused by the vitiation of blood.

Rakta varga, 390, 391
Group of red drugs.

Rakta pitta, 63, 125, 272, 274, 320, 365, 398, 445, 451
An ailment characterised by bleeding from different parts of the body.

Raktikā, 13, 14
Unit of weight; equivalent to two *dhānya māṣa-s;* approx. 125 mg./ml.

Rañjana, 292
Coloration.

Rasa(-s), 27
Juice.
47
Meat-soups.
47
Taste.
10, 118, 127, 276
Recipes containing mercury.

105
Mercury and other metals.
236
Metals.
340, 377, 378, 431, 462
Minerals.
162
Transmutation of basic metals into noble ones.
Rasa bandha, 342, 344, 350
-*bandhana*, 344, 354, 365, 367, 370, 371, 396, 397, 440
Making mercury solidified, non-volatile and heat-resistant.
Rasa dhātu, 163
Plasma, one of the seven tissue elements *(dhātu-s)*.
Rasa kriyā, 27, 51, 53, 79
Solid extract of drugs.
Rasanigaḍa yantra, 168
An instrument for a special process called *nigaḍa*.
Rasa piṣṭi, 156
Paste of mercury.
Rasa vāda, 422
Process of mercury.
Rasa vedha, 412
Transmutation of base metals into noble ones.
Rasa vidyā, 142
Science of mercury and Alchemy.
Rasāyana, 112, 118, 161, 243, 396
Which causes rejuvenation of the body and cure of diseases.
162
Rejuvenating effect of mercury.
276
Rejuvenating recipes.
Rāśi, 4, 17
Unit of weight; Syn. of *droṇa;* approx. 12.288 kg./ltrs
Rasībhavanti, 294
Endowed with the property of penitrability.
Rātra, 16
Unit of weight; Syn. of *prakuñca* according to Caraka, approx. 48 gm./ml.
Rātri, 403
Night - darkness.
Rattī(s), 18, 19, 117, 181, 185, 196, 217, 418
Unit of weight; Syn. of *guñjā;* approx. 125mg./ml.
Ravi, 441
Sun.
Reṇu, 49
Powder, Syn. of *cūrṇa*.
Retas, 158, 278
Secretion of the bartholin gland or menstrual blood.
Rodhana saṃskāra, 158, 159
A process of mercury by which potency-reduction of mercury is protected.
Roditīva, 399
Solace of crying.
Ramāntikā, 371
Measles.
Ropaṇa, 79, 80, 82, 83
Variety of collyrium which helps in the healing of ulcers in eyes.
Roṭikā, 287
Thin and round shape.
Ṛṣyajihva, 336
A type of *kuṣṭha* (obstinate skin disease).
Rudra bhāga, 116
Rudrāṃśa, 116
1/11th of purchaed drugs (for patient) given to physician.
Ṣaḍbindus, 431
Six insects.
Sādhāraṇa rasa-s, 342, 372
General metals.
Sahaja, 236
Type of gold in combination with other metals.
Śaila doṣa, 144, 145
One of the five defects of mercury.
Śaila toya, 414
Śailodaka, 411-414
Water from mountain spring.
Śakti, 16
Sulphur and mica.
Śālagrāma, 276
A type of stone.
Śalākā, 80
Rod.
Śālukā yantra, 158
N. of an instrument.

Śamana, 36-37
A type of decoction which alleviates the aggravated *doṣa-s*.
Sammitā, 189
Fine wheat-flour.
Sampātana yantra, 238
N. of an instrument.
Samputa, 258
A special earthen vessel used for cooking.
Saṃskāra-s, 149, 151, 159-162, 202, 220, 267
Special methods of processing mercury and other metals, minerals, etc.
Samudra, 384
Sea.
Śāṇa, 4, 7, 14, 15, 17, 40, 42, 66
Unit of weight; equivalent to 4 *māṣa-s;* approx. 4 gm./ml.
Ṣaṇḍha, 148
Impotency of mercury.
Sandhāna, 27, 424
An alcoholic preparation.
Sandīpita, 162
Ignited of digestive power.
Saṅgrahaṇī, 369
Sprue syndrome.
Śani, 441
One of the nine *graha-s* (planets), known as Saturn.
Sañjīvana jala, 410
Life-giving water.
Sanmukha jāraṇa, 174
A type of *jāraṇa* process.
Sannipāta, 90, 111, 291, 418, 421, 423, 447
Simultaneous vitiation of all the three *doṣa-s*.
Sānnipātika, 416
Disease caused by the simultaneons vitiation of all the three *doṣa-s*.
-udara, 416
An abdominal disease caused by the simultaneous vitiation of all the three *doṣa-s*.
Santānikā, 56
Formation of scum.
Santarpaṇa, 67
Nourishing.
Sāraṇa, 68
Which causes salivation.
398, 415
Increasing permeability.
-saṃskāra, 168, 415
A process by which permeability of drugs increases.
Śarāva(ka), 4, 16, 192
Unit of weight; approx. 384gm./ml.
Śarāva samputa, 258, 279, 281, 287, 291, 361, 362
Recipe enclosed inside two earthen plates and sealed.
Sarkarā, 327
Presence of sand in the urine.
Śārkara, 73
An alcoholic drink prepared with the decoction of *dhātakī* and *śarkarā* (sugar).
Sarṣapa, 3, 17, 108, 110
Unit of weight; equivalent to three *rājikā-s*.
Sarvatomukha mudrā, 189
Water-proof seal.
Śatavedhi, 401
A process which helps in the transmutation of base metals into noble ones for one hundred times.
Sātmya, 288
Wholesomeness or appropriateness.
Sattva, 11, 114, 128, 164, 195, 211, 218, 220, 252, 271, 315, 316, 318, 320, 322, 328-332, 337-339, 341, 344, 347, 348, 353-355, 364, 371, 373, 374, 377-383, 427, 431, 432, 434, 437, 462
Essence or metallic essence.
-pātana, 176, 291, 319
Taking out the essence from metals.
Satya age, 356
The first age among four ages *(Caturyugī)*, others being *tretā*, *dvāpara* and *kali* ages. It is a period of seventeen lakh and twenty eight thousand (17,28,000) years.
Saurāṣṭra, 110, 264, 356
N. of a kingdom in ancient India.
Sauvīra, 99
(ka), 77
Suvīrāmla, 77
A sour drink prepared by fermenting

Trasareṇu, 3,13
Unit of weight, equivalent to 30 atoms; also Sny. of *vaṃśī*.

Tretā age, 356
The second age among four ages *(caturygas)*. This period is of twelve lakh and ninety six thousand (12,96,000) years.

Tristhalī, 412
N. of a place.

Tṛṇodaka, 413
Grass-water.

Truṭi, 12, 17
Unit of weight; equivalent to six *aṇu-s* (atoms).

Tulā, 4, 5, 17, 19, 52, 71
Unit of weight; equivalent to hundred *pala-s;* 4.800 kg./ ltrs.

Tulā yantra, 158
Balance instrument.

Tuṣāmbu, 77
A fermented liquid.

Udara, 33, 91, 111, 125, 144, 254, 256, 259, 264, 324, 327, 367, 416, 418, 423

-roga, 111
Obstinate abdominal diseases including ascites.

Udumbara, 4, 14
Unit of weight; Syn. of *karṣa;* approx. 12 gm./ml.

Umāyoni, 106
Liquefied form of equal quantity of mercury and sulphur.

Unmāṇa, 4
Unit of weight; Syn. of *droṇa;* approx. 12. 288 kg./ltrs.

Unmatta doṣa, 144, 145
One of the defects of mercury.

Upadhātu-s, 310, 339
Subsidiary metals.

Upaloha, 235, 297, 309
Subsidiary metals.

Upanāha, 65
Type of ointment; which is wrapped with the half of a cloth over the skin.

Uparasa-s, 340, 341, 353, 377, 378, 383, 431, 462
Subsidiary minerals.

Uparatna-s, 441
Subsidiary gems.

Upaviṣa-s 150, 328, 388, 417, 418
Subsidiary poisons.

Ūrdhva pātana, 117, 152, 155, 158
Upward sublimation.
-yantra, 161
An instrument used for upward sublimation.

Uṣṇa, 79
Hot or sharp type of collyrium.

Uṣṇa toya, 414
Water obtained from hot spring.

Uṣṇodaka, 78, 413, 414
Boiled water free from bubbles and foam.

Utkledī, 277
Chipping.

Uttama, 105
Excellent.

Utthāpana, 106
Retrieved or a process by which calcined powder comes back to its original metallic form.
152
Revived.

-saṃskāra, 152
A process for reviving mercury.

Uttarāyaṇa, 104
Northern solstice.

Uttarīya, 452
Sacred thread.

Vāha, 4, 17
Unit of weight; Syn. of *droṇī;* approx. 49.152 kg./ltrs.

Vāhlīka, 75
N. of an ancient kingdom of India.

Vahni, God, 235
God of fire.

Vahni doṣa, 144, 145, 151
One of the defects of mercury because of which mercury causes burning sensation.

Vahnisthāyī, 172
Which does not evaporates when kept over fire.

Vaira giri, 356
N. of a mountain.

Vairecanika, 80
A type of collyrium which causes lachrimation.

Vajra, 210
Thunder bolt.
-kāñjika, 62
A type of vinegar.
-mūṣā, 120, 166, 167, 220, 379, 429, 433, 434, 436
A type of crucible.
Vajrodaka, 99
A type of vinegar.
Vaka nāla, 382
An instrument like the neck of crane.
Vakkasa, 75
The lowest layer of alcoholic preparation, containing the paste of drugs.
Vakra nāl(i), 167, 379, 382
Bent pipe.
Valikā, 83
Application of paste over eyes; Syn. of *piṇḍi*.
Vālukā yantra, 182, 189, 192, 194, 252, 335
See *sikatā yantra*.
Vaṃśī, 3, 13
Unit of weight; Syn. of *trasareṇu*.
Vaṅga, 109
N. of a place.
Vaṅga doṣa, 143, 201
One of the *kañcuka-s* (layers of adluterants) of mercury.
Vārāha, 411
One of the incarnation of Lord Śiva.
Vāritara; 282, 286
Which floats over water.
Vātika, 65, 83, 85, 193, 219, 370
Disease caused by the vitiation of *vāyu*.
Varṣa purī, 415
N. of a place.
Varti, 50, 61, 79, 102
Elongated pill.
172
Wick.
Vasā, 97, 389
Muscle fat.
Vāsanāmukha jāraṇa , 174
A type of *jāraṇa* process
Vāta, 43, 251, 448
One of the three *doṣa-s*, others being *kapha* and *pitta*. Ref. Glossary in p. 625 of Basic Principles of Āyurveda.
Vaṭaka, 4, 14
Unit of weight; Syn. of *kola;* approx. 6 gm./ml.
50
Large size pill.
190
A cooking preparation; also called *baḍā* in vernacular.
Vāta rakta, 272
Gout.
Vātika, 45, 65, 83, 85, 193, 219, 370
-diseases, 57
Diseases caused by the aggravation of *vāyu*.
Vaṭuka, 102
Student of *gurukula;* also called *brahmacārī*.
Vayas, 6
Age.
Vāyu, 40, 44, 51, 63, 64, 85, 89, 93, 124, 125, 142, 146, 163, 198, 212, 217, 243, 247, 260, 270, 284, 289, 295, 321, 324, 327, 333, 349, 366, 369, 371, 443
One of the three *doṣa-s;* other two beings *kapha* and *pitta*. Ref. *Vāta* in p. 625 of Glossary in Basic Principles of Ayurveda.
-alleviating drugs, 57
Drugs which alleviate the *vāyu*.
-diseases, 274
Diseases caused by the aggravation of *vāyu*.
Vedhana, 163
Transmutation of basic metals into noble ones.
Vetāla, 235, 443
Vampire.
Vicarcikā, 336
Eczema.
Vidāhī, 125, 324
Which causes burning sensation.
Viḍāla (ka), 82, 84
External application of paste over eyes excluding eye-lashes.
Viḍāla padaka, 4, 14
Unit of weight; Syn. of *karṣa;* approx. 12gm./ml.

Vidyut, 235
  Lightening.
Vihita, 449
  Having proper colour only in half.
Vikāśi, 326
  Expansive.
Vilepi, 46
  A preparation which is very sticky.
Vindhya, 324, 327, 345, 412
  A mountain range.
Vipāka, 247, 255, 311, 324, 327, 344
  Taste that emerges after digestion.
Vīrya, 235
  Potency or semen.
Vīrya hāni, 144
  Destroy of semen.
Viṣa-s 112, 150, 328, 423. 462
  Poisonous drugs.
  430, 453
  Aconite.
Viṣa doṣa, 145, 151, 153
  Defect of mercury.
Viṣama jvara, 125, 193, 205, 274, 424, 449
  Irregular fever.
Visarpa, 62, 336
  Erysipelas.
Viṣa vāda, 422
  Treatment with poisons.
Viṣodaka, 409
  Poisonous water.
Viśoṣi, 37
  Decoction which dries up the tissues.
Vistīrna, 381
  Diameter.
Vitasti-s 120
  Unit of measurment.
Vraṇa, 62
  Ulcer.
Vṛddha jāraṇā, 174
  Old type of digestion (a process) of mercury with sixteen times of sulphur.
Vṛddha vaidya, 49
  Experienced physicians.
Vrīhi, 93
-dhānya-s, 98
  Cereals.
Vṛntāka mūṣā, 330
  A type of crucible.
Vyāghra pura, 412
  N. of a place.
Yavāgū, 46
  Thick gruel, which is semi-solid in consistency.
Yāma(-s), 83, 151, 153, 155, 166, 175, 178, 179, 181, 183, 185, 195, 197, 238, 253, 263, 285, 314, 334, 337, 369, 428, 434
  Period of time; three hours.
Yantra, 165, 186, 189
  Instrument.
Yauvana jāraṇa, 174
  A type of *jāraṇa* process (youthful) of mercury with four times of sulphur.
Yava 3, 17, 110, 111, 417
  Unit of weight; equivalent to the weight of barley grain.
Yoganidrā, 310
  Deep sleep by yogic practice.
Yogavāha(ī), or *(in)*, 180, 215, 217, 290, 317, 327, 417
  A therapeutic property of drug which enhances the effect of drugs added to it.
Yojana, 397
  Unit of measurement for distance; equivalent to eight miles or 12.872 kilometers.
Yūkā, 12, 17
  Unit of weight, equivalent to six *likṣā-s*.
Yūṣa, 28, 46-48
  Vegetable soup prepared with eighteen times of water.

APPENDIX-I
(Tables of Weights and Measures Described in these Texts According to Māgadha & Kāliṅga Schools)

(A) Māgadha School

(A) (Weights and measures which were prevalent in the ancient state of Magadha)

30 paramāṇu-s (atoms)	1 trasareṇu (Vaṃśi)
6 vaṃśī-s	1 Marici
6 Marici-s	1 Rājikā
3 Rājikā-s	1 Sarṣapa
8 Sarṣapa-s	1 Yava (weight of barley grain)
4 Yava-s	1 Guñjā = 166 mg.
6 Guñjā-s (raktikā-s)	1 māṣa (syn.= dhānyaka) = 1gm.
4 Māṣa-s	1 śāṇa (syns. - dharaṇa, ṭaṅka) = 3 gm.
2 Ṭaṅka-s	1 Kola (syns. = kṣudramo(ko), vaṭaka, draṅkṣaṇa = 6 gm
2 Kola-s	1 Karṣa (syn. akṣa, picu, pāṇitala, viḍāla pādaka, haṃsapada, kavalagraha, udumbara) = 12gm.
2 Karṣa-s	1 Ardhapala (syns. = śukti, aṣṭamikā) = 24 gm.
2 Śukti-s	1 Pala (syns. = muṣṭi, āmra, caturthikā, prakuñca, ṣoḍaśi and bilva) = 48 gm.
2 Pala-s	1 Prasṛti (syn. = prasṛta) 96 gm/ml.
2 Prasṛti-s	1 Añjali (syns. = kuḍava, ardha śarāvaka and aṣṭamāna)=192 gm./ml.
2 Kuḍava-s	1 Mānikā (Syns. = śarāva and aṣṭapala) = 384 gm./ml.
2 śarāva-s or	1 Prastha = 768 gm.
4 Prastha-s	1 Āḍhaka (Syns. = bhājana, kaṃsa, pātra, catuḥ ṣaṣṭi palas) = 3.072 kg./ltrs.
4 Āḍhaka-s	1 Droṇa (syns. armaṇa, ghaṭa, kalaśa, nalvaṇa, rāśi, and unmāna) = 12.288 kg.
2 Droṇa-s	1 Śūrpa (Syns. = catuḥ ṣaṣṭi śarāvakas, kumbha) = 24. 576 kg.
2 Śūrpa-s	1 Droṇī (syns. = goṇi, vāha) = 49. 152 kg.
4 Droṇi-s	1 Khārī (equivalent to 4096 pala-s) = 196.608 kg.
2000 Pala-s	1 Bhāra = 96 kg.
100 Pala-s	1 Tulā = 4.800 kg.

(B) Kāliṅga School

(Weights and measures prevalent in the ancient state of Kaliṅga)

12 Gaura Sarṣapa	1 Yava = 62.5 mg.
2 Yavas	1 Guñjā = 125 mg.
3 Guñjās	1 Balla = 375 mg.
8 Guñjās	1 Māṣa = 1 gm.
4 Māṣas	1 Sāṇa (syn. = niṣka and ṭaṅka) = 4 gm.
6 Māṣas	1 Gadyāṇa = 6 Gm.
10 Māṣas	1 Karṣa = 10 gm.
4 Karṣas	1 Pala (10 śāṇa) = 40 gm/ml.
4 Palas	1 Kuḍava = 160 ml.

Note : Subsequent units of weights and measures are in accordance with Māgadha School.

In the case of liquids, the metric equivalents would be the corresponding litre and mililitre.